Women As They Age:
Challenge, Opportunity, and Triumph

Women As They Age: Challenge, Opportunity, and Triumph

J. Dianne Garner
Susan O. Mercer
Editors

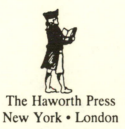

The Haworth Press
New York • London

Women As They Age: Challenge, Opportunity, and Triumph has also been published as *Journal of Women & Aging*, Volume 1, Numbers 1/2/3 1989.

The Haworth Press, Inc., 10 Alice Street, Binghamton, NY 13904-1580
EUROSPAN/Haworth, 3 Henrietta Street, London WC2E 8LU England

Library of Congress Cataloging-in-Publication Data

Women as they age.

"Has also been published as Journal of women & aging, volume 1, numbers 1/2/3 1989" — T.p. verso.
    Includes bibliographies and index.
    1. Aged women — United States. 2. Aged women — Services for — United States. I. Garner, J. Dianne. II. Mercer, Susan O.
HQ1064.U5W598 1989   305.4′0973   88-34803
ISBN 0-86656-805-0
ISBN 0-86656-873-5 (pbk)

Women As They Age: Challenge, Opportunity, and Triumph

CONTENTS

Women As They Age: Challenge, Opportunity, and Triumph

About the Contributors

June Axinn, PhD, is a Professor of Social Welfare at the University of Pennsylvania School of Social Work. She is the co-author of *Social Welfare: A History of the American Response to Need, The Century of the Child*, and, most recently, *Dependency and Poverty: Old Problems in a New World*. Her articles on family policy, social security, poverty, aging, and women have appeared in a wide variety of books and journals. During 1987 and 1988, she was a Visiting Professor of Economics at Temple University Japan and did research on aging and poverty in the Far East.

Cornelia Beck, RN, PhD, is a Professor in the College of Nursing and an Assistant Professor in the Department of Psychiatry, College of Medicine at the University of Arkansas for Medical Sciences. She is co-editor of the psychiatric nursing textbook *Mental Health Psychiatric Nursing: A Holistic Life-Cycle Approach*, which is in its second edition. Dr. Beck authored and co-authored numerous other professional publications. Presently she is principle investigator on an National Institute of Mental Health project in geriatric mental health.

Irene Burnside, RN, MS, is a Professor Emeritus at San Jose State University and currently a doctoral student in gerontological nursing at the University of Texas, Austin. She has authored *Nursing and the Aged*, now in its third edition, and *Working with the Elderly: Group Process & Techniques*, currently in its second edition. In addition, she has written 20 book chapters and 46 professional articles. Her books have won "Book of the Year" awards from the *American Journal of Nursing*, and the American Writer's Association awarded her "best book of the year on a medical subject by a nonphysician." She is a Fellow in the American Academy of Nursing and the Gerontology Society of America.

J. Dianne Garner, DSW, is an Associate Professor of Social Work at Washburn University. Her areas of teaching include both practice and research. Dr. Garner has been the Director of Social Work at Cedars-Sinai Medical Center in Los Angeles and St. Vincent Infirmary Medical Center in Little Rock. She has authored and co-authored numerous articles in the field of aging and has served on editorial boards for professional journals. Dr. Garner is currently the editor of the *Journal of Women & Aging* and the chair of the National Committee on Women's Issues of the National Association of Social Workers.

Susan A. Gaylord, PhD, is with the Department of Medicine at the University of North Carolina at Chapel Hill. Previously she was a research associate and Coordinator of the Program on Aging of UNC School of Public Health. She is the co-editor of *Aging and Public Health* and has published numerous articles in the field of aging with emphasis on health and long-term care issues. In addition to her professional publications, Dr. Gaylord has pursued her interest in wildlife and has published in *Wildlife in North Carolina*.

Naomi Gottlieb, DSW, is a Professor in the School of Social Work at the University of Washington in Seattle, where she is Coordinator of the Concentration on Women, a curriculum sequence for Master's students. During the 1987-88 academic year, she held the Belle Spafford Chair in Women's Studies at the Graduate School of Social Work at the University of Utah. She serves as National Coordinator of the Association for Women in Social Work and is a founding member of the editorial board of *Affilia, Journal of Women in Social Work*. Her books include *Alternative Social Services for Women* and, with Dianne Burden, *The Woman Client*.

Ketayun H. Gould, PhD, is a Professor of Social Work at the University of Illinois at Urbana-Champaign. Her major areas of interest are issues related to women and/or minorities, particularly the development of feminist models of education and practice related to these populations. She is also involved in a major research project on the fertility behavior of an ethnic-minority community in India. Her recent publications include "Life Model Versus Conflict Model: A Feminist Perspective," "Feminist Principles and Minority Concerns: Contributions, Problems, and Solutions," and "Asian and Pacific Islanders: Myth and Reality."

Laura Hubbs-Tait, PhD, is an Associate Professor of Psychology at Washburn University in Topeka, Kansas. From 1981 to 1982 she was an NIMH postdoctoral fellow at the University of Texas at Austin. Her current research interests are the development of the expression and understanding of anger, the psychosocial correlates of anger and hostility across the life span; and the development of emotional responses to stress. She has published articles in a variety of professional journals including *Contemporary Psychology* and the *American Journal of Orthopsychiatry*.

Lou Ann B. Jorgensen, DSW, is the Acting Associate Dean at the Graduate School of Social Work at the University of Utah. She teaches in Administration/Community Planning and Organizational Behavior. Her field of specialization is mental health and women's issues. Dr. Jorgensen directs the PhD program at the School of Social Work. In addition to her doctorate at the University of Utah, she completed postdoctoral work at Harvard University in educational administration. She has held leadership positions in the National Association of Social Workers and the Council of Social Work Education including a recent term on the Council of Social Work Education's Women's Commission.

Toba Schwaber Kerson, DSW, PhD, is a Professor in the Graduate School of Social Work and Social Research at Bryn Mawr College. She holds doctorates in both social work and sociology from the University of Pennsylvania. She is the author of *Medical Social Work: The Pre-Professional Paradox, Understanding Chronic Illness: Medical and Psychosocial Dimensions of Nine Diseases* and *Social Work in Health Settings: Practice in Context*. Dr. Kerson is currently an editorial board member of *Health and Social Work* and the *Journal of Women & Aging*.

Cheryl Kinderknecht, ACSW, is currently a staff writer and researcher in the Research and Development Department of Health Care Education Associates in Laguna Niguel, California. She has practiced social work in both hospitals and home health care agencies prior to beginning her career as a writer. Ms. Kinderknecht has authored over 20 manuals for professionals working in health care settings.

Susan A. McDaniel, PhD, is an Associate Professor of Sociology at the University of Waterloo in Ontario, Canada. She is the author of more than 50 articles and book chapters on family, childbearing, adoption, aging, and women's health issues. Her books include *Canada's Aging Population* and a co-authored book, *Social Problems Through Conflict and Order*. In 1987-88, she became the first Therese Casgrain Research Fellow, which is enabling her to complete her third book. She was the recipient of the University of Waterloo's Distinguished Teacher Award in 1981.

Susan O. Mercer, DSW, is a Professor of Social Work at the University of Arkansas at Little Rock Graduate School of Social Work. She teaches in the areas of clinical practice, aging, health, and women's issues. She has been on the editorial board of *Health and Social Work* and is currently on the editorial boards of the *Journal of Gerontological Social Work*, *Arete*, and the *Journal of Women & Aging*. Dr. Mercer has authored or co-authored numerous articles and book chapters in the areas of aging and long-term care. She consults in long-term care facilities in Arkansas and serves on the Governor's Long Term Care Advisory Board.

Kathleen E. Nuccio, PhD, is an Assistant Professor of Social Work and Women's Studies at The Ohio State University. She has studied the normative foundations of the Civil Rights Act of 1964 and the problems inherent in the implementation of its provisions barring sex discrimination in employment. She has recently received a grant to study the effects of the interaction of sex and race on the employment discrimination experiences of black women.

Barbara Pearson, RN, MN, is a Professor in the College of Nursing at the University of Arkansas for Medical Sciences in Little Rock, Arkansas. Her interest in nursing care of geriatric clients began in her graduate nursing major in rehabilitation and has continued as a part of her teaching role with students.

Susan Rice, DSW, is currently an Associate Professor of Social Work at California State University at Long Beach. She is the author and co-author of numerous articles including "Love and Intimacy Needs of the Elderly: Philosophical and Intervention Issues" and "The Aged in Helping the Sexually Oppressed." Dr. Rice teaches casework and groupwork intervention with the elderly. In addition to her teaching, she has worked with the elderly population for the past ten years and is currently coordinating a program of support groups for a retirement community in Seal Beach, California.

INTRODUCTION AND INTERNATIONAL OVERVIEW

Introduction

J. Dianne Garner, DSW
Susan O. Mercer, DSW

This is a publication about aged and aging women. It is for students, practitioners, administrators, and educators. The multidisciplinary approach includes social work, nursing, psychology, sociology, gerontology, and economics. It is written by women, many of whom are feminists, and all are, by definition, aging. Although much of the current literature focuses on older persons or older men, equal time in this volume is not given to both sexes.

The focus on older women is viewed as an appropriate response to a demographic imperative and the special needs of the majority of our present and future older population. The unique and frequently troublesome situation of older women is not just the result of growing older. It is the result of invasive and historical patterns of socioeconomic and gender stratification in societies.

Although there has been little research on the history of aging

---

J. Dianne Garner is Associate Professor, Department of Social Work, Washburn University, Topeka, KS 66621.

Susan O. Mercer is Professor, University of Arkansas at Little Rock, Graduate School of Social Work, Little Rock, AR 72204.

7

women, it is clear that older women have frequently been disadvantaged and/or victimized by the societies in which they lived. Nor has it been infrequent over time and place for women to be considered nothing more than property to be discarded when old and worn. The origins of this disadvantaged status reside in institutions, the structures of family and caregiver roles, the job market, and social policies (Arendell & Estes, 1987).

In more recent history, older women have begun to stand up against the disadvantages of being both old and female. It is, therefore, important to adjust our lens and realize that the images of older women are not always of gloom and doom. Appraise your own accomplishments, the changes you have seen in your lifetime. Appraise the accomplishments and changes you have seen in your great-grandmother, your grandmother, and your mother. Look at the world around you for the triumphs of older women. The examples that follow represent but a few of the accomplishments and contributions of older women.

After her retirement, former teacher Dr. Ethel Percy Andrus saw the need to change views of retirement. In 1947, she founded the National Retired Teacher's Association and in 1958, the American Association of Retired Persons (AARP). Through her efforts, teacher pensions were increased and health insurance for persons over age 65 became a reality. She inspired thousands to take on second careers, extend their education, and participate in government and community service. Today, AARP represents 27 million members 50 years of age and over (AARP, March, 1988).

In April, 1987, 81-year-old Muriel Clark, retired social worker and member of the Gray Panthers, came out from her undercover job with the New York special prosecutor's office. She had been investigating the state's nursing home situation and her work concluded with two nursing home officials admitting that they took payoffs to accept residents (McNamara & Burkett, 1988).

In June, 1987, Margaret Thatcher, age 62, was reelected to her third term as Prime Minister of Britain. Frequently dubbed an "Iron Lady," she is the longest-serving Prime Minister of Britain in the twentieth century. This grocer's daughter is also the longest-serving of any current Western leader.

In July, 1987, a 91-year-old woman, Hulda Crooks, reached the top of Mount Fuji. With that achievement she became the oldest climber to reach the highest peak in Japan. She is said to have begun mountain climbing in her 40s to regain her health after a serious bout with pneumonia (McNamara & Burkett, 1988).

In August, 1987, a septuagenarian named Molly Yard was elected president of the National Organization for Women. NOW continues the battle for equal rights for women and Ms. Yard travels the United States speaking out for women both young and old.

In November, 1987, Tish Sommers and Laura Shields, representing the Older Women's League, published their book and formally proclaimed "caregiving" as a women's issue (McNamara & Burkett, 1988).

Ivans (1988) told us the courageous story of Beulah Mae Donald's victory over the Ku Klux Klan. This elderly black woman now owns the building that housed the headquarters of the Ku Klux Klan in Alabama. With strength and perseverance, she went after the murderers of her 19-year-old son. It took years and a civil suit for Donald to finally triumph over the Klan. Yet, as she knows only too well, nothing can ever substitute for the life of her child.

Maggie Kuhn, age 82, is the founder of the Gray Panthers, an advocacy group for the elderly. She was recently mugged on a Philadelphia street but continues to refuse to give in to old age (Lewis, 1988). She also refused to live with other older people and has opened her home to younger housemates who provide companionship, assist with chores, and have a place to live at a reasonable rate. She is quoted as saying that "retirement communities are glorified playpens where wrinkled babies can be safe and out of the way" (Bradley-Steck, 1987).

Ester Peterson, age 81, heads a national education program on long-term care health care and insurance. She is considered a pioneer in the consumer movement. Her advice to consumers may also be an appropriate philosophy of life. She says to "compare policies, shop around, read the fine print, and get some help. Don't be afraid to ask questions" (Franckling, 1987).

Wilma Maude Roebuck, age 96, refused to live any place except in her own home. She arose one morning in July for her usual 5 a.m. cup of coffee, had a heart attack, and died exactly where she wanted: in her home. During her lifetime, she witnessed the evolution of transportation from horse and buggy to jet, Carrie Nation was a guest in her home, and she fought for women's suffrage. She raised her five children and three of her grandchildren. She was proud of both her age and of being a woman. To us she left a legacy of independence and determination.

There are hundreds of thousands of older women the world over whose accomplishments are not so newsworthy, but they continue to live life to the fullest and daily debunk the myths that surround aging women. Their lives attest to the scientific fact that "senility" and "infirmity" are not normal processes of aging.

It is important to keep in mind that disorientation among the old, commonly referred to as "senility," occurs in the presence of brain disease, chemical imbalance (frequently the result of overmedication), or depression and that only a small percentage of the elderly show any signs of disorientation. The vast majority of older women continue to meet the challenges of living with clarity of thought, perception, and wisdom born of experience. Older women are entering our universities in droves. They do not believe that "you can't teach old dogs new tricks"; nor does their performance reflect difficulty in learning the most modern theories and skills. Steinem (1983) wrote that one day an army of gray-haired women may quietly take over the earth. Demographics and the growing accomplishments of older women lend support to her words.

Keeping in mind the strength and progress of those older women who have gone before us and those who are currently struggling with the dilemmas of being old and female, this collection attempts to provide information of assistance to those whose profession or lives include providing services to older women.

The collection begins with an international demographic overview of older women, who represent the majority of the aging population worldwide. The "state of the art" and developmental perspectives across the professions of sociology, psychology, social work, and nursing are then explored. Next, a closer examination is provided of the unique issues facing older minority women. The relationship of older women to family, including the effects of family responsibilities on other roles, is then discussed. Issues of sexuality and intimacy faced by older women are explored, and the use of groups as one approach for enhancing the quality of life of older women is presented. Public policy, employment discrimination, and social program adequacy and equity are critical issues for older women and each is explored in separate sections. The common thread for these sections is the picture of governmental responses to aging and aged women. The collection concludes with a practical resource guide that explores the services available to older women, and the material is written in a "where to go and how to get it" format.

There is much to say and too little space to say it. Each section highlights the challenges older women present to professionals whose job it is, directly or indirectly, to provide assistance to that vast array of women who have entered and are entering old age.

Butler stated it well a decade ago when he said that "the problems of old age in America are largely the problems of women" (Butler, 1979). In viewing aging women from an international perspective, Butler's statement has been found to be true in other parts of the world as well. In other words, all of the issues of aging are women's issues. Some are more critical than others and have a more profound effect on women. Longevity, widowhood, chronic health problems, mental health difficulties, and the feminization of poverty have resulted in older women becoming significant consumers of health care and human services. These women present both challenges and opportunities to professionals and to those planning to enter human service fields.

REFERENCES

American Association of Retired Persons (1986). *A portrait of older minorities*. Washington, DC: Author.

American Association of Retired Persons (1988, March). *Reclaiming the past . . . rewriting the future*. Washington, DC: Author.

Arendell, T., & Estes, C. (1987, Spring). Unsettled futures: Older women . . . economics and health. *Feminist Issues*, pp. 3–27.

Bradley-Steck, T. (1987, March 8). Open house. *Arkansas Gazette*.

Butler, R. N. (1979). Preface, U.S. National Institute on Aging. *The older woman: Continuities and discontinuities*. Washington, DC: U.S. Government Printing Office.

Franckling, K. (1987, December 20). Long term care draws interest. *Arkansas Gazette*.

Ivans, M. (1988, January). Beulah Mae Donald. *Ms. Magazine*.

Lewis, C. (1988, January 3). America is graying gracefully. *Arkansas Gazette*.

Lewis, M. (1985). Older women and health: An overview. In S. Golub & R. Freedman (Eds.), *Health needs of women as they age* (pp. 1-15). New York: Haworth Press.

McNamara, M., & Burkett, K. (1988, January). 1987 . . . the laughter, tears, and triumphs. *Ms. Magazine*, pp. 34-37.

Steinem, G. (1983). *Outrageous acts and everyday rebellions*. New York: Holt, Rinehart & Winston.

An International Overview
of Aged Women

Susan O. Mercer, DSW
J. Dianne Garner, DSW

The demographic emphasis in aging has historically been placed on men or aggregate data. To be more specific, the focus has primarily been on the experiences of the older white man. This male-dominated orientation has partly occurred because of available data; it has primarily occurred because gender-differentiated questions have frequently not been asked by scholars and demographers. As recently as the early 1970s, older women were basically invisible within the population of women and the elderly. Older women were, in the main, simply not considered a distinctive group meriting attention. This omission and imbalance of emphasis on gender differences is particularly critical considering the ever-increasing number and percentage of aged women living in the world. It is also critical when one ponders the realization that old age represents a significant proportion of the average woman's life span . . . predictably 15 to 25 years beyond the age of 65 (Conable, 1986; Feinson, 1985; Norton, 1979).

It is finally dawning on us that women constitute the majority of the world's growing numbers. Fortunately, in the past decade more international and national attention has focused on aged women as a discrete population. About 12 years ago, the United Nations opened what was called the "Decade on Women." Five years into this

Susan O. Mercer is Professor, Graduate School of Social Work, University of Arkansas at Little Rock, Little Rock, AR 72204.

J. Dianne Garner is Associate Professor, Department of Social Work, Washburn University, Topeka, KS 66621.

"Decade on Women" there was an international forum in Denmark that had workshops on older women. These well-attended sessions provided a starting point for organized international discussions of the issues. The British Society of Gerontology sponsored an important conference on "Women in Later Life" in 1981. In 1982, The Older Feminists' Network in Great Britain was established. One of its goals included campaigning against the misrepresentation of older women in the media and the formation of an effective lobby around issues such as housing, health, work conditions, pay, and pensions. In 1985, there was a forum in Kenya; more issues emerged and older women came forward as a concern to be reckoned with. In fact, so many proposals for activities for older women were received in advance of the Kenya conference that the American Association for International Aging (AAIA) was created as the coordinating organization.

Recognition of issues of aged women was also growing in the United States during this period. The Older Women's League was formed in 1980 and the National Coalition on Older Women's Issues evolved in 1981. In 1981, the White House Conference on Aging included a special section on older women for the first time in its 30-year history. During the conference, the Committee on the Concerns of Older Women adopted a bill of rights. This bill specifically mentioned the following rights: self-esteem, freedom from a stigma if one lives alone, the expression of sexuality, economic support and equal employment opportunities, an adequate level of health care, positive representation in the media, and ridding oneself of dependence on others. Ironically, this bill of rights was similar in intent to the Women's Declaration of Independence, passed by U.S. feminists in Seneca Falls, New York, in 1849 . . . to guarantee equality and equality of life for women and men (Final Report, 1981; Markson, 1983; Peace, 1986).

The United Nations "Decade on Women" has drawn to a close but the coalescing and increasing recognition of older women as a discrete population with particular needs and contributions continues to grow (Conable, 1986). Older women the world over make significant, perhaps immeasurable, contributions to the social, economic, and political development of nations through their contributions to the labor force, the family, and the community. Older women are often the primary careproviders of grandchildren, spouses, frail parents, and other relatives. It is estimated that women provide almost 100% of the volunteer work around the globe.

The life expectancy of women continues to increase, and they continue to be more likely to be widowed, poor, and alone. The resources they have available in their later years are generally quite different from those of men. Aged women also experience what is referred to as "double jeopardy"; that is, in addition to experiencing discrimination based on age, they may also face discrimination based on gender. Minority females may confront triple jeopardy with discrimination based on race. Too often policies that are developed to serve the entire older population or even women in general will fail to take into account the special concerns of older women (*Women and Aging Around the World*, 1985).

The purpose of this discussion is to summarize international demographics, socioeconomic statistics, and trends on aged women. Older women are viewed in diverse ways around the world, but they remain vulnerable to some universal problems. This big picture of older women on our planet will reveal their marvelous diversity, special needs, myriad roles, living arrangements, education, employment and income status, and health care needs. International demographics trends are presented first in each section, followed by statistics from the United States. This disaggregation of the data shows important gender differences that must be reckoned with at all levels of policymaking and planning.

OUR PLANET IS AGING

The elderly population of the world is growing at a rate of about 2.5% each year, and this rate of growth in numbers and as a proportion is greater than the rate of the global population as a whole. This translates to more than 410 million elderly in the world by the year 2000 as compared with 290 million today. These numbers are expected to continue to grow into the twenty-first century. By the year 2020 it is predicted that in developed countries one out of every five persons will be age 60 or older, as will one out of every ten residents of developing nations. The proportion of elderly is lower in developing rather than developed nations but it is growing at a much faster rate (75% compared with 35% between the years 1980-2000). Developed, or "more developed," nations include all of Europe, the Soviet Union, North American, Japan, Australia, and New Zealand. The remaining nations are considered to be developing or "less developed" (Torrey, Kinselle, & Taeuber, 1987; *Women and Aging Around the World*, 1985).

Older women significantly outnumber older men in most nations of the world. In developed nations, the ratio of males to females in 1980 was 93 to 100; in developing nations, there were only 66 males per 100 females. This imbalance is even more dramatic as advanced ages are examined. For individuals aged 70 and over, the ratio dropped to 58 males per 100 females in developed countries in 1980 and 86 males to 100 females in developing countries. By 2020, the imbalance between the sexes is predicted to increase to some extent in developing nations and lessen in developed nations (*Women and Aging Around the World*, 1985).

The "old old," those 85 years or older, now constitute more than 14% of the world's elderly population. In the main, this age group will be the fastest-growing segment of the older population through the middle of the next century in almost all nations. And, yes, older women constitute the majority of persons in this "old old" group. The most rapid growth is occurring in developing nations. Specifically, the "old old" will increase a staggering 131% in developing countries between the year 2000 and 2025. Some suggest that these estimates are understated. Because this age group generally represents the major consumers of health and social services, policymakers should wake up with concern.

In the United States, the 1980 census documented more than 25 million Americans over the age of 65, which represented about 11% of the population. White elderly outnumber minority elderly. This is most likely a reflection of the socioeconomic discriminations experienced earlier in life, which increase the risks of substandard housing, poverty, malnutrition, poor education, and less access to health care.

Although white elderly currently outnumber minority elderly, the recent trend of a faster growth rate among elderly minorities is expected to continue. In 1980, over 10% of the population 65 and older were black, Hispanic, Asian/Pacific Islanders, and Native

Americans. Approximately 2.1 million or 8% of the black population in the United States are 65 years or older. The aged black population increased about 34% between 1970 and 1980 whereas the total black population increased only 16%. About 5% of the Hispanic population (persons who share a common language but come from diverse cultures such as Mexico and Cuba) are 65 years of age or older, and some 6% of Asian/Pacific Islanders are age 65 or greater. Between 1965 and 1975 there was a fourfold increase in the number of Asian/Pacific Islander elderly. The Asian/Pacific Islanders include a number of distinct cultural groups: Asian Indian, Cambodian, Chinese, Filipino, Hawaiian, Japanese, Korean, Samoan, Vietnamese, and others. Many of these persons migrated with their families to the United States from Southeast Asia in the 1970s. Of the Native American population (this includes Indians, Eskimo, and Aleut) 5% are 65 years of age or older. The proportion of elderly among Native Americans has grown faster than other minority groups. In fact, between 1970 and 1980, their population grew by 65%. This rate is about twice that of white or black elderly (*A Portrait of Older Minorities*, 1986; Torrey et al., 1987; *Women and Aging Around the World*, 1985).

The majority of the elderly in the United States are women, and the imbalance in the sex ratio is dramatic. In 1982, there were 16.6 million women 65 years or older, in contrast to only 10.7 million older men (Lewis, 1985).

The "old-old" segment of the elderly in the United States now numbers more than 6 million or 22% of all elderly. This is likely to expand to more than 14 million by the year 2020. By the time women reach age 85 or older, there are 220 women to every 100 men. Does one need to ask if demography shapes, in part, the destiny of older women (Markson, 1983; *Women and Aging Around the World*, 1985)?

LONGEVITY:
A NOT SO DELICATE BALANCE
BETWEEN THE SEXES

The level of life expectancy varies both within and among nations. There are stark extremes. Japan, for example, has an average life expectancy of 77 years, which is the highest among the developed nations; in contrast, Bangladesh and some African countries south of the Sahara have yet to achieve a life expectancy at birth of 50 years. Improved health services and nutrition have, nevertheless, made an enormous difference in closing the gap between many developed and developing countries.

Women, on the average, outlive men in almost all parts of the world. Not only do women have higher life expectancies at birth, but female death rates are lower than male death rates at all ages in essentially all nations. As a result, as the population ages, the percentage of women in each age cohort steadily increases. This pattern is quite impressive in developed countries where the proportion of older women among the old reaches as high as 70%. The female advantage in life expectancy is greater than 7 years in North American and several European countries, whereas the difference between female and male life expectancy in most developing countries is narrower. In a developing country, a female born between 1975 and 1980 can expect to live about two years longer than a male born during the same time span. By age 60, women in developing nations can expect to live an additional 16 years. The gap in female and male life expectancy is expected to widen in all developing nations in the next few decades and to narrow slightly in developed countries. It is probably too early to determine if this will occur (*Women and Aging Around the World*, 1985).

The typical pattern of women outliving men is reversed in a few developing countries in South Asia and the Middle East. In these societies, there is an interplay of cultural factors such as low female social status and a preference for male rather than female newborns, and these factors contribute to a higher male life expectancy at birth. This preference for male offspring is carried to its extreme in the form of female infanticide in China. Although female infanticide is illegal, some China "watchers" suggest it is again on the rise and the result is a nationwide outnumbering of female infants by males. The act of killing female infants is officially condemned and the topic is not a popular one for visiting professional groups to bring up for discussion during a visit to China (Xiao, 1984).

It is unclear precisely why women outlive men, and the subject continues to stir controversy and generate continued research. The gap will perhaps never completely close because of a basic biological advantage of women. There are, however, a number of life style patterns that may contribute to part of the differences. These include life style-related causes of higher male mortality such as a higher rate of accidents, alcohol consumption, and cigarette smoking (*Aging America*, 1984; *Women and Aging Around the World*, 1985). Nevertheless, women clearly have different biological strengths as well as vulnerabilities. And apparently a great majority of the female animal world also have a longer life expectancy (Lewis, 1985).

In the United States, a person born around the 1900s could expect to live an average of 49 years. Even as early as 1930, there were relatively equal numbers of females and males aged 65 and over. Women now live decidedly longer than men. There remain variations in life expectancy according to race, although advances have occurred in the last four decades. In fact, after whites and blacks achieve age 65, the differences in life expectancy are smaller. Racial differences in life expectancy have been generally attributed to socioeconomic status that has adversely affected quality of life in all dimensions. By 1983, the average life expectancy for a white female was 78.8 years, 73.8 years for a black female, 71.6 years for a white male, and 65.2 years for a black male. These differences in life expectancy are predicted to continue to increase until 2050 and then level off. By that time, life expectancy for women will be about 81 years in contrast to 71.8 years for men (*Aging America*, 1984; Cox, 1988; *A Portrait of Older Minorities*, 1985).

MARITAL STATUS

Trends in marital status, including widowhood, are integral components in the analysis of the older woman because the role of family is intimately linked to her social, economic, and emotional well-being. Marriage, including common-law unions, is the most common status among adult populations in our world. However, widowhood increases substantially with age. The rates of widowhood among persons 65 years and over range from 31% to 47% and vary little between developed and developing countries. Among persons 75 years and older the range is from 46% to 61% (Torrey et al., 1987).

The proportion of widowed older women is many times greater than for older men in practically all developed and developing nations. Widowhood is a fact for a significant number of older women the world over for a number of reasons. Women live longer than men, and they are more likely to marry men older than themselves. Older men are also more likely to remarry than are older women. Because men generally marry women younger than themselves, they have a larger pool of persons from which to choose a mate. In some countries, there are even social norms that strongly discourage older women from remarrying. It is, therefore, easy to understand that the older a woman becomes the more likely she is to become a widow. Among the countries that maintain data on the marital status of the "old old," the median rate of widowhood for women 80 years or older is a dramatic 75%. This same data base for the male median in all countries is 39%, or almost half the level for older females (Torrey et al., 1987; *Women and Aging Around the World*, 1985).

Gender differences in remarriage rates are also reflected in the percentage of older women who are divorced or separated. In most developed and developing countries, there are more divorced or separated older women than older men. Although the absolute numbers of older women who are divorced or separated is small in comparison to the demographics on widowhood status, the proportions are increasing and merit attention.

In the United States, the international patterns also hold true. The majority of older women are widowed and the majority of older men are married. This is true among whites and all minority groups. According to 1986 statistics, 40% of older women are married in contrast to 77% of older men. One half of all older women were widows in 1986. This translated to 8.1 million older women who were widows and only 1.5 million older men being without spouses.

Divorced persons represented only about 4% of all older persons in 1986. Their numbers (1.1 million), however, had increased almost four times as fast as the older population as a whole in the preceding decade. With persons 65 years or older, the single (never married) and divorced rates are about equal for men and women. There is a difference in this trend among minorities, however, that is noteworthy. More than twice as many older black males as whites are divorced or separated, and the proportion of widowed is also slightly higher. The divorced or separated rate for the older black woman is also slightly higher than her older white female cohort (*A Profile of Older Americans*, 1987; *A Portrait of Older Minorities*, 1985).

The high level of widowhood is not surprising in view of women's greater life expectancy. Neither is the high rate of marriage surprising considering that contemporary older women were socialized to view marriage as the optimal, standard, and enduring organization for adulthood. And yet these same women are statistically more likely to be the sole survivers of marriages terminated by the death of a spouse.

There are a number of current trends that may portend dramatic shifts in the lives of future older women. Some of these trends include an increase in the incidence of divorce, an increase in the number of unmarried persons who live together, a delay in the incidence of first marriages, a delay in childbearing, an increase in the number of couples remaining childless, increasing numbers of women entering the work force, earlier sexual experiences, greater acceptance of older women choosing and perhaps marrying younger men, and a somewhat greater tolerance in our society of variant forms of sexual expression and life styles such as homosexual couples.

Some of these trends offer a form of preparatory experience that may help future older women with being more adaptive and coping with the losses. We have more options today than our mothers or grandmothers had. These options may provide a training ground for building self-sufficiency and a more self-directed life style. Women today are less likely to be satisfied with either sublimation or abstinence. Although there is "good news and bad news" with respect to these trends, they probably signal that older women of the future have increased choices and a greater chance of surviving with a stronger sense of self.

These increases in choices will probably also lead to an extension of family supports through friendships. Although older women have always found satisfaction in companionship with women friends, these friendships may be even stronger in the future. As contemporary younger women increasingly feel free to participate in a range of activities without a male escort or mate, the suggestion that a man-less activity carries a social stigma or represents a social failure or personal vulnerability will hopefully lessen or become obsolete (Abu-Laban, 1987). The end result should be a strengthening of relationships, within and without marriage, for both women and men.

LIVING ARRANGEMENTS

Historically, the family has been the basic societal structure that provided care, economic assistance, and other needed support for the older family members. This assistance used to be short term; it is now potentially very long term. Urbanization and economic development have also affected the family unit, and there is generally a present-day shift from an extended family to a nuclear family structure. Living alone is becoming increasingly common throughout the world, and it is certainly becoming the norm in developed countries.

In developed countries, the majority of older women, even in the old-old category, live alone or in the community rather than with families or in institutions. And they are, in the main, able to function relatively independently. The United States Current Population Survey revealed that half of all women aged 75 or older lived alone in 1985, in contrast to only one-fifth of men in the same category. Current census data from our neighbor to the north, Canada, revealed similar findings. There over one-fourth of the elderly, and a third of those 75 years or older, lived alone. This figure is even higher in Great Britain, where 80% of all elderly persons who live alone are women.

The pattern of living arrangements in Japan is quite different from that of the United States, Canada, and Great Britain. In Japan, about 75% of the elderly live with relatives, and about a half of these live in three-generation households. This pattern is true for both older women and men. Multigenerational families are still quite common in rural areas of Eastern Europe, such as Poland, Romania, and the Soviet Union. As in other developed countries, however, older women are still two to three times as likely as older men to live alone.

In the West, when older women do live with their families, it is generally with an adult daughter. The tendency to live alone frequently seems to stem from a desire on the part of the older woman to maintain her privacy and independence and "not be a burden" on her children rather than from evidence that families do not care for their elderly. Research from Sweden indicated that many older women assess living alone positively because of their freedom from marital and family obligations. Apparently, in Sweden more older women than older men attend the theater and belong to literary clubs and educational activities.

Nevertheless, living alone frequently has a darker side. From a psychosocial perspective, living alone contributes to isolation and diminished socialization. Researchers in Germany reported that the level of isolation increases with advancing age, the duration of the time a person lives alone, and declines in health and income. Information from the 1983 American Housing Survey reported that older persons tended to live in older homes that are more likely to have defective conditions and lacked adequate facilities. The home may be defective because the older person is physically and financially unable to maintain the property (Torry et al., 1987; *Women and Aging Around the World*, 1985).

In developing nations, fewer older persons, including women, live alone. For example, in the Phillippines and Singapore, only 2% and 6%, respectively, of all the elderly live alone. In these countries, as is true for many developing countries, the family still provides the major economic support for the older person, including housing. In some nations, it would not be uncommon for an older woman to move into her daughter or son's households, or rotate her stays among several children. In some developing countries, the tradition is for an older woman to live with her son, particularly the eldest, and his family. This is common in some African countries and some Asian countries such as Bangladesh, India, Pakistan, and the People's Republic of China. In China, a son is still a form of "social security" in old age. Women in these cultures who have no son will either live alone or live with a married daughter (Torrey et al., 1987; *Women and Aging Around the World*, 1985). In fact, China is one of the few countries in the world where children are bound by law to provide for their parents. China's Family Law stipulates that children have the duty to support and assist their parents and that parents have the right to demand that their children pay for their support. Furthermore, this law is passed down to grand-children if there are no living children (Butterfield, 1982).

And yet traditional patterns are breaking down in many develop-ing countries as they experience the demographic and social forces similar to those of developed countries of urbanization, industrial-ization, and increasing mobility. When the young make massive migrations from rural to urban areas, there are inevitably many wid-ows who are left behind with few or no close kin (*Women and Aging Around the World*, 1985). Some call this progress.

Institutional Care

The frail elderly are more likely to be cared for by family mem-bers than in nursing homes in most countries. Nursing home place-ment is more likely to occur in the United States than in other coun-tries, but it is still relatively low even in the United States. We know that the institutionalized elderly are disproportionately very old, very female, and very widowed or unmarried. Otherwise, little is known about the institutionalized elderly in most countries.

Throughout the world, middle-aged women, adult daughters or daughters-in-law, are the primary careproviders to the chronically ill elderly residing in the community or at home. These careprovi-ders generally do not have the same level of care and support when they require it in their own old age or during illness. In Hungary, for example, a study reported that one out of three older women reported that no family member was available to care for her during illness, whereas only one out of ten men reported this lack of avail-able care.

It is noteworthy that although the majority of institutional resi-dents are older women, relatively little is known about the qualita-tively different experiences of women and men within institutions. Some research from Great Britain has shown quite different profiles for women and men. For example, men are admitted to nursing homes at a younger age, are generally in better health, and are more ambulatory. In national surveys in Great Britain, institutionalized women have also expressed less satisfaction than men primarily because of feelings of uselessness and isolation. This is perhaps because the relocation is a loss of a domestic role for women as well as a loss of contact with the community (*Women and Aging Around the World*, 1985).

In the United States, the majority of our elderly, about 94%, live in the community rather than in an institutional environment. The profile for noninstitutionalized elderly is generally similar to that of other developed countries. In 1986, about 57% of older women, or 9.1 million, lived in families in contrast to approximately 83%, or 9.3 million, older men who resided with families. The proportion of the elderly residing in a family setting decreased with advancing age. About 18% of older women and 7% of older men were not living with a spouse but were living with a child, siblings, or other relatives. An additional 2% of older women and 3% of older men lived with nonrelatives. In teasing out the demographics more, we learn that in 1986 about 41%, or 6.6 million, older women lived alone and only 15%, or 1.7 million, older men lived alone (*A Profile of Older Americans*, 1987).

Minority Americans present a somewhat different profile. A slightly higher proportion (96%) of blacks reside in the community. Because relatively more blacks are widowed, divorced, or separated, it follows that a smaller proportion are living with their spouses. Some data suggest that sharing a home with a grown child, frequently an adult daughter, is a common living arrangement. About 97% of the Hispanic elderly live in the community . . . either alone, with a spouse, family members, or with nonrelatives. The Asian/Pacific Islander older woman is more likely to be married than her white cohorts and thus a smaller proportion remains single in the later years. they are also less likely to be living alone . . . only 19% in contrast to 30% of their white cohorts. About 96% of Native American elderly live in households in the community, and a majority (66%) of these live with family members. About a fourth of the elderly live on American Indian reservations or in Alaskan Native villages (*A Portrait of Older Minorities*, 1986).

Institutional Care in the United States

In 1985, we had 1,491,400 persons living in 19,100 nursing homes in the United States. According to the 1985 National Nursing Home Survey, only 5% to 6% of our nation's elderly are residents in a nursing home on any given day. This statistic is consistent with the findings from previous national nursing home surveys conducted in 1973-74 and 1977. This figure is misleading, however, without examining the data in more detail because age is an important factor. The rate of institutionalization is less than 2% for those 65 to 74 years of age. This rises to about 7% for those age 75 to 84. The number then jumps to 20% for those 85 years of age or older. Longitudinal studies predict that people age 65 have between a 25% and 40% chance of spending some time in a nursing home before they die (Hing, 1987; Kane, Ouslander, & Abrass, 1984; Vincente, Wiley, & Carrington, 1979).

Nursing home residents in the United States are likely to be old, female, and white. Of the residents in 1985 75% were female and 93% were white. Of the remaining numbers, only 6% were black and less than 1% were other races. Elderly white residents had an average age of 83 (84 for women, 81 for men). Although the use of a nursing home increased as both women and men aged, women used nursing homes at significantly higher rates than men regardless of the age level. In 1985, one in four women 85 years or older lived in nursing homes, compared with only 1 in 7 men in the same age group. Females were generally more functionally dependent than males. The greater utilization of nursing homes by elderly women than men is an artifact of women's greater life expectancy and a greater tendency among persons without spouses and with poor health to enter nursing homes. It is also an artifact of caregiving norms. It seems that caregiving for women is an expectation, a duty, whereas caregiving for men is often an unexpected demonstration of compassion. It is suggested that men do not have the "knack" for caring for the infirm, but perhaps a woman's "knack" is just a lifetime of societal expectations (Shields, 1988).

As stated previously, white elderly are more likely to reside in nursing homes than black persons and those of other races. This is particularly true in the old-old group of persons 85 years of age or older. In this "old-old" group, 23% of whites, compared with 14% of blacks, resided in nursing homes. The 1982 Long-Term Care Survey data suggested that a higher proportion of elderly blacks and other races were more functionally impaired than white elderly and yet they remained in the community. This lower use by elderly blacks and other races appears to result from more informal care-providing in the home and in family units. In other words, elderly blacks are more likely to receive care at home than within an institution (Hing, 1987).

One particular shift from the 1977 study of nursing home residents to the 1985 study is noteworthy. In general, in 1985, nursing home residents in the United States were more dependent with respect to performing activities of daily living (ADLs) than in 1977. Elderly black residents, both females and males, tended to be more functionally dependent than elderly white residents, both females and males. Functional dependency is determined, in part, by the extent to which a person requires assistance in performing the basic activities of daily living. ADLs are a measure of functional dependency and include bathing, dressing, using the toilet, transferring in and out of bed, continence, and eating. A partial explanation for this shift toward increased functional dependency is the shift in the age distribution of nursing home residents to the old-old group of 85 years and older. An additional explanation is the impact of Medicare policy on nursing home care. The Medicare prospective payment system was instituted in 1983, and this reimbursement system rather forcefully encourages hospitals to reduce patient lengths of stay. It is possible that the elderly person released earlier under this new system may require a higher level of care in the nursing home than would have been necessary had he or she been able to remain longer in the hospital environment. In general, however, it is accurate to say that functional dependency increases with increasing age (Hing, 1987).

One further caveat on nursing homes is noteworthy. For some elderly women the nursing home is the only solution, and perhaps even the best solution. Then the problem becomes not only how to finance the care, but how to get them into a facility. The poor, minority, and "difficult to care for" elderly are discriminated against and often have a difficult time locating a nursing home. For instance, a recent New York City study of state records found that white elderly were accepted at better nursing homes, and blacks and Hispanics were relegated to poorer facilities. Potential nursing home residents may also be discriminated against on the basis of income. The nursing home industry is increasingly going for private-pay residents rather than Medicaid residents because the income is greater. Some suggest that the shortage of nursing home beds, particularly for Medicaid residents, is expected to reach a critical point by the end of this century (Sidel, 1986). The preferential treatment of private-pay residents over Medicaid residents is already a major ethical dilemma.

EDUCATION

Education is important for many reasons . . . not the least of which is that it is a major example of how events in the lives of young people affect their lives as older people. Education provides a broader knowledge base and a potentially greater level of skill relative to employment opportunities. Education generally increases a person's capacity to prepare for the economics of old age by enhancing occupational capabilities to accumulate resources as one ages. The more resources a person has, the less likely that person is to be dependent on society for care in the "twilight" years (Torrey et al., 1987).

Although the United States is in a favorable position compared with many of the developed nations, as a general guideline the level of education attained by the elderly in the world is well below that of the younger population. This educational gap is, however, narrowing. In most developed nations, about 90% of persons aged 15 to 34 have completed primary level school. Among the elderly, this rate is considerably lower. Women and men are equally likely to have completed school at the primary level. A small proportion of all age groups have completed secondary school, and it is here that the differences between the elderly and the young become more pronounced. Gender differences also become more pronounced at this level as older men are more likely than older women to have completed secondary school.

Even though older women of today in developed countries are considered better educated than those of the past, there are still major disparities. For example, among Canadian women in 1976, one half of all women age 65 and over had completed no more than primary school, compared with only 13% of women aged 25-34. In the United States in 1981, only 28% of women aged 65 and over had completed high school, compared with about one-half of those aged 45-54 (Torrey, Kinsella, & Taeuber, 1987).

It is perhaps even more significant to look at literacy rates. Not surprisingly, literacy is much higher among men than women. In 1980, greater than one-half of the female population in Asia and Africa was illiterate. The proportion rises to 80% in African countries. The proportions of illiterate women are about one third in Latin America. It is further bad news that this disparity has remained constant for about 20 years even though female illiteracy is decreasing in most developing nations. This area is such a concern that a recent report from the Secretary General of the United Nations concluded that female illiteracy is "one of the priority problems in developing nations" (*Women and Aging Around the World*, 1985).

In the United States, the educational level of the older population has steadily increased. This is particularly true for the years between 1970 and 1986, when the median educational level advanced from 8.7 years to 11.8 years (11.9 years for females, 11.7 years for males). The percentage of the older population who completed high school increased from 28% to 49%. In 1986, approximately 10% had four or more years of college.

The educational level attained varied considerably, however, by race and ethnic origins among older persons. Affirmative action programs instituted in the last 20 years should cast a different light on future generations of older minorities, but they have not particularly benefited the black elderly of today. Although only 6% of black elderly have had no formal education (compared with 2% of whites), only 17% have completed high school as compared with 41% of the white elderly. The median number of years of school completed by blacks in 1986 was 8.3 years (12.1 for whites).

The picture is considerably different among those minority elderly of Hispanic background. They are, in fact, the least educated, with the proportion with no formal education being eight times as great as for elderly whites. Of Hispanics 65 years and older 16% have had no education and only 19% graduated from high school. The median number of years of school completed for Hispanics was 7.2 years in 1986.

The Asian/Pacific Islanders have the greatest proportion of high school graduates (26%) of all minority elderly. This percentage, however, is still lower than for white elderly. The most recent Asian/Pacific Islander migrants have more well-educated professionals than any other migrant group, yet 13% of their elderly lacked formal education.

About 12% of Native American elderly have no formal education, and about 22% of their numbers have graduated from high school. Native American elderly have been educated almost exclusively within the U.S. school systems, both on and off reservations (Agree, 1987; Fowles, 1987).

EMPLOYMENT

In all parts of the world, participation in the labor force declines as persons approach retirement age. The proportion of the elderly still active in the paid labor force is generally a small portion relative to the corresponding number of persons age 25 to 54 years. Changes in the educational system and technology give younger persons a competitive edge over their older counterparts, and many older persons are squeezed out of the labor force. At the same time, many private businesses and governments have established lower retirement ages and policies that make it economically possible for older persons to opt for retirement rather than continued employment.

Although older men significantly outnumber older women in the work forces of the world, total economic activity rates among older women in developed nations have been rising or are at least holding steady. A record level of increasing participation is seen among women aged 55 to 59 (and younger) and future trends will undoubtedly reflect this pattern (Torrey et al., 1987).

In developed regions of the world, less than 8% of older women are in the labor force, a relatively small number. About one in three middle-aged women (55 to 64) were in the work force in 1980 in developed countries. This pattern varies, of course, with some nations. For example, about one-half of the middle-aged women in Great Britain and Denmark were in the work force by the late 1970s. This same percentage of employed middle-aged women was true of Japan by 1983. Not only were these middle-aged women working in record numbers, but surveys in both Europe and the United States reflected their strong preference to continue working when compared with attitudes of men in the same age group. This pattern remained true even if the middle-aged women felt they could afford to retire.

In developing nations as a whole, the proportion of middle-aged women economically active in 1980 was generally similar to that of developed nations. There is a major difference, however. The participation rate of women 65 years and older is more than twice as high as that of their cohorts in developed countries (16% to 7%). It is not surprising to note relatively high participation rates at older ages in developing countries. These rates are influenced by a number of factors: less prevalent pension and retirement supports, a large number of self-employed persons, the inappropriateness of the concept of retirement in some countries, and the nature of the work itself.

Furthermore, these numbers dramatically underestimate the economic contributions of older women to their country. The rate is underestimated because much of what women "do" throughout the world is essentially invisible by the standards recorded in censuses or surveys. Much of the labor is in agriculture, small-scale trading, and the informal labor sector and is not counted (*Women and Aging Around the World*, 1985). Furthermore, as every homemaker in the world knows, her work within the home makes an enormous contribution to the family, and yet this role has little to no economic recognition.

In many African nations, women provide the dominant agricultural labor force, even up to 80% of the workers. Older women in these societies generally continue to do this strenuous work as long they are physically able. With the recent migration of the young to the urban areas and the introduction of cash crops, many of these older women now have even less help than they previously had. And yet their needs are seldom spoken to in rural development plans in these countries. In South Asia, about a third of women aged 55 to 64 and about 14% of women 65 years and older are classified as in the active labor market. Their occupations also tend to cluster around agriculture, domestic help, and small-scale trading. Fewer older women appear to be economically active in the Latin American countries. One explanation for the sharp decline in older women working in these countries is that many are forced out of the labor market in urban areas in favor of younger, better educated workers (*Women and Aging Around the World*, 1985).

It is not new information that "women's jobs" are clustered in a fewer number of occupations relative to men and that these "women's occupations" pay less. It, therefore, follows that there is a significant earnings gap between women's and men's work; that is, women earn generally less than men all over the world. This discrepancy is more severe in developing countries than in developed nations, but the United States has nothing to boast of relative to pay equity. In 1987, U.S. women cracked the 70% barrier for the first time on record in narrowing the pay gap. That means the median weekly earnings for women working full time was 70 cents for every $1.00 earned by men. This earnings gap cannot be justified soley by the standard explanations that women have less work experience, more interruptions in their careers, do not have equivalent education, and tend to work in nonunionized jobs. The reasons go much deeper and include employment discrimination, a history of "protective legislation" that excluded women's full economic participation, disincentives in the tax and social security systems in some nations, sexism, racism, ageism, and a general devaluing of "women's work" and thus of women, by society. There is another appalling trend known as "occupational resegregation." This process occurs when women move into a male-dominated field only to realize that their growing female presence has caused wages to drop. If this trend is really an extensive problem, then women may continue to confront gaping wage disparities regardless of the fields they enter. It is noteworthy that so many middle-aged women have reentered the work in the face of all of the above. Perhaps only when all women are given equal value in our world will their work be given equal value (McClure, 1988; Sidel, 1986; Staff, 1988; *Women and Aging Around the World*, 1985).

In the United States in 1986, there were about 3 million older Americans in the work force or actively seeking work, including 1.2 million women and 1.8 million men. This represented about 2.6% of the U.S. labor force and some 3% of this number were unemployed. Also in 1986 about 54% of the workers over age 65 were employed part-time and the majority (61%) of these were women. About 26% of older workers in 1986 were self-employed and three quarters of this number were men (Fowles, 1987).

Generally, about the same percentage of minorities and whites continue to work after age 65. However, among Hispanic and native American elderly who are seeking work, the percentage of unemployment is nearly twice as great (9%) as among whites (5%). A greater number of Asian/Pacific Islanders remain in the labor force than any minority group (approximately 16% of those 65 years or older). Many of these, about 25%, are self-employed.

Blacks, however, are more likely to have experienced periods of unemployment, are more likely to accumulate less work experience, and are also more likely to leave the work force earlier. It is suggested that black women have had a very different experience. From the beginnings of their lives in the United States, one group of women have worked outside their homes on a full-time basis: slave women. They worked as farm workers and domestics in the "big house," and pregnancy apparently made little difference in their work assignments (Agree, 1986; Sidel, 1986). An ex-slave, Frederick Douglass, poignantly describes his mothers's work and how her family and nurturing role had to be sacrificed to her slave job:

> I never saw my mother . . . more than four or five times in my life . . . she was hired by Mr. Stewart, who lived about twelve miles from my home. She made her journeys to see me in the night . . . on foot . . . after the performance of her day's work. She was a field hand, and a whipping is the penalty of not being in the field at sunrise . . . I do not recollect of ever seeing my mother by the light of day. She was with me in the night. She would lie down with me, and get me to sleep, but long before I waked she was gone . . . She died when I was seven years old . . . I was not allowed to be present during her illness, at her death, or burial. (Wertheimer, 1977, p. 6)

INCOME: THE HAVES AND HAVE NOTS

When a person retires, he or she is, in the main, more economically vulnerable because income and ability to replenish assets are diminished. In developed countries, the major sources of income for older persons are personal savings, public and private pensions, Social Security benefits, and "transfer payments" such as Supplemental Security, unemployment, and veteran's benefits. As a nation's population ages, the public resources that must be contributed to the economic security of its elderly generally rise. All of this sounds fine on the surface, but the subtle and not so subtle discriminations directed toward older women in all nations continue and the area of level of income is no exception. The reality is that older women in developed and developing countries are more likely to fall below the poverty level than older men and are more likely to be dependent on their families for support than older men. The reasons for this have been discussed throughout: greater longevity, increased likelihood of widowhood, devalued earnings from work and little or no economic recognition for "work in the home," distinctive labor force patterns that are commonly interrupted by the nurturance of child and infirm family elderly, pension inequities, and so forth. Some progress has been made in recent years in developed nations in increasing overall pensions for women and men, but benefits for women generally have not kept pace with those of men in the last two decades.

Developing countries have sparse data on the economic positions of older women. One can safely conclude, however, that their status is frequently precarious. Few older women in developing countries are protected by pensions and thus they are more likely to be dependent on their children or other close relatives. This dependency becomes even greater for widows and the very old. Those childless older women are especially vulnerable.

A 1982 study of older person in eight settlement colonies in India provides an example. In the survey, almost three-fourths of the older women reported they were totally dependent on others for support. This is in contrast with only two out of five men reporting the same level of dependency. Studies from Bangladesh have similar findings.

Some African countries have made agrarian reforms that have frequently failed to take into account the needs of older women. For example, widowed women in Tanzania have traditionally had rights to use their father's, brother's, and husband's land. Recent land laws have taken away these women's rights and the "reforms" established exclusive male ownership. In Kenya, widowed women are able to inherit land from sons, and thus having "only" daughters means they are virtually landless.

In most developed countries, older women are also more likely to fall below the poverty level than older men. Those older women particularly at risk are the widowed, separated, and divorced. Because older women live longer, it is not uncommon for them to exhaust their economic resources before the end of their lives. This is particularly true if their spouse has a prolonged health problem prior to death. What else accounts for this higher level of poverty?

In most developed countries, the majority of older women depend on Social Security or "welfare" through means-tested benefits for their primary income. Such benefits continue to be inadequate in most developed countries (and essentially nonexistent in developed countries). Social Security benefits are almost always developing in reference to full-time workers, who are usually males. They also frequently exclude or penalize the homemaker, domestic worker, part-time employee, and the agricultural worker. It is important to remember that many of today's older women have not been in paid employment for major portions of their lives. If an older woman has never worked, she is in further jeopardy as in most nations she will receive only a fraction of the pension to which her husband was entitled. Therefore, when an older woman's husband dies, her income is reduced but her living expenses remain essentially the same.

Even those women who have worked for substantial portions of their lives generally receive significantly lower pensions than men. A four-country comparison of average earnings in the manufacturing industry illustrates this point. In 1980, women's benefits as a proportion of men's in the United States were 61%, 79% in France and Switzerland, and 83% in Sweden. There has been some progress made. In 1980, there were five developed countries where women's benefits equaled men's: Australia, New Zealand, Great Britain, the Federal Republic of Germany, and the Netherlands. In most nations that have parity between women's and men's pensions, some form of "universal flat-rate pension" system is used. That means that all persons who reach a certain chronological age receive a certain amount of pension whether they have been in the labor force or not. Short of this strategy becoming a universal one, the other solution is for women's wages to become comparable to men's or to revise benefit formulas to take into account women's lower salaries. Comparable pay for comparable work is a more self-esteem building process for all women (Torry et al., 1987; *Women and Aging Around the World*, 1985).

In the United States in 1986, the median income of older women ($6,425) was substantially lower than that for older males ($11,544). About 3.5 million older persons, or 12.4%, were below the poverty level in 1986. An additional 2.3 million, or 8%, were classified as "near-poor." Nine southern states had the highest poverty rates for older persons: Mississippi (34%); Alabama, Arkansas, and Louisiana (28% each); Georgia (26%); South Carolina and Tennessee (25% each); North Carolina (24%); and Kentucky (23%). The rate of poverty for older women (15%) was almost twice as great as for older men (8%). Keep in mind that the official 1986 definition of the poverty level was $5,255 for an older person living alone and $6,330 for an older-couple household.

Families headed by persons age 65 or greater had a median income in 1986 of $19,932. About 15% of the families with an elderly head of household had incomes less than $10,000 and 38% had incomes of $25,000 or more. The major source of income for older families (and individuals) in 1985 was Social Security (35%), income from assets (25%), earnings (23%), public and private pensions (14%), and "transfer payments" (Supplemental Security, unemployment, and veteran's payments). The median net worth, which is assets minus liabilities, of older households in 1986 was $60,300. This is considerably above the U.S. average in 1984 of $32,700. Of older households, 16% had a net worth of $5,000 or below, and 7% had a net worth of $250,000 or more. Older persons living alone or with nonrelatives were more likely to be poor (25%) than were older persons living in families (6%). Older women are statistically more likely than older men to be living alone or with nonrelatives (Fowles, 1987).

Blacks, as is true of other minorities, are more likely to work low-paying, sporadic jobs with limited employment opportunities. They are also more likely to be in jobs not covered by Social Security prior to the 1950s. And they are less likely to accumulate adequate assets and pension benefits, which makes them more dependent on Social Security for the majority of their retirement income than whites. The median income for black women age 65 to 69 in 1984 was $4,477 (this drops to $3,850 for black women 70 years and older) and $7,097 for black males 65 to 69 (this drops to $5,114 for black men 70 years and older) (Hooyman & Kiyak, 1988).

The black elderly in the United States are the most economically disadvantaged of any of the minority groups. Over 35% live with incomes below the poverty level in contrast with about 13% of the white elderly. The most disadvantaged groups are older black women, those living in rural areas, and the "old old" (85 years or older). Almost 70% of rural black women live in poverty, making them the most impoverished of any group of elderly (Agree, 1987).

For an excellent discussion of working conditions for black and white women, and how social welfare policies from colonial times to the present have regulated the lives of women, see Abramovitz (1988).

HEALTH

It is generally true that throughout the world the health care industry is dependent on women; that is, women are the majority of the "patients" and, at all but the top levels, are the majority of the providers of health care. Women certainly provide the vast majority of the extra market caretaking or the unpaid home care for sick family members. Other general facts of women's health are that women report higher morbidity than men and have lower mortality rates; women are, as a group, hospitalized more often than men; they receive the majority of surgical procedures; consume more drugs than do men (especially psychotropics); and are institutionalized more often than men (Marieskind, 1980).

A number of factors impede a comprehensive and accurate assessment of women's health status. Many countries do not collect or report health data separately by sex or age. When women are reported as a discrete group, data frequently do not differentiate among ethnicities, age, marital status, education, economic status, employment, sexual preference, and so forth. It is widely accepted that these socioeconomic factors have a significant impact on morbidity and morality and health status in general. Furthermore, there are other factors that may introduce a sex bias. For example, it is believed that women engage in more help-seeking behaviors and are more cooperative than men in complying with survey requests. It is possible that this factor may inflate figures regarding their reported illnesses. It is also more socially acceptable for women to report illness. In spite of the above, attempts are being made by the United Nations and other organizations to provide a more realistic and comprehensive assessment of women's health status in our world and one that is more free of sex-based stereotypes (Marieskind, 1980).

There are surveys that suggest that the most common health problems affecting older women in some developing countries may be quite different from those of older women in developed countries. According to some research, the health problems of older women in developing countries tend to be illnesses induced or aggravated by social factors such as physically strenuous labor, poor nutrition, frequent reproductive activities in their youth, inadequate environmental conditions, lack of proper sanitation, and inadequate health services. It is clear that socioeconomic conditions and health are interdependent.

Data from India illustrate the frequently poor nutritional status of older women. In a survey of over 300 older persons in Delhi, significantly more older women (30%) than older men (18%) expressed dissatisfaction with their diet and the quality of their food. An additional one-third reported an inadequate quantity. A survey of older women in Sierra Leone in West Africa reported that almost one-half of the women over age 65 said that health was their most important problem. They also reported that none of the older women looked to their husbands for help in this area, although some husbands expected help from their wives when they had health problems (*Women and Aging Around the World*, 1985).

Although poverty is an enormous variable in malnutrition, cultural patterns also play major roles. In some African and Asian countries, the more valued sources of energy and nutrition are reserved for the males in the family. There are even cultural restrictions in some countries that make some foods like meat, fish, and poultry forbidden to women. A number of countries go beyond these external controls. For instance, some tribal societies in Ethiopia have a ritual of pulling several crucial teeth as a sign of a young girl's entry into adulthood and her state of marriageability. The ritual is in the name of beauty but it also serves to make eating meat, a rare and valued food, a permanently difficult task. Steinem (1983) referred to these acts as the sexual politics of food.

In developed countries, older women pay the health consequences of greater longevity. Older women are more likely than older men to have to cope longer with chronic illnesses and experience the risks of serious impairments in physical functioning. Even though there are sex differentials in mortality rates, women in developed countries die from the same primary illnesses as men: cardiovascular disease, cancers, cerebrovascular disease, and respiratory disorders. Older women around the world are more likely than men to suffer from certain chronic health conditions such as osteoporosis, arthritis, hypertension, and diabetes (*Women and Aging Around the World*, 1985).

Data from a number of developed countries indicate that older women experience significantly greater mobility problems than older men. Studies from Great Britain, Spain, and Hungary reported that older women are more likely to be bedfast or unable to perform essential self-care tasks or activities of daily living (ADLs) and could only infrequently leave their homes because of their immobility. Accidents, especially falls, are another leading cause of illness and disability among older women and are related to the increase in immobility. In Great Britain, the incidence of hospital-treated falls is four times greater among women 75 years or older than among their male counterparts (*Women and Aging Around the World*, 1985). Cardiovascular diseases can predispose an older woman for a fall. Syncope or fainting due to cardiac arrhythmias (very slow or fast heart rates) also account for a number of the falls (Markson, 1983). Frequently, these falls result in hip injuries that further restrict the older woman's mobility. Osteoporosis and arthritis are also important contributing factors.

In the United States, more data is collected according to sex, age, and ethnicity. Unfortunately, this greater variability of data has not necessarily led us to set world-class standards in health care relative to older women.

According to 1984 statistics, about 6 million (23%) older, community-based persons (25% women and 19% men) reported health-related difficulties with one or more activities of daily living. Less than half of these persons reported receiving personal help. Of course, the older the person becomes the more likely he or she is to need assistance in activities of daily living as well as home-management activities.

Older persons accounted for 31% of all hospital stays and 42% of all days of care in hospitals in 1986. Older persons in the United States also averaged more visits to a physician in 1986 than did persons under age 65 (9 visits in contrast to 5 visits) (Fowles, 1987). Older men spend more days in the hospital than older women but older women are more likely to spend time in a nursing home or to need home care services (Lewis, 1985). Nursing homes are at least twice as likely to be filled with older women than older men (Hooyman & Kiyak, 1988).

Hospital expenses in 1984 were projected to account for the largest share, some 45%, of health expenditures for older persons. Hospital expenses were followed by nursing home care (21%) and physician costs (21%). Federal programs, including Medicare ($59 billion), Medicaid ($15 billion), and others ($7 billion), were projected to cover abut 67% of these health expenditures (Fowles, (1987). The proportion of elderly men eligible for health care through the Veteran's Administration is growing rapidly. This may result in an "issue of competition" for federal dollars supporting long-term care of the elderly. More pressure will likely be put on private insurance, yet little is known about the role that private insurance coverage plays in the health expenses of older women. It is known that millions of older women have no private insurance because of ineligibility or an inability to pay the costs. In any case, these plans currently mean little assistance with respect to long-term care coverage (Rathbone-McCuan, 1985).

It is estimated that older women spend about one-third of their median income on medical expenses. In addition to this financial burden, many married older women must worry about ways of coping with a spouse's need for medical care and how to pay for that care. This becomes the wife's primary problem since she is more likely to outlive her husband. The emotional and financial costs can be devastating, particularly when institutional care is required. Too frequently older women are forced to "spend down" their meager incomes to achieve Medicaid eligibility, if they are not already at this level. Many middle-income older women become the "new poor" or near-poor as a result of their own or their spouse's illness (Sidel, 1986).

The black elderly in the United States fare even less well in the health care system. They are more likely to be sick, disabled, and perceive themselves as being in poor health than their white elderly counterparts. Black elderly do have higher levels of chronic disease, functional impairment, and hypertension. All of these conditions put them at greater risk. At age 65 to 75, the mortality rates of blacks are higher than whites. Blacks that are age 75 or older have lower mortality rates but significantly higher rates of poverty and poor health (Agree, 1987). Black women are particularly prone to have hypertension, obesity, heart disease, diabetes, nutritional deficiencies, and digestive problems such as ulcers, gastritis, and cirrhosis of the liver. Lower income black women have higher mortality rates from cervical and breast cancer than are reported in the general population. In general, it is accurate to state that blacks, both women and men, have less access to health care than their white counterparts. This is particularly true for rural black women, whose conditions are likely to be even more debilitating because of grinding poverty, inadequate water supplies, and poor sanitation (Marieskind, 1980).

Hispanic elderly tend not to use formal, long-term care services even though 85% of those Hispanics 65 years and older reported at least one chronic condition (Agree, 1987). Not only do they suffer from arthritis, hypertension, cardiovascular conditions, obesity, and anemia, but the problems of poverty as it relates to health may be compounded by the large numbers of women in this group who are, or have been, migrant farm workers. Through this work, they are exposed to potentially harmful pesticides that put them further at risk (Marieskind, 1980).

Asian/Pacific Islander elderly experience certain types of cancers, hypertension, tuberculosis, malnutrition, eye failure (from working in poorly lighted conditions), and alcoholism as major health concerns. Some of these conditions are associated with crowded, substandard housing and poverty. Little is actually known of their utilization of health services. What is known indicates that they are less likely to use formal health care services. Language and cultural differences, a distrust of western medicine, and a reliance on nontraditional medicine are possible explanations (Agree, 1986; Marieskind, 1980).

Many Native Americans are poor and, therefore, have health problems associated with poverty. The major health problems include tuberculosis, alcoholism, diabetes, liver and kidney disease, hypertension, pneumonia, and malnutrition. A majority of elderly Native Americans rarely see a physician. This is true, in part, because many live in isolated areas with unreliable transportation and limited resources. They also bring their own cultural perspectives and tribal customs to assessing and treating illness. If these cultural differences are ignored or overlooked by health care professionals, then a further schism is created (Agree, 1987).

CONCLUSION

We have examined international and national demographics and socioeconomic trends impacting on older women relative to gender differences in longevity, family life, living arrangements, education, work, income, and health. The effort, while exhausting, is not exhaustive and has only highlighted key issues that will be addressed in greater depth in the following sections of this volume. It is difficult to summarize "the problem," and so it follows that it is difficult to develop solutions. The causes for the inequities are complex; the solutions are equally as complex.

What is clear, however, is that older women are, in the main, more likely to live longer, be alone more of the last quarter of their life, be poorer, less well educated, and have serious health problems. It also seems apparent that these same older women are more likely to be at risk over and over again throughout their lifetimes. This risk is potentially even greater for divorced women, minorities, and women who have never married (Sidel, 1986).

Women of all ages and ethnic backgrounds have certainly made progress. Future cohorts of older women will be better educated, more likely to have worked outside the home, more likely to have managed their own finances, and to have interests outside the home. Hopefully, women of all ages will continue to learn how to be better friends and to engage in even more effective networking. These changes ought to translate to more independence, more control over one's life, and a greater sense of self. Will this occur? The crystal ball is cloudy but there is much to be optimistic about and much to be done.

Addressing the needs and inequities faced by older women should be a priority for human service professionals in both practice and public policy. Increased longevity can and should be a positive for women worldwide. It is reasonable to visualize the future with professionals joining hands with older women to make a difference in the quality of life experienced in later years. We close by taking liberties with an idea put forth by Bella Abzug and adapting it to what the future may well bring to aged women the world over:

> Some will run with a torch, some will run for office, and some will run for equality. But let us hope that none will need to run for cover.

REFERENCES

Abramovitz, M. (1988). *Regulating the lives of women*. Boston, MA: South End Press.

Abu-Laban, S. (1987). Women and aging: A futurist perspective. *Psychology of Women Quarterly, 6*(1), 85-98.

Aging America (1984). Washington, DC: American Association of Retired Persons.

Agree, E. M. (1987). *A portrait of older minorities*. Washington, DC: American Association of Retired Persons, Minority Affairs Initiative.

A portrait of older minorities (1985). Washington, DC: American Association of Retired Persons, Minority Affairs Initiative.

A portrait of older minorities (1986). Washington, DC: American Association of Retired Persons, Minority Affairs Initiative.

A profile of older Americans (1987). Washington, DC: American Association of Retired Persons.

Butterfield, F. (1982). *China...alive in the bitter sea*. New York: Bantam Books.

Conable, C. W. (1986). *Conversations in Nairobi*. Washington, DC: American Association for International Aging and the American Association of Retired Persons, Women's Initiative.

Cox, H. G. (1988). *Later life...the realities of aging* (2nd ed.). Englewood Cliffs, NJ: Prentice-Hall.

Feinson, M. C. (1985). Where are the women in the history of aging? *Social Science History, 9*(4), 429-452.

Final Report: The 1981 White House Conference on Aging (1981). Washington, DC: U.S. Government Printing Office.

Fowles, D. G. (1987). *A Profile of Older Americans: 1987.* Washington, DC: American Association of Retired Persons, the U.S. Administration on Aging, and the U.S. Department of Health and Human Services.

Hing, E. (1987, May 14). *Use of nursing homes by the elderly: Preliminary data from the 1985 National Nursing Home Survey* (DHHS Publication No. 135, PHS 87-1250). Washington, DC: Vital and Health Statistics.

Hooyman, N. R. & Kiyak, H. A. (1988). *Social gerontology...a multidisciplinary perspective.* Newton, MA: Allyn & Bacon.

Kane, R. L., Ouslander, J. G., & Abrass, I. B. (1984). *Essentials of clinical geriatrics.* New York: McGraw-Hill.

Lewis, M. (1985). Older women and health: An overview. In S. Golub & R. Freedman (Eds.), *Health needs of women as they age* (pp. 1-15). New York: Haworth Press.

Marieskind, H. I. (1980). *Women in the health care system...patients, providers, and programs.* St. Louis: Mosby.

Markson, E. W. (1983). *Older women: issues and perspectives.* Lexington, MA: Lexington Books.

McClure, L. (1988). Wage gap between sexes is unchanged. *New Directions for Women, 17*(1), 1-24.

Norton, M. B. (1979). The myth of the golden age. In C. R. Berkin & M. B. Norton (Eds.), *Women in America: A history* (pp. 15-38). Washington, DC: Houghton Mifflin.

Peace, S. (1966). The forgotten female: Social policy and older women. In C. Phillipson & A. Walker (Eds.), *Aging and social policy...a critical assessment* (pp. 61-85). London & Vermont: Gower Publishing.

Rathbone-McCuan, E. (1985). Health needs and social policy. In S. Golub & R. Freedman (Eds.), *Health needs of women as they age* (pp. 17-28). New York: Haworth Press.

Shields, L. (1988). Who will need me...who will feed me...when I'm 64? *New Directions for Women, 17*(1), 1-24.

Sidel, R. (1986). *Women and children last...the plight of poor women in affluent America.* New York: Viking Penguin.

Staff (1988, February 2). Aging. *Arkansas Gazette.*

Steinem, G. (1983). *Outrageous acts and everyday rebellions.* New York: Holt, Reinhart & Winston.

Torrey, B. B., Kinsella, K., & Taeuber, C. M. (1987). *An aging world* (International Population Reports, Series P-95, No. 78). Washington, DC: U.S. Department of Commerce and Bureau of the Census.

Vincente, L., Wiley, J. A., & Carrington, R. A. (1979). The risk of institutional-ization before death. *The Gerontologist, 19,* 361-366.

Wertheimer, B. M. (1977). *We were there: The story of working women in America*. New York: Pantheon.

Women and aging around the world (1985). Washington, DC: The International Federation on Aging in cooperation with the American Association of Retired Persons.

Xiao Lu (1984). China (People's Republic of China). In R. Morgan (Ed.), *Sisterhood is global* (pp. 142-151). Garden City, NY: Anchor Press/Doubleday.

Women and Aging:
A Sociological Perspective

Susan A. McDaniel, PhD

The sociological perspective is unique in its direct focus on society and on individuals as social beings. The sociological perspective on women and aging emerges from a blend of the sociologies of aging and of women, two subfields that come to the study of women and aging with different assumptions about the social world, about aging, about women, and about how sociology should proceed. Despite the differences, however, a new sociology, one that looks at women and aging, is emerging. Much more sociological work, both in research and theory, remains to be done in order to understand the problems and the opportunities women experience as they age in society. Considerably more work needs to be done to explain the connections between the place of older women in society and socially structured gender inequality.

In this article, an overview of the sociological approach to women and aging is provided. To set the stage for understanding women and aging in contemporary society, the situation of older

Susan A. McDaniel is with the Department of Sociology, University of Waterloo, Waterloo, Ontario Canada N2L 3G1.

women in the past is briefly reviewed. The basic orientation of the sociological perspective is highlighted, with particular attention to the similarities and differences between the sociologies of aging and of women. Recent steps toward integration into a sociology of women and aging are discussed and a critical assessment of the "state of the art" of this emerging subfield is provided. The article concludes with speculation about what the future holds for older women in society, as well as for enhanced sociological understanding of women and aging and of women's situations in an aging society.

OLDER WOMEN IN THE PAST

Little is known about older women in the past. History's tendency is to exclude both older people and women, on the assumption that history (or at least what matters in history) is made largely by young or middle-aged men (de Beauvoir, 1970). Older people in the past tend to be lumped into the general category of adults. There is little doubt now that understanding of women in history has been hampered by the omission of women from historical accounts, both as actors and as thinkers (Spender, 1982). Older women are virtually nonexistent in written history.

Despite the lack of detailed information on older women in the past, the little that is known suggests that much of what older women experience in today's society may not be new at all. In most societies in the past, women's social status was not high and tended to decline with age. In some societies, old women were thought to possess supernatural powers, in part because they tended to outlive men, but even this was a mixed blessing since older women were more often regarded as witches. There are societies, such as China, in which the status of women grew with age (de Beauvoir, 1970), but old women there tended to reinforce male domination of younger women (usually daughters-in-law) by treating them harshly and requiring firm obedience to both husband and mother-in-law or grandmother-in-law.

The tendency to romanticize the past has led to the widespread belief that old people were revered for their wisdom. There is truth in this to the extent that past societies were premised on the accumulation of experience, thus requiring collaboration between old and young to survive and move forward. Modern society, by contrast, tends to think that knowledge does not accumulate with the years, but grows out of date (de Beauvoir, 1970).

Paralleling social beliefs, and guiding them, is economic change. Once property replaces strength as the source of status, the old tend to have more power than the young. The system of inheritance of accumulated wealth means that the old may lose status because they have wealth wanted by their offspring. This quite often resulted in elder abuse (de Beauvoir, 1970, p. 219) as well as in destitution and homelessness among the old (de Beauvoir, 1970; Haber, 1983) as older parents were driven off their land and their wealth taken by the children. Since women tended to outlive men and have less firm connections to the developing industrial order of the early and middle nineteenth century, they became even more likely candidates for poverty and homelessness. The feminization of poverty (the concept that poverty is more often a woman's problem than a man's) is thus not a new phenomenon.

Interestingly, the poverty of older people, particularly women, in the nineteenth century was in fact abetted by social workers, sociologists, and the charities (Haber, 1983). In their writings and public comments, it became clear that these professionals saw aging as associated with weakness and decline and hence saw poverty as a probable outcome. Although publicity to the link between poverty and old age may have resulted from the early work of professionals in social welfare, this may not have been their intention. Nonetheless, the effect was the growing belief that poverty might be inevitable among the old and possibly something about which little could be done.

WHAT IS THE SOCIOLOGICAL PERSPECTIVE ON AGING?

The sociological perspective is a different way of seeing familiar social reality. Our familiarity with society may make the sociological perspective appear indistinguishable from common sense, thus ordinary. The surprise in the sociological perspective is that what was thought to be familiar becomes unfamiliar and sometimes even uncomfortable as assumptions and myths are torn away and we discover that things are not what they seem. The sociological perspective expands each individual's own experiences with the social world to reveal how wider social forces such as economic change, belief systems, and class structure affect and are affected by individuals. As Mills (1970) suggest, the sociological imagination enables us to understand the relationship of social history and personal biography, so that we can simultaneously see how the individual is constrained by society and how we can use social forces to bring about different social ends.

The sociological perspective, at its best, asks fundamental questions about the way we live, the way we treat others and see ourselves, and the future of society. This means that sociology does not remain abstract or academic, but is involved with the pressing social issues of the day (McDaniel & Agger, 1982). Because of this, sociology tends toward the controversial, or even the subversive. Allied disciplines such as psychology, economics, and social work also focus on society and on social issues, but do so in a way that is less wide-sweeping than sociology. For example, psychology tends to be more focused on individuals, asking questions about perceptions, thought processes, personality or individual development over time. Economics, in its concern with income and financing, is also more sharply focused than sociology, but in a different way than psychology. Social work is applied sociology and psychology, focused on individuals, families, and communities. These, like any short definitions, are overly simple; the complexities involved in these perspectives are discussed in articles specific to them elsewhere in this volume.

The sociology of aging is at once in its infancy and as old as sociology itself. The focus of sociology has always been on change over time — how society arrived at the present from the past and where we are heading in the future. In this large sense, all of sociology is the study of aging, transition, and change. What is typically thought of as the sociology of aging, however, is a newly emergent subfield in sociology (Binstock & Shanas, 1985; Gee & Kimball, 1987; McPherson, 1983). It was not until the 1940s that sociologists began to study age as a variable in social behavior and social structure (Linton, 1942; Parsons, 1942). Until that period, sociology focused largely on topics such as social structures, classes, religions, or the division of labor. To the extent that sociologists were concerned with individual life-course issues, their focus tended to be on childhood, particularly socialization in childhood, or adolescence rather than on older people (McPherson, 1983). The original preoccupation of sociology of aging was, and largely continues to be, with older people (Binstock & Shanas, 1985; Gee & Kimball, 1987; McPherson, 1983), but recently it has broadened to include the process of aging throughout life, with specific attention to life-course issues.

Within sociology, there tends to be a divergence between an individual focus (called micro-level) and a societal focus (macro-level). The micro-level of analysis is concerned with individuals and social interactions of individuals, whereas the macro-level focuses on social structure, social processes and problems, and their interrelationships. In sociology of aging, the micro-level has been emphasized (Binstock & Shanas, 1985; Chappell & Driedger, 1987), with research attention focusing on individual adjustment to aging, including deteriorating health, exits from social roles (such as retirement and widowhood), well-being (both subjective and objective), and social support. It has been estimated that approximately 30% of journal space in social gerontology (a field of which sociology of aging is only one part) is devoted to well-being among the old (Chappell & Driedger, 1987). Macro-level issues in sociology of aging have received, until recently, limited attention, as have micro-level issues other than adjustment or well-being. Examples of recent macro-level concerns are age stratification (related to the fact that older people may form a kind of class with fewer resources and lower status than younger people), the causes of poverty among the old, gender discrimination as a factor in older women's life circumstances, the role of values or ideology in defining aging as a social problem, and pension funds as a source of power in an aging society, among others.

The sociology of aging, perhaps as a result of its relative youth as a subdiscipline, is not as theoretically developed as other subdisciplines in sociology. Most of the theories it employs, when theory is used at all, are tentative, insufficiently developed, and not well integrated with established sociological theories. One persistent critique of the sociology of aging has been its focus on data collection to the neglect of theory building (Binstock & Shanas, 1985; Chappell & Driedger, 1987; McPherson, 1983). One reason for this is that research in the sociology of aging has tended to be oriented to specific social problems rather than to understanding the social process of aging. This results in much research in the sociology of aging having an applied common-sense "feel" to it, lacking in the surprise of discovery mentioned above. It also means that the sociology of aging has not been engaged as much as other sociology subdisciplines, with the larger social questions of the day. Aging as a social process is thus less well understood than it might be.

The prevalent theoretical approaches in the sociology of aging are the normative perspective and the interpretative, both with a macro and micro component. The normative perspective focuses on social order premised on cooperation, interdependence, and shared values, adjustment by the individual to society, and societal equilibrium. By contrast, the interpretative perspective gives primary attention to societal conflicts, social relations between dominant and subordinate groups, the ways in which dominant groups prevail in values and control, and social change (McDaniel & Agger, 1982). These are the basic theoretical orientations in sociology and they are not particular to the sociology of aging. In the sociology of aging, these perspectives have not been as fully utilized as they could be to enable sociological insights about aging women. In the examples that follow, it is imagined how these perspectives might be more fruitfully applied to women.

An example of a normative macro approach is age stratification theory (Riley, Johnson, & Foner, 1972), which holds that role changes accompany age changes, so that women of 80 are expected to behave differently from women of 50. Older women are thought to form an age class with shared interests and a common history. This approach has the advantage of studying age groups not in isolation, but in relation to other age strata. The focus is on how social structure affects individuals within age groups and the importance of chronological age as a determinant of behavior in providing social roles and opportunities on the basis of age. Gender has not been emphasized to the extent that it might be by this approach. Differences in the interests and histories of women and of men might be more fully analyzed, rather than presuming a universal and inevitable series of stages in the aging process. Despite its limitations in its preoccupation with social order and mechanistic social relations age groups, the macro normative perspective might have untapped potential for better understanding of how similar historical experiences might produce different consequences for women and men in the same age group.

Disengagement theory (Cumming & Henry, 1981), a landmark theory when it first appeared, is an example of a normative micro approach. Normal aging is seen as a gradual process of disengagement from society by the aging individual and from the individual by society. In this way, the old make way for the young, without intergenerational conflict. Disengagement, in enabling the aging person to be relieved of social expectations and constraints, can be satisfying and contribute to well-being. What the theory overlooks is that some disengagement is involuntary, such as mandatory retirement and widowhood, and thus may not necessarily enhance well-being. Also insufficiently emphasized is the fact that disengagement from society may not take the same pace or pattern for all people. For example, men might disengage earlier than their wives because they tend to be older and have lower life expectancy. Women may have mor involuntary disengagement experiences as they more often outlive their relatives and friends.

Macro-level interpretative approaches, although not common in the sociology of aging, are gaining in popularity and newsworthiness. One example is Davis and van den Oever's (1982) analysis of aging populations in which gender and age groups engage in fierce competition for scarce resources. Population aging, this approach contends, necessitates a shift in resources from the young to the old, which creates strife between generations. Davis and van den Oever argue that this might result in resentment and abuse of the old, particularly of women. Old women may be viewed as even less deserving and more demanding (because of their greater longevity) of available resources than old men. This approach is reminiscent of what occurred in the nineteenth century.

An alternative macro-level interpretative approach, called the political economy of aging, argues among other things that it is corporate capitalism that accounts for the diminished status of older people, particularly women. Proponents of this approach, such as Myles (1984), see the diminished social status and economic circumstances of the old in western society as being due in part to the fact that the state assumes responsibility for their maintenance. Thus, the issues of public pensions, pension accessibility, and public burden become salient. Women's lesser economic independence and resources throughout their lives combined with their greater longevity means that women are more often economically dependent on government in old age for subsistence as well as for health care.

At the micro-level, the interpretative perspective sees individuals and groups of individuals as creators of social change through social action. Conflict between groups, according to this approach, is seen as beneficial to society because it can result in changes for the better. Groups such as the Gray Panthers in the United States, who lobby for changed images of older people and improvements in rights, could be analyzed with this approach. In Canada, there are many activist seniors groups that have been successful in turning back government initiatives to de-index pensions. Insufficient research attention has been devoted to the role of women in these movements for change, but there hare hints that their role may be central.

SOCIOLOGY OF WOMEN/SOCIOLOGY OF AGING:
TOWARD AN INTERFACE

The sociology of women, like the sociology of aging, is at the same time old and new. The question of women's place in society goes back almost as far as sociology itself, although the answers provided vary substantially (Engels, 1902; Parson, 1955). Despite the long history of sociological interest in women's roles, a sociology of women *per se* began to develop only in the 1970s (Delamont, 1980; Eichler, 1985; Mackie, 1983; Stacey & Thorne, 1985). The concept of gender, meaning socially determined aspects of behavior rather than biologically determined aspects denoted by sex, has emerged, thus intertwining the sociology of women with the sociology of social life. The perspective used in the sociology of women is essentially that of the sociological imagination — putting individual experience (particularly the experience of women) into social context, and thus revealing how the personal is political and social as well as how understanding of social forces gives individuals power to change society and themselves (Oakley, 1980). The sociology of women, feminist sociology in particular, has a commitment to social issues, often from a social change standpoint. Gender has come to be seen as a central organizing feature for social life.

Since the 1970s, there has been an extraordinary amount of sociological work in gender (Stacey & Thorne, 1985). The sociology of women has been path-breaking in both its attention to previously unresearched topics and in its perspective and orientation (Delamont, 1980; Eichler, 1985; Stacey & Thorne, 1985). Topics researched either for the first time or in distinctly new ways include childbirth and mothering (Chodorow, 1978; Oakley 1980), housework (Oakley, 1974), rape, sexual assault, and wife battering (Holmstrom & Burgess, 1978), contraception (Luker, 1975), marriage (Bernard, 1974), and divorce (Weitzman, 1981). Attention has turned, to a limited extent, to issues of women and aging with research on widowhood (Lopata, 1973), the life course (Rossi, 1980), abuse of older women, and women's experiences with aging (Abu-Laban, 1981; Barnett & Baruch, 1978; Bart, 1975; Beeson, 1975).

The basic orientation of the sociology of women is in sharp contrast with that of the sociology of aging. Whereas the sociology of aging tends to be data oriented, the sociology of women is more theoretical. The sociology of aging focuses on micro-level issues of adjustment and well-being, while the sociology of women attempts to understand the macro-level issues affecting women's (and men's) lives. The sociology of women is more action and social change oriented than the sociology of aging, which often emphasizes individual adjustment to existing social structures. Even the methods used by the two subdisciplines are different: the sociology of aging tends to be survey dominated and largely quantitative, whereas the sociology of women is interview oriented and more qualitative. This means that there is a tendency in the sociology of aging to observe behavior outside its social context, while research in the sociology of women tends to contextualize. It is, in fact, difficult to imagine two subdisciplines that are more divergent in approach and orientation.

It is not surprising, in light of the difference in the basic approaches of the two subdisciplines, that women have not been particularly central in sociological studies of aging (Burwell, 1984; Sinnott, 1986) or that aging has not been a high priority for sociological studies of women (Burwell, 1982). The title of a 1972 article (Lewis & Butler), for example, asks "Why is women's lib ignoring older women?" Attempts at an interface between the sociology of aging and the sociology of women have, in fact, only occurred quite recently (Abu-Laban, 1981; Burwell, 1982, 1984; Chappell & Haven, 1980; Cohen, 1984: Dulude, 1987; Gee & Kimball, 1987; Hess, 1985; Rossi, 1986; Sinnott, 1986), although clearly some sociological research has been done prior to the 1980s on women and aging. This earlier research, as mentioned in the preceding section, was focused less on women *per se* than on sex as one of many variables in studies of aging. It must be emphasized that very little was known about women and aging, with the exception of widowhood experiences (Lopata, 1973), until the past few decades. The distinction in recent efforts at integration is the shift of focus specifically to women, rather than applying male or general perspectives, as these often are inappropriate to women's experiences. For example, both women's and men's poverty in old age may be analyzed using the interpretative perspective, but the factors contributing to women's poverty may be different.

One example of fruitful integration of the sociologies of aging and women is research on women's and men's different life-course experiences. It has long been known that women, on average, outlive men and that women tend to marry men slightly older than themselves, but the implications of these realities for older women's socioeconomic well-being and life experiences had not been analyzed. A growing body of recent research (Dulude, 1987; Fenwick & Burresi, 1981; Gee, 1986; Gee & Kimball, 1987; Marcil-Gratton & Legare, 1987; McDaniel, 1986; Stewart & Platt, 1982) is showing that many of the problems faced by older women are a function of their spending more of their later years alone. This might explain older women's greater poverty, since pensions often cease on the death of the husband unless there are specific survivor's provisions, which many private pensions do not have. In addition, women are much more likely to be poor in their later years because their inadequate pensions, if they have pensions at all other than basic public pensions, which were never meant to be any more than supplements, must be stretched over a longer period (McDaniel, 1986; Myles, 1984).

Given the fact that women are more often widowed than men, and the death of one's spouse has been found to be the most critical life experience, women more often experience life disruption (Dulude, 1987; Lopata, 1983; Martin-Matthews, 1982). That women, through the combined effects of greater longevity and marriage to older men, are more often left without a mate to potentially care for them at home when they become ill or disabled means that women are more often institutionalized and, not unrelatedly, more often experience problems in maintaining a home and control over their own lives (Dulude, 1987; Martin-Matthews, 1982). Women's poverty and aloneness in old age makes them more dependent on adult children, with potential for the kind of conflicts that can result in negligence and emotional or even physical abuse. On the positive side, women's stronger ties of friendship are carried into old age with beneficial results on well-being and support.

A second example of the combined approaches of the sociology of aging and of women is "double-jeopardy" research. Since this approach is discussed in other articles in this volume, the discussion here will be brief and limited to sociological aspects. Essentially, double jeopardy holds that old women may experience what Posner (1977) calls a "double whammy" in being discriminated against on two fronts — for being old and for being female. Research has confirmed that old women do experience combined effects greater than the effects of being either old or female alone, for objective indicators of mental health, but not for subjective well-being (Chappell & Haven, 1980). Another way to see double jeopardy is to picture the accumulated effects of secondary status (being a woman) in old age, combined with negative images of the elderly and the fact that women are seen to be older sooner than men (Cohen, 1984; Gee & Kimball, 1987). Recent evidence suggests that double jeopardy may have the social effect of adding not only to fear of aging at the individual level among both women and men, but to collective fears about population aging that are associated with moving toward a society comprised of old, sick, dependent, and poor women (Cohen, 1984; McDaniel, 1986, 1987).

A third useful integration of the sociologies of aging and women is the "sandwich generation" research done largely by social workers (Brody, 1981; Brody, Johnson, & Fulcomer, 1984; Brody & Schoonover, 1986), which has found that contrary to popular belief about abandonment of the elderly by family members (Shanas, 1979), caretaking by family members is quite common (Brody, 1981; Shanas, 1979). Caretaking patterns of older family members, however, are highly gender specific, falling disproportionately to middle-aged daughters and daughters-in-law (Brody, 1981), whether or not these "women in the middle" work outside the home (Brody & Schoonover, 1986), or have children still at home, or have more than one generation of older family members requiring care (Marcil-Gratton & Legare, 1987). The combined effects of major demographic shifts to an older population (McDaniel, 1986) and increased work-force participation among women, regardless of marital or parental status, means that middle-aged women add most of the responsibility, if not the direct care, for older family members to an already full agenda of work, childcare, and home responsibility. This research has clear implications not only at the individual level in its revelations about the ways in which women are sandwiched in the social structure, but for policymakers who must address these issues in the development of priorities for home care or support programs for caretakers of the elderly (Hess, 1985).

A fourth example of insightful integration of the sociologies of aging and of women is research on poverty among old women. The general impression is that the economic circumstances of older people has generally improved recently (Gee & Kimball, 1987). Although this may be true, on average, older women, particularly those who are widowed or who have spent their entire lives as homemakers or working on the family farm or in small business, are not well off and, in fact, may quickly fall into poverty on the death of their husbands. Women without men, and hence access to men's greater earning power, constitute the bulk of the poor in North America. Single mothers and old women are the poorest in both Canada and the United States. The sociology of women has long recognized that this is due to disparities between men's and women's earning power as well as, and related to, discrimination against women.

These economic inequities tend to accumulate in old age and are exacerbated by a pension system that is not workable for many women. Research in the sociology of aging has discovered that women have no homemaker's pensions, seldom have pensions of their own because they work in jobs with few or no benefits or have insufficiently long service in the job to be eligible, or that their husbands' pensions die with him (Gee & Kimball, 1987). Thus, women's greater likelihood of poverty in old age can be clearly understood only with simultaneous reference to the sociologies of women and aging.

THE STATE OF THE ART/SCIENCE

Recent efforts, some of which have been outlined here, to integrate the sociology of aging with the sociology of women are welcome, not only because they address obvious gaps in our knowledge about women and aging, such as limited knowledge of gender differences in the experience of aging, of women's life experiences and how these accumulate in old age, of poverty as a women's issue in old age, and of the effects of stereotypes in the situations faced by old women, but also because these efforts reveal the extent to which aging *is* a women's issue. Women predominate among the older populations in both the United States and Canada and will gain in numerical predominance in the future (Gee & Kimball, 1987; McDaniel, 1986; Rossi, 1986). At the individual level, women, for a variety of reasons (some of which are simply the result of their greater longevity) tend to experience more social, economic, and health problems as they age than men do.

Significant strides have been made recently in research on women and aging, although the very fact of this recent research interest reveals the enormity of the need for further research.

What are some of the strengths of the sociological research and thinking about women and aging? The demographic knowledge base is solid, although more research needs to be done on the implications of demographic changes for women. Given good demographic data, life-course changes and differences for men and for women are beginning to be better understood, as discussed previously. Some of the differences between men's and women's later years spent alone are also well understood, although, again, the social implications for pensions, health care, informal and formal caregiving, nursing home planning, and volunteer services may not have been fully explored. More is known about older women's family circumstances than any other aspects of their lives (Burwell, 1984; Gee & Kimball, 1987; Shanas, 1979). Given the primacy of family to most women and many women's economic imbeddedness within the family, this emphasis may not be inappropriate. Alternatively, it has been argued that concentration of research on women as primarily familial may be a result of male bias — the assumption that women become widows, whereas men retire, for instance (Burwell, 1984).

Additional strengths of sociological research on women and aging are found in evidence about women's roles, both in earlier and later life, being constrained by social expectations and by larger social forces (such as population aging and increased female labor-force participation), over which women may have limited choices. All four examples discussed previously reveal this, although in different ways. New research on women and aging has enhanced our understanding of women's experiences with aging by asking women themselves what they feel about their lives and their own experiences. The surprise has been that despite the objective problems they face, older women are relatively happy with their lives (Brody & Schoonover, 1986; Chappell & Haven, 1980; Gee & Kimball, 1987; among others). New research has measured both subjective and objective well-being among older women, providing a good basis on which to assess health needs and problems.

Despite the strengths of recent research efforts, gaps remain, not only in what we know sociologically about women and aging, but also in how we conceptualize the issues to be studied. In terms of gaps, not enough is known about the complete spectrum of women's lives as they age. Research has focused on family and women's well-being, or adjustment to old age, or on health issues, to the exclusion of women's work and retirement, social relationships and sexuality, the social meanings of living on limited income or experiencing stereotypes, older women's political and social values, attitudes toward social change, and, very important, the diversity of experiences among women with aging.

As the integration of the sociology of aging and the sociology of women develops further, it is likely that less research on women and aging will be of the descriptive type that characterizes the sociology of aging. More theoretically oriented research typical of the sociology of women needs to be done. The possibilities here are almost boundless, since so little theory exists about women and aging. Enticing suggestions arise from work by Sinnott (1986) on changing gender roles, attitudes, and expectations with age. The preliminary conclusion Sinnott reaches based on research done thus far is that both women and men, but particularly men, seem, as they age, to dispense with the divisive and sharply divergent roles specialized by gender that characterize youth. Older people tend to become more androgynous or gender-similar (Rossi, 1986). There is surprisingly scant research on gender-role shifts with age. This is a potentially fruitful theoretical area of research.

Equally enticing hints from an almost untouched theoretically important area come from a study by Berger (1982), another social worker, on the experience of gays and lesbians with aging. Berger's conclusion contains that element of surprise that is part of good application of sociological imagination. Lesbians, in particular, report an easier aging experience than heterosexual women. The theoretically important explanation offered by Berger is that older lesbians have prior experience with the deviant label and so may have less difficulty in dealing with the social stigma when they become old women. Essentially, lesbians have lived their lives as exceptions to what is socially expected, so when they become older women, they appear to have less trouble than heterosexual women in living their lives as they see fit, regardless of society's stereotypes of old women. This is interesting because it may have relevance to other deviant groups as well, such as possibly women of greater-than-average achievement, or the childless, to name just a few.

Sociological research on women and aging could benefit from the theoretical models and insights developed by feminist sociologists in studying reproduction (Oakley, 1980), for instance, or sexual assault (Holmstrom & Burgess, 1978), or wife abuse. The strengths of these theories, and others in feminist sociology, rest on asking new and fundamental questions about the relationships between women's everyday experiences and wider social structures and forces. The answers offered are sometimes unexpected, even shocking, but reveal previously unnoticed connections between individuals and social structures, so they must be posed, no matter how difficult. Reproduction, for example, previously considered a largely biological private process, has been found to contain elements of wage labor and to be firmly within the most public of all realms, politics (Oakley, 1980). Sexual assault, similarly, previously seen as an act of lust, was discovered to be related more to social power than to biological urges (Holmstrom & Burgess, 1978), as well as being a product of a social system of gender inequality.

Most of the challenging theoretical questions about women and aging remain to be asked. Two examples of important areas that need to be fully explored are abuse of older women and women's experiences with retirement. It is not known whether dynamics similar to wife abuse or child abuse are operant in abuse of old women, who are the common victims, or whether additional factors come into play. Retirement as an important life experience for women has also been neglected as a research area. Generally, it has been assumed that women become widows and men retire. Even the effects of husbands' retirement on wives have not been examined as fully as they should be. As more women work, potential conflicts over retirement timing and plans between spouses might occur.

WHAT LIES AHEAD?

The future holds great promise for the sociological study of women and aging for two quite different reasons. First, the process of discovering social truths about women and aging has only begun. Possibilities still to be explored far exceed what is already known. There are few remaining areas of research in any realm about which this kind of statement can be made with much confidence. Second, the future quite literally belongs to older women. As the American and Canadian populations continue to age, older women will constitute greater proportions of the totals. This could mean a shifting balance of power from youth to older people and from men to women, accompanied by a variety of changes on political and social agendas.

Among research areas likely to be given priority in the future, in addition to those mentioned previously, are linkages between private and public caretaking and between formal and informal caregiving, connections between family work and wage labor, redefinitions of chronic and long-term care, relationships between pension systems and social status of older women, innovations in home care and community living, and the nature of transition from one status to another. All of these areas have been underresearched; all are crucial to policymaking and planning for the future; and all more central to older women that older men because of women's different patterns of aging and different social roles throughout life. Paralleling pursuit of these research priorities would be the advancement of theoretically informed research questions and the development of systematic theories of women and aging, so that knowledge building can proceed along with data collection.

Aging women of the future may have some distinct advantages over aging women today. There are clear trends suggesting that tomorrow's old women will be better educated, more likely to have worked outside the home for a significant part of their lives, have access to better pensions and health care, perhaps experience menopause as a less salient event in their lives due to compressed childbearing and the decreased centrality of reproduction in their lives, have more experience with making transitions from work to home or married to divorced status, have wider "family" circles including more friends and surrogate family members, and perhaps best of all, become more political as they age. Tomorrow's old women may also be more physically fit, more independent, and less willing to be stereotyped, although class differences will no doubt continue to exist.

Despite the good reasons for optimism about the future of women and aging, practical and policy challenges remain. The need for decent pensions for all women, including homemakers, remains a priority in the policy realm. Without secure incomes, old women will find it difficult to be healthy and active. Programs and policies giving priority to enabling old women to remain in their own homes as long as possible should be explored. There is no question that choice in one's living arrangements and control over one's immediate environment are important preconditions for healthy and happy aging. Independent living has the additional bonus of being far less costly than institutionalization, a factor that should provide incentive to policymakers.

Attention might also be given by governments to deliberate campaigns to educate people about the diversity and energy of old women in an attempt to dispel labeling and stereotyping. Small-scale campaigns such as this have been launched in Canada but the results have not yet been reported. Encouraging more social contact across generations (less age segregation) is also important for reducing stereotyping and enhancing real understanding of aging. Last, in a far from definitive list, policymakers and the public might make a transition in their thinking from seeing aging, both individual and collective, as something to be feared to seeing aging as an opportunity.

In individual terms, aging is clearly an opportunity, if one remembers Mark Twain's comment that aging is far better than dying young. Collectively, too, population or societal aging may be an opportunity for previously disadvantaged groups such as women to gain in political and social power. The gender gap in politics in the United States today suggests that older women with political clout might go some distance to contributing to a better world, with their concerns about world peace, the environment, and decency toward our fellow women (and men).

REFERENCES

Abu-Laban, S. M. (1981). Women and aging: A futuristic perspective. *Psychology of Women Quarterly*, *6*, 85-98.

Bankoff, E. A. (1983). Social support and adaptation to widowhood. *Journal of Marriage and the Family, 45*, 827-839.

Barnett, R. C., & Baruch, G. K. (1978). Women in the middle years: A critique of research and theory. *Psychology of Women Quarterly*, *3*, 187-197.

Bart, P. B. (1975). Emotional and social status of the older woman, in *No longer young: The older woman in America* (Occasional Papers in Gerontology No. 11). Ann Arbor, MI: University of Michigan Institute of Gerontology.

Beeson, D. (1975). Women in studies of aging: A critique and suggestion. *Social Problems, 23,* 52-59.

Berger, R. (1982). The unseen minority: Older gays and lesbians. *Social Work, 27,* 236-242.

Bernard, J. (1974). *The future of marriage.* New Haven: Yale University Press.

Binstock, R. H., & Shanas, E. (Eds.). (1985). *Handbook of aging and the social sciences* (2nd ed.). New York: Van Nostrand Reinhold.

Brody, E. M. (1981). Women in the middle and family help to older people. *The Gerontologist, 21,* 471-480.

Brody, E. M., Johnson, P. T., & Fulcomer, M. C. (1984). What should adult children do for elderly parents? Opinions and preferences of three generations of women. *Journal of Gerontology, 39,* 736-746.

Brody, E. M., & Schoonover, C. B. (1986). Patterns of parent-care when adult daughters work and when they do not. *The Gerontologist, 26,* 372-381.

Burwell, E. J. (1982). The handwriting is on the wall: Older women in the future. *Resources for Feminist Research, 11,* 208-209.

Burwell, E. J. (1984). Sexism in social science research on aging. In J. M. Vickers (Ed.), *Taking sex into account* (pp. 185-208). Ottawa: Carleton University Press.

Chappell, N., & Driedger, L. (1987). *Aging and ethnicity: Toward an interface.* Toronto: Butterworths.

Chappell, N. L., & Haven, B. (1980). Old and female: Testing the double jeopardy hypothesis. *The Sociological Quarterly, 21,* 157-171.

Chodorow, N. (1978). *The reproduction of mothering.* Berkeley: University of California Press.

Cohen, L. (1984). *Small expectations: Society's betrayal of older women.* Toronto: McClelland & Stewart.

Cumming, E., & Henry, W. (1981). *Growing old: The process of disengagement.* New York: Basic Books.

Davis, K. & van den Oever, P. (1982). Demographic foundations of new sex roles. *Population and Development Review, 8,* 495-511.

de Beauvoir, S. (1970). *Old age.* Harmondsworth, England: Penguin.

Delamont, S. (1980). *Sociology of women: An introduction.* London: Allen & Unwin.

Dulude, L. (1987). Getting old: Men in couples and women alone. In G. H. Neimiroff (Ed.), *Women and men: Interdisciplinary readings on gender* (pp. 323-339). Toronto: Fitzhenry & Whiteside.

Eichler, M. (1985). And the work never ends: Feminist contributions. *Canadian Review of Sociology and Anthropology, 22,* 619-644.

Engels, F. (1902). *The origins of the family, private property and the state.* Chicago: Kerr & Company.

Fenwick, R., & Burresi, C. M. (1981). Health consequences of marital status and change among the elderly: A comparison of cross-sectional and longitudinal analysis. *Journal of Health and Social Behavior, 22,* 106-116.

Gee, E. M. (1986). The life course of Canadian women: An historical and demographic analysis. *Social Indicators Research, 18,* 263-283.

Gee, E. M. & Kimball, M. M. (1987). *Women and aging.* Toronto: Butterworths.

Haber, C. (1983). *Beyond sixty-five: The dilemma of old age in America's past.* Cambridge: Cambridge University Press.

Hess, B. B. (1985). Aging policies and old women: The hidden agenda. In A. S. Rossi (Ed.), *Gender and the life course.* New York: Aldine.

Holmstrom, L. L., & Burgess, A. W. (1978). *The victim of rape: Institutional reactions.* New York: Wiley.

Lewis, M. I., & Butler, R. N. (1972). Why is women's lib ignoring older women? *International Journal of Aging and Human Development, 3,* 223-231.

Linton, R. (1942). Age and sex categories. *American Sociological Review, 7,* 589-603.

Lopata, H. Z. (1973). *Widowhood in an American city.* Cambridge, MA: Schenckman.

Luker, K. (1975). *Taking chances: Abortion and the decision not to contracept.* Berkeley: University of California Press.

Mackie, M. (1983). *Exploring gender relations: A Canadian perspective.* Toronto: Butterworths.

Marcil-Gratton, N., & Legare, J. (1987). Vieillesse d'aujourd'hui et de demain: Un meme age, une outre realite? *Futuribles International, May,* 3-22.

Martin-Matthews, A. M. (1982). Review essay — Canadian research on women as widows: A comparative analysis of the state of the art. *Resources for Feminist Research, 11,* 227-230.

McDaniel, S. A. (1986). *Canada's aging population.* Toronto: Butterworths.

McDaniel, S. A. (1987). Demographic aging as a guiding paradigm in Canada's welfare state. *Canadian Public Policy, 13,* 330-336.

McDaniel, S. A., & Agger, B. (1982). *Social problems through conflict and order.* Toronto: Addison-Wesley.

McPherson, B. D. (1983). *Aging as a social process.* Toronto: Butterworths.

Mills, C. W. (1970). *The sociological imagination.* New York: Oxford University Press.

Myles, J. (1984). *Old age in the welfare state: The political economy of public pensions.* Boston: Little, Brown.

Oakley, A. (1974). *The sociology of housework.* Bath, England: Pitman.

Oakley, A. (1980). The sociological unimagination. In A. Oakley, *Women confined: Towards a sociology of childbirth* (pp. 70-91). London: Martin-Robertson-Oxford.

Parsons, T. (1942). Age and sex in the social structure of the United States. *American Sociological Review, 7,* 601-616.

Parsons, T. (1955). Sex role and family structure. In T. Parsons & R. Bales, (Eds.), *Family socialization and interaction process.* New York: Free Press.

Posner, J. (1977). Old and female: The double whammy. *Essence, 2,* 41-48.

Riley, M. W., Johnson, M., & Foner, A. (1972). Elements in a model of age stratification. In M. W. Riley, M. Johnson & A. Foner (Eds.), *Aging and society: Vol. 3. A sociology of age stratification* (pp. 3-26). New York: Russell Sage.

Rossi, A. (1980). Life span theories and women's lives. *Signs: Journal of Women in Culture and Society, 8,* 471-489.

Rossi, A. (1986). Sex and gender in an aging society. *Daedalus, 115,* 141-169.

Shanas, E. (1979). Social myth as hypothesis: The case of the family relations of older people. *The Gerontologist, 19,* 3-9.

Sinnott, J. (1986). *Sex roles and aging: Theory and research from a systems perspective.* Basel: Karger.

Spender, D. (1982). *Women of ideas – and what men have done to them from Aphra Behn to Adrieene Rich.* London & Boston: Routledge & Kegan Paul.

Stacey, J., & Thorne, B. (1985). The missing feminist revolution in sociology. *Social Problems, 32,* 301-316.

Stewart, A. J., & Platt, M. B. (1982). Studying women in a changing world: An introduction. *Journal of Social Issues, 38,* 1-16.

Weitzman, L. J. (1981). *The marriage contract.* New York: Free Press.

Women and Aging:
A Psychological Perspective

Susan Gaylord, PhD

INTRODUCTION

What is a Psychological Perspective?

Psychology is defined as the science of the mind and mental processes. The mind itself—that nebulous entity that perceives, thinks, feels, knows, and remembers—is often difficult to study directly. Instead, psychology often becomes the study of the tangible output of mind, behavior, with the goal of psychology being "to describe, understand, predict, and control" the behavior of individuals (Williams, 1977, p. 13).

Humans exhibit a vast array of behaviors; accordingly, psychology covers a broad range of topics: perception, cognition, psychophysiology, personality, motivation, mental health, and others. The causes of behavior are multifactorial, involving genetic, social, cultural, and environmental determinants. Psychology's interactions with the neighboring disciplines of biology, sociology, anthropology, and physics serve to enrich its understanding of behavior.

A psychological perspective on aging and women is thus potentially broad in scope and addresses not only the behavior of older women, but the behavior of others toward them. This article provides a brief overview of research findings and issues in some but not all of the relevant areas. First, the history of psychological study

---

Susan Gaylord is with the Department of Medicine, University of North Carolina at Chapel Hill, Chapel Hill, NC 27599.

69

of older women is overviewed. Next, psychological study is placed in the context of biological, social, and cultural factors. A brief discussion follows concerning the need for circumspect interpretation of the research literature to be presented. The main body of the article covers aspects of the wide-ranging psychological literature pertaining to older women. Topics include information processing and cognition, intelligence, creativity, personality, and life satisfaction. Some major topics are not discussed here because they are addressed by other authors in this volume. Omitted are descriptions of sensory changes with age, issues of stereotyping, sexuality, and mental health, as well as the large body of psychoanalytic literature.

Historical Overview

Psychological research has often ignored women and neglected women's issues. The roots of experimental psychology are in 19th-century Western Europe, converging from the disciplines of philosophy and physiology. In academic settings, where ideas were born and nurtured, most of the researchers were men (Boring, 1950), with women only gradually entering the field, often to study child or educational psychology.

Early, basic experimental studies of perception, cognition, learning, and memory frequently used only male subjects but generalized their findings to the entire population. One rationale was that male subjects were easier to obtain, a situation due in part to the common use of the "college sophomore" as study population. Another rationale is that combining males and females in a sample added unwanted variability to the experimental outcome. Often, a hidden assumption was that males represented the norm in behavior for the species; data on females that did not correlate with this norm tended to be explained away or disregarded. This trend continued with research on psychological aspects of aging, where frequently only male subjects were used or sex of subject was not reported.

Interest in individual differences in the mid to late 1800s led to research on sex differences. Here, early studies seemed bent on proving what was commonly held to be true: that women were not only physically but mentally the weaker sex. Anatomists argued that the brains of women were inferior in size and structure to that of men, thus verifying women's obvious inferior intellectual and creative capacity (Shield, 1975). Statisticians pointed to what they perceived to be the wider range of mental capacity in men — from greater numbers of mentally deficient to greater numbers of intellectually prominent — as proof that women could not hope to aspire to genius.

Early experimental studies often reached erroneous conclusions because of sample biases that favored the generally better-educated male. A notorious example is Galton's inference, based on anthropometric and psychometric measures on a large sample of men and women attending his health exhibit, that women tend to be inferior to men in all their capacities (Boring, 1950). Such "evidence" was used to bolster arguments that girls should receive separate and lesser educational training than boys. To the extent that such arguments were persuasive, they only reinforced the prevailing view.

Fortunately, when intelligence testing in schools became widespread, it became apparent that neither sex was superior overall; however, sex differences remained, with females generally superior in verbal skills and males superior in mathematics and spatial relations. More recently, studies have found the gap closing on most of these sex differences (Feingold, 1988).

This pattern of research closely parallels that of research in aging, where seeming age differences in a number of variables have been found to represent differences in cultural upbringing or education. Progress in the psychology of aging, as in the psychology of women, has involved foregoing stereotypical views in order to focus on the wide range of individual differences. The following two sections describe some of the biological as well as sociocultural influences that affect the behavior of older women.

Biological Influences

Aging has a strong genetic basis, most readily observed in the fact that various species mature, grow old, and die at vastly different rates, even under optimal environmental circumstances. Not only physical traits but behavioral characteristics may have a strong genetic component. For example, studies of aged mice show differences betweens strains in degree of activity decline, sensory loss, and behavioral rigidity (summarized in McClearn & Foch, 1985). A longitudinal study of aging human twins found greater similarity in cognitive performance in one-egg than in two-egg twin pairs (Bank & Jarvik, 1978).

Although men and women share many aspects of the human condition, they differ biologically in obvious and subtle ways that differently affect their physical, psychological, and social experience of living, and thus of aging. Beginning in utero, chromosomal differences in the developing organism produce differing hormonal ratios, leading to differential developmental of sexual characteristics. From birth onward, differing sexual characteristics such as the male's generally greater physical strength and the female's ability to bear offspring have a profound influence on roles and behavior. It is a matter of debate as to how, once sexual differentiation has occurred, biological, psychological, and sociological factors interact to produce these resulting sex differences.

One obvious male-female difference is the female's greater longevity, found in most species. In humans, this biological superiority in survival capability is seen even in the prenatal phases and weighs more heavily in favor of females with each succeeding age decade. A combination of genetic and social factors may account for this difference. One biological theory is that the presence of an additional X chromosome is a stabilizing influence, screening out potentially harmful recessive genes. Another theory involves that fact that the development in utero of a male is essentially an add-on process, and thus more vulnerable to error. A social factor involved in the greater fatality rate is the male's generally greater propensity for risk taking. This phenomenon, too, may have a biological basis: in terms of reproductive capacity, males are superfluous in comparison with females, since one male can inseminate numerous females.

Superior female survival has psychological and sociological ramifications. Reduced numbers and proportions of aging men mean that the aging experience is predominantly a female aging experience. In this society, where women most often marry men older than themselves, the state of widowhood is common, and older women are most often called upon to make psychological adjustments toward greater independence at a time when they are increasingly functionally dependent and in need of support.

Social and Cultural Influences

Human beings are highly social animals. Much of their behavior is influenced by their perception of their role as a member of a group. A life-span perspective on aging is necessary to provide a complete picture of the psychology of aging women. While the biological foundation as females provides a common core of experience, different environmental and societal influences provide unique psychological perspectives for different cohorts of women throughout their life span, resulting in different experiences of aging (Riley, 1979).

For example, cross-cultural studies (e.g., Townsend & Carbone, 1980) have revealed enormous variation in the experiences reported at menopause. The only universal events are cessation of menstruation and decreased estrogen production. Hot flashes and sweats are common but not inevitable, and other symptoms, such as depression, irritability, fatigue, dizziness, headaches, and loss of libido, vary in frequency of occurrences both within and between cultures.

Caveats About the Research Literature

Before drawing conclusions from the research findings to be described below, one should be aware of several points:

1. Solid research focusing on older women or describing male-female differences with age is scanty. In much of the research literature, only male subjects were used, either because they were more readily available or because there was no theoretical basis for assuming that sex differences might exist. Thus, reports describing the performance of "older people" may or may not be referring to older men and women.

2. The majority of conclusions described here have been reached through cross-sectional studies and thus have the potential for unwitting measurement of cohort effects such as education level and familiarity with the stimuli presented, rather than true age effects. There is less of a possibility of such biases occurring in studies of simpler biological processes than more complex, culture-bound tasks such as are involved in studies of concept formation and memory. Longitudinal studies are more likely to be measuring true aging effects, but subject attrition and repeated testing of the subject pool creates another set of biased outcomes. Cross-sequential studies, a

combination of cross-sectional and longitudinal measures, are more successful in eliminating the above problems, but they are more costly to perform in terms of time and money. A good description of methodological issues is found in Botwinick (1984).

3. In perceptual and cognitive studies, it is often difficult to know whether one is measuring discriminative capabilities or response processes. One example of potential response bias is elderly people's tendency to be more cautious, unwilling to make a mistake in judgment than younger people. Although this trait has survival value in real-life situations, in experimental settings it may further bias results in favor of the young, making the older subjects look slower and less discriminating than they actually are. Certain experimental techniques, such as signal detection paradigms, can help to uncover any differences in response processes between old and young subjects.

4. In comparing outcomes of studies with older and younger groups of people, one should be aware of the ecological validity of those studies and the measures contained in them. Responses of older people, when they differ from those of young people, may not reflect deficits except according to the "youth-centered standards adopted by researchers" (Labouvie-Vief, 1985, p. 505). Rather, they may reflect an aspect of adaptation to environmental demands, a learning process that occurs with age. For example, older people tend to remember better concrete, rather than abstract, items on memory tests, reflecting their interest, based on a lifetime's experience, in the practical, manifest world, rather than the youth-oriented world of abstract ideas. An excellent exposition of this complex issue is found in Labouvie-Vief (1985).

INFORMATION PROCESSING AND COGNITION

Speed of Processing

That older people tend to be slower than younger people in processing sensory information is a well-replicated finding. Slowing seems to involve both central and peripheral processes. There is little experimental evidence to suggest that older women differ from older men in this regard. Findings are reviewed briefly below. For in-depth coverage of the topic, an excellent reference is Botwinick (1984).

Strong evidence that peripheral processes are involved in slowing is shown by age differences in the critical flicker fusion point, the point at which two or more elements separated in time are experienced as one. For vision, it is the point at which a flashing light appears to stay on continuously; in audition, the point where clicks fuse; in touch, the point where separate shocks merge. It is a measure of a system's ability to track change. Older people experience stimulus fusion at greater time separations (Axelrod, Thompson, & Cohen, 1968; Coppinger, 1955; Misiak, 1947). Other evidence that stimuli persist longer in the older nervous system is the finding that old people are better than younger people at identifying words in which one-half of each letter of a word is presented as the first stimulus and the other half is presented as the second stimulus (Kline & Orme-Rogers, 1978). Another supporting study involves the phenomenon of color fusion: when red and green lights are presented sequentially to the eye at certain rates, yellow is perceived. Older people see yellow with greater distance in time between flashes (Kline, Ikeda, & Schieber, 1982). Also, afterimages last longer in the old than the young (Kline & Nestor, 1977).

Time taken to perceive stimuli is longer in older than in younger people. For example, in one study it took longer, by 20 to 40 msec, for old people to detect gaps in circles (Eriksen, Hamlin, & Breitmeyer, 1970). Another group of experiments has shown that older people have more difficulty identifying stimuli that are spread out, fragmented, or disguised (e.g., Axelrod & Cohen, 1961).

These and other studies point out why older people are at a disadvantage in quickly paced tasks. Compensatory adjustments in behavior may occur to make use of skills or abilities that are still relatively strong. The increased cautiousness observed in older people may be a compensatory mechanism. One study has shown that older people value accuracy and will sacrifice speed to achieve it (Salthouse, 1979).

That slowing is a central nervous system phenomenon is illustrated by the general finding that whereas older people tend to be slower than the young on cognitive tasks, they are even more so when judgments are more complex (Gaylord & Marsh, 1975; Sternberg, 1969). With practice, older people improve, often, more than do the young. However, they do not reach the speed of the young.

Concept Formation

Cross-sectional studies have found that older people are generally inferior to young people in learning and using concepts. Poor logical abilities, rather than memory, seem to be the reason for differences in these tasks. When tasks are made concrete, rather than abstract (e.g., Arenberg, 1968), the elderly do better, although they never perform as well as younger age groups. Differences in educational level and intelligence may be the primary factors involved here, rather than age per se. Kesler, Denney, and Whitely (1976) gave a large variety of problem-solving tasks to people age 30 to 50 and 65 to 81. Results indicated that both education and intelligence were related to problem solving, but age was not.

Some studies have found evidence that older people are less flexible in their thinking than younger people on problem-solving tasks (e.g., Hartley, 1981). Wetherick (1965) found that, even when matched for intelligence, older people adhered more rigidly to a previously established concept, even when it was shown to be incorrect. Other studies question the conclusion that rigidity per se is the problem. Instead, they point to a difficulty in forming concepts (e.g., Nehrke & Coppinger, 1971). Again, differences in education, not only in number of years of training but in recency of exposure, should be considered in accounting for these results.

Learning and Memory

Information processing involves three phases: getting information into the system, keeping it in, and getting it out again. These processes may be termed encoding, storage, and retrieval, respectively. The encoding process is commonly called learning. Storage and retrieval are part of memory.

Traditionally, studies comparing learning between older and younger adults have found older adults to be poorer learners. For older people, encoding an equivalent amount of information takes more time and requires more effort than for younger people. More recent studies have discovered that factors involved in increasing learning include instructing the older person in how to organize information, making tasks meaningful, rewarding the person just for responding, and augmenting visual information with auditory input (Botwinick, 1984). When information has been encoded equally well in young and old subjects, memory storage is similar in the two groups (Hulicka & Weiss, 1965).

Two common types of memory tasks involve recognition and recall. Recall involves search and retrieval of information from storage; recognition involves matching information in storage with information in the environment, thus bypassing the retrieval process. Research shows that recognition is superior to recall for all ages, with recall worsening with each increasing age decade and recognition showing little decline (Erber, 1974; Schonfield & Robertson, 1966). Recognition deteriorates as there are increased responses from which to choose. Young people are no better than old people on recognition tasks in which there are only two responses from which to choose, but are better when there are four or more possible responses (Kausler & Kleim, 1978).

Memory Storage

Sensory memory, often called iconic memory in vision and echoic memory in audition, lasts much less than a second. It is harder to find, takes longer to develop, and lasts longer in old people than in young. Thus, older people are already at a disadvantage at the first stage of information processing (Botwinick, 1984). Primary, or short-term, memory lasts only a few seconds. It is often measured by the length of a list of randomly presented digits that can be recited back without error. By tests such as this, primary memory has been shown to decline with increased age (e.g., Parkinson, Lindholm, & Inman, 1982).

Secondary, or long-term, memory is what most people mean by the term "memory." It is said to decline with age, as a result of poorer encoding. Tertiary memory is very long-term memory, over months or years. In one study, subjects' "total knowledge," defined as "information that is relatively permanent, acquired during a lifetime of formal education and day-to-day experience" (Lachman & Lachman, 1980, p. 287, quoted in Botwinick, 1984, p. 329), was found to increase from age 20 to 52 and remain constant to age 71.

How do these changes affect older women in a practical sense? Many of these changes, although *experimentally* significant, are small in terms of their effect on the behavior, or well-being, of normal, older women. Usually, the *fear* of memory loss, for example, is much greater than the loss itself. Most older women learn to adapt to those changes that do occur, often by compensatory behavior such as slowing down motor movements, increasing rehearsal of elements to be committed to memory, or avoiding unfamiliar environments unless properly prepared. A particular deficit may not be noticed until a new challenge occurs, such as a move out of familiar surroundings or the death of a spouse. Unfortunately, in the lives of older women, one unwanted change often precipitates another. For example, the loss of a husband may lead one to move, perhaps under pressure from family members, from a familiar neighborhood, with a well-established social network, to a novel environment, where social ties are as yet unformed.

Intelligence

The issue of whether intelligence declines with age has been hotly debated (e.g., Baltes & Schaie, 1974; Horn & Donaldson, 1976, 1977). In cross-sectional investigations, older people perform less well than young people on most standard intelligence tests, whereas longitudinal studies show comparatively little decline (Schaie & Labouvie-Vief, 1974). The classical aging pattern, seen in cross-sectional and to a lesser degree in longitudinal studies, is that tests in the verbal grouping (e.g., information, vocabulary, and comprehension) hold up fairly well with aging, but that tests in the performance grouping (e.g., digit symbol, which measures speed of copying, and a picture arrangement task, which measures logical ability) show declines with increased age. These effects are seen for both men and women.

What are the rationales for the changes seen, and what are the aruguments concerning their interpretation? Verbal functions in large part measure what people already know, reflecting stored information or general intellectual achievement. The term for this is "crystallized intelligence." Performance functions call for manipulative skills, with unfamiliar materials, involving figural and logical relations and emphasizing speed. These tasks are a measure of fluid intelligence, which is said to be a function of the state of the brain.

A number of objections have been raised to traditional intelligence tests and their interpretation as a measure of intellectual function in older adults (see Botwinick, 1984). First, intelligence measures usually heavily weigh speed of response. As we have seen previously, older people are at a disadvantage in speeded tasks. The question of whether cognitive slowing can be equated with decreased intellectual capacity has not yet been resolved. A second argument concerns the dependence of test scores on subjects' acquired and stored knowledge. Not only are the aged likely to have had less formal education, but they are more remote from their school days at the time of testing. Birren and Morrison (1961) found that educational level, but not age, contributed to intelligence test scores. Such findings account for the objection to cross-sectional as opposed to longitudinal studies described earlier. An important final criticism of most intelligence tests concerns the issue of ecological validity, the extent to which tests are relevant to the daily lives of older people. Some investigators (e.g., Schaie, 1978) have argued that adult intelligence tests should measure competence in dealing with the problems of daily life. Demming and Pressey (1957) designed a test containing practical informational items, including use of a telephone directory. Older adults scored better than younger adults, even when scoring more poorly on a conventional test.

Such findings should be reassuring to older women. Most healthy elderly persons continue to gain, rather than decline, in the ability to manage their daily affairs. Again, it is usually only in times of stress or loss (which is itself a major stressor) that the normal adaptive mechanisms may be pushed to their limits. At that point, social support represents an important, external, compensatory mechanism.

Creativity

Two broad areas of research on creativity are relevant to the study of older women: the study of male-female differences and the study of age differences. These areas will be discussed briefly, followed by implications for the little-researched area on older women and creativity.

Research findings as to whether creativity increases, decreases, or just changes in form with age have depended upon the subjects, the definition of creativity, and the methodology used in various studies. Lehman (1953), in a massive study of creative output in many fields of endeavor, found that creativity tended to peak in the early 30s. There have been a number of critics of his conclusion, primarily because of his use of people who died young. When people who lived long lives were analyzed, creativity was found to peak much later or to continue at a high plateau (Dennis, 1966). Creativity in older women has not received much discussion in the literature, although there are a number of outstanding examples. Georgia O'Keefe was a superb artist who produced steadily and prolifically throughout her long life (1887-1986).

As described previously, early theoretical frameworks did not support the view that women possessed a high degree of creative abilities. However, research with primary school children has found no male-female differences in creativity. Interestingly, women themselves downplay their creative contributions in comparison with men. For example, Barren (1972) interviewed men and women art students who had been rated by their teachers as equally creative. When asked, "Do you think of yourself as an artist?" 76% percent of women and only 34% of men said no. Of the men, 40% felt that their work was superior when compared with others at the art school, and only 14% felt their work was inferior. For women, only 17% felt their work was superior, and 40% felt it was inferior. Thus, there is a lack of self-esteem and confidence expressed by these women.

Other theories have emphasized a "creative force" that is the province of males, not females. Helson (1978) found, however, in her studies of creative and noncreative mathematicians and writers, that creative personalities, males or females, possess similar intensity with regard to the creative act. Rationales for women's lesser visibility in creative efforts may be due more to social factors. First, men, as well as boys, are rewarded more for their creative efforts, from grade school onward. Second, a woman's creative genius is often secondary to the time-consuming, though itself creative, activity of raising a family. In fact, it may be in older women, who possess a greater sense of mastery and self-esteem as well as freedom from distractions than their younger counterparts, that latent talents can flourish.

PERSONALITY

How do people's self-perceptions and behavior—what can be called personality—change as they age? There is little agreement as to whether personality remains stable to changes throughout the life span. As in most cases of research, the answer is somewhere in between. Much of the disagreement comes from differences in methodology used. The limitations of cross-sectional and longitudinal designs, discussed earlier, apply here, as well as the criticisms raised by the life-span and life-course developmental approach: much of what may seem to be biologically based, universal features of behavior may in fact be cohort or culturally bound and thus true for only a small segment of the population.

Stage theories are compelling schemata for viewing personality development, because they offer an overarching view of the life span. A well-known example is Erickson's (1963) eight stages of development: the first five stages cover the period from childhood through adolescence; the sixth involves early adulthood and focuses on the task of developing intimacy; the seventh covers middle adulthood and focuses on the task of generativity, teaching, or guiding the next generation (failure in this effort leads to overindulgence); the eighth covers old age and focuses on the task of self-acceptance and ego integrity (failure in this task leads to despair).

There is some supporting evidence for this stage model. For example, studies of life satisfaction have shown that those who accepted their aging had a high degree of life satisfaction, whereas those who had not accepted themselves as aging were unhappy. One problem with the cross-sectional studies used to obtain these results is that it is impossible to know whether such personality traits as happiness and unhappiness were specifically connected with success or failure in a particular stage or whether these were stable traits throughout the life span. In fact, there is evidence that life satisfaction, though influenced somewhat by external circumstances, is a relatively stable trait (Larson, 1978).

Other studies of personality have focused on the stability or change of particular characteristics. These will be discussed below.

Sex-Role Changes

There is evidence of a lessening of sex-role identity with aging. The traditional male role is one of dominance, aggression, and independence, whereas the traditional female role is one of submission, nurturing, sensitivity, and dependence. Neugarten and Gutmann (1958) found in a cross-sectional study that with increased age people incorporated more attributes of the opposite sex into their self-perception. Older women, for example, saw their position as one of dominance and that of older males as submissive, in certain cards on the Thematic Apperception Test. They also were more tolerant of their aggressive impulses, compared with younger women. Older men were more tolerant of their nurturant impulses.

Gutman (1975, 1987) has suggested that traditional sex roles are connected with the need for role division during active parenting — the mother must nurture offspring and inhibit competitive impulses that would detract from parenting, while the father must be aggressive and achievement oriented. Later, as these roles are no longer needed, both parents revert to their basic characters, which incorporate both masculine and feminine traits. Partial support for such a hypothesis was given by a study by Feldman, Biringen, and Nash (1981). Men and women at eight stages throughout the life cycle were asked to rate themselves in terms of masculine and feminine characteristics. Although women saw themselves as more compassionate and tender than men during most of the periods of life, during the married-childless stage and the grandparent stage, men and women saw themselves as equally tender.

Monge (1975) found similar evidence for sexual-attribute changes with later age. Although men scored higher overall in the dimension of masculinity, differences between males and females lessened with increased age. Females scored higher overall on congeniality/ sociability, but showed no difference from males in the oldest (65-89 years) age group.

An analysis by Troll and Parron (1981) concluded that over the life span, each sex continues to maintain self-perception of its sex role as a dominant model, but in later life, integrates more of the qualities of the opposite sex. For example, older women may see themselves as having greater autonomy and assertiveness than previously.

More studies should be made of how such traits change over the life span of difference cohorts and subsets of women. For example, will women who in younger years cultivate the traditionally more masculine traits of assertiveness and competitiveness in order to rise to the top in business or academia find themselves more tolerant of their nurturant qualities in later years?

Self-Esteem

Surprisingly, self-esteem tends to rise or remain stable with age. Bengtson, Reedy, and Gordon (1985) reviewed 17 studies of self-esteem and aging. Eight studies showed a positive relationship between age and self-esteem, seven showed no age differences, and one showed self-esteem peaking in the fourth decade. Only one study found older groups to be lower in esteem than young. Because all studies were cross-sectional, it is impossible to state definitively that these are effects of age rather than cohort. However, since publication dates of those studies with positive results ranged from 1954 through 1980, a span of 26 years, reflecting samples of different cohorts, the effect seems somewhat generalizable. Of the eight positive studies, five used both male and female subjects, two used only females, and one used only males. Of the seven studies that showed no relationship between self-esteem and age, two used only female subjects.

One study found self-esteem significantly related to life events and finances (Kaplan & Pokorny, 1969). Another found self-esteem related to health (Ward, 1977).

Control

There are few investigations of change in perceived control over the life span. Ryckman and Malikiosi (1975) used a scale of internal-external locus of control to study 400 men and women aged 21 to 79. They found that perceived internal control increased with each decade until the seventh. Again, cohort effects must be taken into account. More attention should be given to uncovering the causal factors involved in perceived control.

Issues of control and well-being will be discussed below.

LIFE SATISFACTION AND WELL-BEING

Life satisfaction is an internal construct having to do with subjective well-being. An excellent review by Larson (1978) of a number of studies of life satisfaction in older ages, using both male and female subjects, found well-being to be most strongly related to health, followed by socioeconomic factors such as income as well as degree of social interaction. Health or degree of physical disability accounted for 4% to 16% of the variance; income or other socioeconomic variables, 1% to 9%; and social activity, 1% to 9%. Marital status, housing, and transportation accounted for very small proportions of the variance, from 1% to 4%. There was no correlation of level of well-being with age, per se, when other variables were factored out. Also, sex as a variable did not correlate with level of well-being. Interestingly, most of the variance (an average of approximately 60%) was left unexplained in these studies. It seems that life satisfaction may be a relatively stable personality characteristic, most highly correlated with one's previous sense of life satisfaction.

Some predictors of life satisfaction in older age may be different for men and women. Mussen, Honzik, and Eichorn (1982) were able to reinterview old men and women who had been in a study 40 to 50 years previously as young parents at about age 30. For men, the strongest predictors of life satisfaction were their wife's emotional characteristics, as well as their own emotional and physical well-being. For women, life satisfaction was correlated most highly with the amount of income and leisure time, rather than their husbands' personalities.

PSYCHOSOCIAL FACTORS THAT INFLUENCE LIFE SATISFACTION

Research has shown that, overall, life satisfaction does not decrease with aging, except for the oldest old. This is surprising, given the fact that a number of events that often accompany aging decrease the degree of life satisfaction of aging women, including decreased health, decreased financial resources, widowhood, loss of friends, and decreased activity. In the following paragraphs, we will briefly consider some of the psychosocial variables that affect well-being and discuss some interventions that have proven helpful.

Adaptation

There is a healthy tendency for humans and other living beings to adapt to changing situations — be they pleasant or unpleasant — to the extent that the situation cannot be altered. Sing aging is a normal part of the developmental process for human beings, it is not surprising that there is adaptation to many of the physical, mental, and social changes that occur. Studies have shown that role shifts that occur "on time" are less stressful than those that occur unexpectedly. For example, women who experience widowhood during old age have less stress than those who are suddenly subjected to widowhood during midlife. Another example of adaptation is the fact that older people often rate their health as "good" or "excellent," whereas physicians' ratings are somewhat lower, although with high correlation (LaRue, Bank, Jarvik, & Hetland, 1979).

Often, researchers and lay people alike have viewed the problems of aging from the perspective of youth-oriented society and have thus placed more weight on certain events than do the elderly themselves. For example, older women tend to be less concerned about loss of physical attractiveness than many younger women.

Stress and Coping

Stress is the body's response to a demand, and it can be triggered by either positive or negative events (Seyle, 1975). Stress produces a variety of psychological and physical outcomes, including anxiety, headaches, ulcers, and other symptoms and illnesses. Coping responses may be healthy, such as exercise or meditation, or unhealthy, such as overeating or alcohol abuse.

A study by Griffith (1983a) of younger and older women found that stressors varied depending on age group. A total of 576 women ranging in age from 25 to 65 years were asked to rate on a scale of 1 to 4 both the importance to them of a particular situation and the degree of satisfaction they were experiencing with regard to that situation. The twenty-two items were factored into six major categories of potential stressors: love relationships (romantic), personal success, physical health, parent-child relationships, personal time, and social relationships. A stressor was defined as the situation in which importance of a particular item was two or more points higher than satisfaction with that item. The highest stressor for the oldest group, age 55 to 65, was physical health (26%), followed by personal time (20%). The highest stressor for the youngest group, age 25 to 34, was personal time (32%), followed by physical health (26%), personal success (12%) and love relationships (8%). The oldest group experienced less stress than any of the younger groups, when stress was measured as importance of a situation minus satisfactions with that particular situation. In part, lack of stress was due to the lower importance attributed to each of the items. For example, oldest and youngest groups ranked equally low in satisfaction with social relationships (i.e., relationships with close friends, coworkers, and social life with significant other). However, the youngest group rated social relationships as highly important, whereas the oldest group rated social relationships as much less important. As the author concluded: "Younger women have higher expectations that are often unsatisfactorily met, while older women have either achieved their valued expectations or place less importance on attaining them" (Griffith, 1983a, p. 325).

In the second part of this study (Griffith, 1983b), younger women reported physical and emotional symptoms of stress more than older women. Common physical symptoms for all groups of women included restless/fidgety, sinus problems, backaches, headaches, and trouble sleeping. Emotional symptoms included feeling fat and overweight, feeling sad or depressed, frequently nervous or tense, anxious or easily upset, sudden mood changes, and often irritable or angry. Coping responses varied with age, with younger women relying on talking, rest/relaxation, and isolation and older women using work, religion, and ignoring the problem.

Further research should include longitudinal studies and should extend the study of stress and coping patterns to older age groups and different subgroups of women.

Control

Personal control may be defined as the ability to manipulate some aspect of the environment (Schulz, 1976). Loss of control can result in the phenomenon of learned helplessness (Seligman, 1973; Seligman & Maier, 1967). In the original experimental paradigm, dogs were forced to undergo repeated shock that they would otherwise avoid, then subsequently exposed to shocks that they could avoid with any action on their part. The result was that the animal's normal escape responses were extinguished, resulting in passive submission to the unpleasant experience. In humans, depression, lack of motivation, and even cognitive deficits may be a manifestation of learned helplessness. Passiveness and hopelessness result from repeated failures to control, escape, or avoid events. Noncontingent positive events may also result in helplessness and depression (Seligman, 1973).

Seligman's revised theory incorporates the notion that one's explanation for an uncontrollable bad event determines the extent to which she will feel helpless or depressed. If events are explained in stable (e.g., this always happens to me), global (e.g., I can't do anything right), and internal terms (e.g., it's all my fault), then hopelessness and depression are more likely than if events are explained in unstable, specific, and external terms. Unfortunately, females, even in grade school, tend to use the internal mode of explanation to a greater degree than boys. Seligman suggests that reprogramming at an early age to avoid such cognitive styles could serve as a preventive measure against depression and hopelessness in later years (Trotter, 1987).

Loss of perceived control often accompanies the aging experience, particularly in cases of disability. Schulz and Aderman (1973) have hypothesized that feelings of helplessness cause adverse reactions to institutionalized older persons, possibly precipitating early death. Schulz (1976) randomly assigned institutionalized aged individuals to one of four conditions: (1) one group could determine the frequency and duration of visits by college undergraduates; (2) a second group was told when visits would be made but had no control over them; (3) a third group was visited on a random schedule, without warning; and (4) data from a fourth group formed a baseline. In comparison with the random and no-treatment groups, both the predict and control groups were rated as healthier, took less medication, perceived themselves as happier, and had higher levels of activity. No differences were found between either the random and no-treatment groups or the predict and control groups. The latter finding suggests, according to Schulz, that the positive outcome is due to predictability alone.

Langer and Rodin (1976) gave one group of nursing home residents a communication emphasizing their responsibility for themselves, as well as freedom to make choices, and the responsibility of caring for a plant. A second group received a communication emphasizing the staff's responsibility for them, and gave them a plant to be watered by the staff. The "responsibility" group improved on measures of alertness, active participation, and general well-being. Moreover, the program had long-term benefits in terms of health and mortality indicators (Rodin & Langer, 1977). Mercer and Kane (1979) performed a similar study in which subjects in a nursing home were encouraged to take responsibility for themselves, were given the opportunity to care for a plant, and were invited to participate in a residence council; subjects in the control nursing home received no intervention. Pre- and post-test measures found significant reductions in hopelessness, increase in activity, and positive changes in behavior for the experimental group. Professionals should be educated as to the power of such supportive environments, and practical work should be carried out to refine strategies for their design and implementation.

CONCLUSIONS

What can we conclude from this broad survey? First, aging may be the ultimate challenge in a woman's life, testing the limits of her resources and capabilities. Second, older women seem to possess the potential for successfully meeting this challenge. Although declines and losses are almost certainly inevitable, adaptive mechanisms, combined with supportive environments, can allow older women to fulfill their lives with dignity and confidence. Evidence suggests that older human beings tend to strive for competence in their environment (Birren, 1985) and develop strong urges to act as protectors and transmitters of the best of their culture (Labouvie-Vief, 1985). Given the optimal sociocultural framework, older women could take their proper place as leaders in society. Gutmann's (1987) cross-cultural studies, for example, show that women in older ages become more adventurous, expansive, and assertive.

A major task of professionals working with older people is to assist in cultivating the optimal supportive environment. Strategies involve educating both professionals and laypeople concerning problems of older women and their potential. Research efforts should seek practical solutions to problems that create unnecessary barriers to self-actualization. Ultimately, such efforts on behalf of older women would benefit the whole society.

REFERENCES

Arenberg, D. (1968). Concept problem solving in young and old adults. *Journal of Gerontology*, *23*, 279-282.

Axelrod, S., & Cohen, L. D. (1961). Senescence and imbedded-figure performance in vision and touch. *Perceptual and Motor Skills*, *12*, 283-288.

Axelrod, S., Thompson, L. W., & Cohen, L. D. (1968). Effects of senescence on the temporal resolution of somesthetic stimuli presented to one hand or both. *Journal of Gerontology*, *23*, 191-195.

Baltes, P. B., & Schaie, K. W. (1974). Aging and IQ: The myth of the twilight years. *Psychology Today*, *7*, 35-40.

Bank, L., & Jarvik, L. F. (1978). A longitudinal study of aging human twins. In E. L. Schneider (Ed.), *The genetics of aging* (pp. 239-252). New York: Plenum Press.

Barren, F. X. (1972). *Artists in the making*. New York: Seminar Press.

Bengtson, V. L., Reedy, M. N., & Gordon, C. (1985). Aging and self-conceptions: Personality processes and social contexts. In J. E. Birren & K. W. Schaie (Eds.), *Handbook of the psychology of aging* (2nd ed.) (pp. 544-593). New York: Van Nostrand Reinhold.

Birren, J. E. (1985). Age, competence, creativity, and wisdom. In R. N. Butler & H. P. Gleason (Eds.), *Productive aging: Enhancing vitality in later life* (pp. 29-36). New York: Springer.

Birren, J. E., & Morrison, D. F. (1961). Analysis of the WAIS subtests in relation to age and education. *Journal of Gerontology*, *16*, 363-369.

Boring, E. G. (1950). *A history of experimental psychology* (2nd ed.). New York: Appleton-Century-Crofts.

Botwinick, J. (1984). *Aging and behavior* (3rd ed.). New York: Springer.

Coppinger, N. W. (1955). The relationship between critical flicker frequency and chronological age for varying levels of stimulus brightness. *Journal of Gerontology, 10,* 48-52.

Demming, J. A., & Pressey, S. L. (1957). Tests "indigenous" to the adult and older years. *Journal of Counseling Psychology, 2,* 144-148.

Dennis, W. (1966). Creative productivity between ages of 20 and 80 years. *Journal of Gerontology, 21,* 1-8.

Erber, J. T. (1974). Age differences in recognition memory. *Journal of Gerontology, 29,* 177-181.

Ericksen, C. W., Hamlin, R. M., & Breitmeyer, R. G. (1970). Temporal factors in visual perception as related to aging. *Perception and Psychophysics, 7,* 354-356.

Erickson, E. H. (1963). *Childhood and society* (2nd ed.). New York: Norton.

Feingold, A. (1988). Cognitive gender differences are disappearing. *American Psychologist, 43,* 95-103.

Feldman, S. S., Biringen, Z. C., & Nash, S. C. (1981). Fluctuations of sex-related self attributions as a function of stage of family life cycle. *Developmental Psychology, 17,* 24-35.

Gaylord, S. A., & Marsh, G. R. (1975). Age differences in the speed of a spatial cognitive process. *Journal of Gerontology, 30,* 674-678.

Griffith, J. W. (1983a). Women's stressors according to age groups: Part I. *Issues in Health Care of Women, 6,* 311-326.

Griffith, J. W. (1983b). Women's stress responses and coping patterns according to age groups: Part II. *Issues in Health Care of Women, 6,* 327-340.

Gutmann, D. (1975). Parenthood: A key to the comparative study of the life cycle. In D. Octan & L. H. Ginsberg (Eds.), *Life-span developmental psychology* (pp. 167-184). New York: Academic Press.

Gutmann, D. (1987). *Reclaimed powers. Toward a new psychology of men and women in later life.* New York: Basic Books.

Hartley, A. A. (1981). Adult age differences in deductive reasoning processes. *Journal of Gerontology, 36,* 700-706.

Helson, R. M. (1978). Creativity in women. In J. A. Sherman & F. L. Denmark (Eds.), *The psychology of women: Future directions in research* (pp. 553-604). New York: Psychological Dimensions.

Horn, J. L., & Donaldson, G. (1976). On the myth of intellectual decline in adulthood. *American Psychologist, 31,* 701-709.

Horn, J. L., & Donaldson, G. (1977). Faith is not enough: A response to the Baltes-Schaie claim that intelligences does not wane. *American Psychologist, 32,* 369-373.

Hulicka, I. M., & Weiss, R. L. (1965). Age differences in retention as a function of learning. *Journal of Consulting Psychology, 29,* 125-129.

Kaplan, H. B., & Pokorny, A. D. (1969). Self-derogation and psychosocial adjustment. *Journal of Nervous and Mental Diseases, 149,* 421-434.

Kausler, D. H., & Kleim, D. M. (1978). Age differences in processing relevant versus irrelevant stimuli in multiple item recognition learning. *Journal of Gerontology, 33,* 87-93.

Kesler, M. S., Denney, N. W., & Whitely, S. E. (1976). Factors influencing problem solving in middle-aged and elderly adults. *Human Development, 19,* 310-320.

Kline, D. W., Ikeda, D., & Schieber, F. (1982). Age and temporal resolution in color vision: When do red and green make yellow? *Journal of Gerontology, 37,* 705-709.

Kline, D. W., & Nestor, S. (1977). The persistence of complementary afterimages as a function of adult age and exposure duration. *Experimental Aging Research, 3,* 203-213.

Kline, D. W., & Orme-Rogers, C. (1978). Examination of stimulus persistence as the basis for superior visual identification performance among older adults. *Journal of Gerontology, 33,* 76-81.

Labouvie-Vief, G. (1985). Intelligence and cognition. In J. E. Birren & K. W. Schaie (Eds.), *Handbook of the psychology of aging* (pp. 500-530). New York: Van Nostrand Reinhold.

Lachman, J. L., & Lachman, R. (1980). Age and the actualization of world knowledge. In L. Poon, J. L. Fozard, L. S. Cermak, D. Arenberg, & L. W. Thompson (Eds.), *New directions in memory and aging* (pp. 285-311). Hillsdale, NJ: Erlbaum.

Langer, E. J., & Rodin, J. (1976). The effects of choice and enhanced personal responsibility for the aged: A field experiment in an institutional setting. *Journal of Personality and Social Psychology, 34,* 191-198.

Larson, R. (1978). Thirty years of research on the subjective well-being of older Americans. *Journal of Gerontology, 33,* 109-125.

LaRue, A., Bank, L., Jarvik, L., & Hetland, M. (1979). Health in old age: How do physicians' ratings and self-ratings compare? *Journal of Gerontology, 34,* 687-691.

Lehman, H. C. (1953). *Age and achievement.* Princeton, NJ: Princeton University Press.

McClearn, G., & Foch, T. T. (1985). Behavioral genetics. In J. E. Birren & K. W. Schaie (Eds.), *Handbook of the psychology of aging* (pp. 113-143). New York: Van Nostrand Reinhold.

Mercer, S., & Kane, R. A. (1979). Helplessness and hopelessness among the institutionalized aged: An experiment. *Health and Social Work, 4,* 90-116.

Misiak, H. (1947). Age and sex differences in critical flicker frequency. *Journal of Experimental Psychology, 37,* 318-332.

Monge, R. H. (1975). Structure of the self-concept from adolescence through old age. *Experimental Aging Research, 1,* 281-291.

Mussen, P., Honzik, M. P., & Eichorn, H. (1982). Early antecedents of life satisfaction at age 70. *Journal of Gerontology, 37,* 316-322.

Nehrke, M. F., & Coppinger, N. W. (1971). The effect of task dimensionality on discrimination learning and transfer of training in the aged. *Journal of Gerontology, 26,* 151-156.

Neugarten, B. L. & Gutmann, D. (1958). Age-sex roles and personality in middle age: A thematic apperception study. *Psychological Monographs: General and Applied, 17* (Whole No. 470).

Parkinson, S. R., Lindholm, J. M., & Inman, V. W. (1982). An analysis of age differences in immediate recall. *Journal of Gerontology, 37,* 425-431.

Riley, M. W. (Ed.). (1979). *Aging from birth to death: Interdisciplinary perspectives.* Boulder, CO: Westview Press.

Rodin, J., & Langer, E. J. (1977). Long-term effects of a control-relevant intervention with the institutionalized aged. *Journal of Personality and Social Psychology, 35,* 897-902.

Ryckman, R. M., & Malikiosi, M. X. (1975). Relationship between locus of control and chronological age. *Psychological Reports, 36,* 655-658.

Salthouse, T. A. (1979). Adult age and the speed-accuracy trade-off. *Ergonomics, 22,* 811-821.

Schaie, K. W. (1978). External validity in the assessment of intellectual development in adulthood. *Journal of Gerontology, 33,* 696-701.

Schaie, K. W., & Labouvie-Vief, G. (1974). Generational versus ontogenetic components of change in adult cognitive behavior: A fourteen year cross-sequential study. *Developmental Psychology, 10,* 305-320.

Schonfield, D., & Robertson, E. A. (1966). Memory storage and aging. *Canadian Journal of Psychology, 20,* 228-236.

Schulz, R. (1976). Effects of control and predictability on the physical and psychological well-being of the institutionalized aged. *Journal of Personality and Social Psychology, 33,* 563-573.

Schulz, R., & Aderman, D. (1973). Effect of residential change on the temporal distance of death of terminal cancer patients. *Omega: Journal of Death and Dying, 4,* 157-162.

Seligman, M. (1973). Fall into helplessness. *Psychology Today, 7,* 43-48.

Seligman, M. & Maier, S. (1967). Failure to escape traumatic shock. *Journal of Experimental Psychology, 74,* 1-9.

Seyle, H. (1975). *The stress of life* (2nd ed.). New York: McGraw-Hill.

Shields, S. A. (1975). Functionalism, Darwinism, and the psychology of women: A study in social myth. *American Psychologist, 30,* 737-754.

Sternberg, S. (1969). Memory scanning: Mental processes revealed by reaction time experiments. *American Scientist, 57,* 421-457.

Townsend, J. M., & Carbone, C. L. (1980). Menopausal syndrome: Illness or social role — a transcultural analysis. *Culture, Medicine, and Psychiatry, 4,* 229-248.

Troll, L. E., & Parron, E. M. (1981). Age changes in sex roles and changing sex roles: The double shift. In C. Eisdorfer (Ed.), *Annual Review of Gerontology and Geriatrics* (Vol. 2) (pp. 118-143). New York: Springer.

Trotter, R. J. (1987, February). Stop blaming yourself. *Psychology Today.*

Ward, R. A. (1977). The impact of subjective age and stigma on older persons. *Journal of Gerontology, 32*, 227-237.

Wetherick, N. E. (1965). Changing an established concept: A comparison of the ability of young, middle-aged, and old subjects. *Gerontologia, 11*, 82-95.

Williams, J. H. (1977). *Psychology of women: Behavior in a biosocial context.* New York: Norton.

Coping Patterns of Aging Women: A Developmental Perspective

Laura Hubbs-Tait, PhD

The meaning or lack of meaning that old age takes on in any given society puts that whole society to the test, since it is this that reveals the meaning or the lack of meaning of the entirety of the life leading to that old age.

Simone de Beauvoir (1977)

The purpose of this article is to provide a conceptual framework for understanding the data on women's psychological coping patterns as they age beyond midlife. There are several factors that complicate this task. First, although theoretical work in life-span developmental psychology has grown rapidly over the past 20 years, it has rarely addressed differences between men and women during the older years. Second, with rare exceptions, neither theoretical nor empirical work has focused on differences among women as they age, even though results relevant to individual differences can be gleaned from recent research. Although integration of data on aging women's coping behaviors is possible within the theoretical framework provided here, the integration is not complete: there are data that do not fit neatly into the framework. This lack of fit emphasizes the fact that much research is needed on the psychology of aging women in general and about elderly women's coping patterns in particular.

Laura Hubbs-Tait is Associate Professor of Psychology, Department of Psychology, Washburn University, Topeka, KS 66621.

The author would like to thank Cara Iwig for her help in locating the research reviewed in this article and for proofreading earlier drafts. Special thanks go to Drs. Dianne Garner and Susan Mercer for their editorial suggestions.

There are several issues that are relevant to a developmental perspective within the field of psychology, as applied to coping patterns of aging women. One is the issue of change versus stability. Do women's coping patterns change as they age beyond midlife or are they stable? Another issue is the source of change, if it occurs. If the differences in coping patterns are between older women and younger ones, as opposed to between the older versus younger years of the same woman's life, then the issue of cohort differences surfaces. That is, if an older woman's coping patterns are different from those of a younger one, this difference may have been there for decades and may be due to the different sociohistorical contexts in which these two women have lived their lives. Alternatively, the difference may be due to the psychological tasks of aging. Only with longitudinal studies or variations on them can these two sources of change be distinguished (Baltes, Reese, & Nesselroade, 1977).

A third issue is whether coping patterns of aging women are nomothetic, that is, universal or true of all elderly women, or idiographic, that is, unique to particular individuals (Baltes & Nesselroade, 1973; Livson, 1973). For the practitioner, nomothetic coping patterns are important because they will be true of all elderly female clients. Idiographic coping patterns are important because they are more likely to be related to individual personality characteristics (McCrae & Costa, 1986) or clinical diagnoses.

The definition of coping patterns used in this article is adapted from one provided by Munnichs and Olbrich (1985). Coping patterns may be either episodic or enduring. They are behaviors that a person uses in dealing with demands that require more than a habitual response. They crystallize when situational demands are similar and the coping behaviors suffice to meet those demands. They also crystallize when individuals continually seek out situations that make similar demands upon them, regardless of whether these demands are constructive or destructive (Smith & Anderson, 1986). Coping patterns need to be modifed when situational demands change.

By defining coping patterns in this way, divergent assumptions made by researchers may be included: the enduring nature and coherence of coping mechanisms (Haan, 1977) as well as the modifiability and independence of coping behaviors (Lazarus & Folkman, 1984). Since this definition of coping includes both the possibility of stability and the possibility of change, it is eminently appropriate to a developmental perspective. Finally, although this definition places coping within the intersecting areas of developmental, clinical, and personality psychology, coping patterns need not be equated with personality characteristics.

The remainder of this article is organized in the following fashion. First, several developmental theories relevant to the coping patterns of aging women are reviewed: those of Erik Erikson, Hans Thomae, David Gutmann, Carol Gilligan, David Bakan, and Jeanne H. Block. Included in this section is the literature on the importance of the feminine developmental experience. Second, the physical and social challenges faced by women as they age are discussed. Third, research on coping mechanisms used by elderly women is reviewed. Finally, some concluding comments are made about research that is still needed, and suggestions are offered about the relationship of research on coping to practice with and provision of social services to aging women.

DEVELOPMENTAL THEORIES

Erik Erikson

Erik Erikson's theory of the eight stages of human life was one of the earliest theories (see also Bühler, 1933) to describe developmental changes beyond childhood and adolescence. Erikson is also eloquent on the subject of the older years of adulthood (Erikson, 1963, 1968, 1978). In part, his theory is maturational; at each stage a particular ego function matures. However, the manner in which that ego function is expressed is influenced by the individual's genes, social and cultural context, and personal history. At each stage of life, there is a crisis as the ego function emerges and attempts to express itself. This crisis is an acute period analogous to a medical crisis in which the individual's psychological functioning takes a turn for the better or the worse. With each passing stage, the influence of the social and cultural context increases as does the influence of one's personal history.

In the older years, the ego function that emerges is wisdom; the crisis is between integrity and despair. For integrity to predominate, an older adult needs to be able to accept her life and feel that, in general, that life has been well spent. Integrity involves accepting human progress, both one's own and that of others. With integrity comes wisdom, "the detached and yet active concern with life itself in the face of death itself" (Erikson, 1978, p. 26). Despair arises when the older adult cannot accept her life and is unable to face death. For Erikson, despair is caused not by feeling that one has made many wrong decisions in one's life but rather by the feeling that one has made no decisions at all. Underlying despair is the avoidance of actively choosing throughout one's life. With despair comes anger that one does not have another chance to make sense of one's life. Despair can also be manifested in a fear of death and a contempt for other people.

Implicit in Erikson's descriptions of elderly adults are two categories of coping patterns. The functional one, integrity, is predicted by a life of actively engaging issues and making choices. The dysfunctional one, despair, is predicted from passivity and disengagement. In samples of normally functioning elderly women, the coping pattern of integrity, of acceptance of one's life as one has lived it, should predominate.

Erikson's theory assumes that biological influences on ego functioning decrease with age and social and cultural influences increase. To the extent that a culture has different expectations for the two genders with regard to a particular adult ego function, then there would be significant differences between men and women in the expression of that ego function. Erikson suggested that for American males the midlife ego function of generativity, being helpful or useful to others, may not be well developed because American males confuse generativity with productivity and acquisition. It does not seem as though the possible existence of different expectations for the integrity of older men and women by contemporary cultures has been investigated. However, Ryff and Heincke

(1983) found no gender differences in integrity among elderly American adults.

Hans Thomae

Hans Thomae's theory of aging (1959, 1970, 1983; Thomae & Simons, 1967) consists of three major assumptions. First, the subjective perception of change rather than objective change is related to behavioral change. For example, positive perceptions of retirement are related to positive adjustments to it. The perceived quality of one's life is a better predictor of satisfaction than are objective measurements of the quality of one's life. Stressors that are perceived as such are those against which coping mechanisms will be mobilized.

The second assumption is that any change is perceived and evaluated in terms of the dominant concerns and expectations of the individual. If a concern about the diminishing possibilities of one's existence is predominant, then any changes in one's situation will be evaluated in light of that concern. Thomae (1983, pp. 70-71, 80-81) finds that among the elderly, there is a highly significant difference in the pleasantness ratings of daily activities between those whose concern is with diminishing possibilities and those who are not concerned about the diminishing possibilities of existence.

The third assumption is that one's adjustment to aging is a function of the balance between the cognitive and motivational structures of the aging individual. Those individuals who perceive change positively and who adapt their self-concepts and motivations so that they are congruent with their perceptions of change will age "successfully." For Thomae (1983) the existence of gender differences in aging is linked to sociohistorical conditions.

David Gutmann

David Gutmann's theory of development (Gutmann, 1985a, 1985b; Neugarten & Gutmann, 1958) suggests that women and men differ during middle and older adulthood as a function of "the parental imperative" or the "chronic emergency of parenthood." According to Gutmann, before and after the parenting period the norm for both males and females is androgyny (1985b). During the parenting period, clear divisions in the sex roles arise for the sake of the children. A female's traits of "agency," "rationality," "aggressivity," and "assertiveness" are minimized so that she may nurture vulnerable infants and children. A man's traits of "communion," "sentimentality," and "nurturance" are minimized so that he may actively provide for his family. Following the parental period, women express a more active mastery or coping pattern than they did while they were nurturing their children. Men, on the other hand, develop a more passive pattern.

Thus, Gutmann's theory predicts consistencies in development within each gender but a reversal of the pattern of change between the two genders from middle to older adulthood. However, Gutmann's labeling the pattern for women as androgyny-femininity-androgyny and the one for men as androgyny-masculinity-androgyny may well obscure the actual nature of the changes that take place. For example, an increase with age in women's assertiveness would be labeled an increase in masculinity; an increase in rationality would be identically labeled. Such labeling obfuscates the distinction between assertiveness and rationality and ignores the possibility that the reasons for increases in these two characteristics might be completely different.

Carol Gilligan

Carol Gilligan (1982) proposes that the developmental experiences of males and females in Western societies are very different. She argues that the childhood experience of males is one that emphasizes separation and individuation, whereas that of females is one that emphasizes attachments to and relationships with others. This difference in socialization accounts for the differences in moral reasoning between men and women. When women confront moral dilemmas, they want to know about the relationships and social resources of the protagonists. Men, on the other hand, impartially weigh the different claims for justice. Women's morality is a morality based on responsibility; men's is based on rights.

David Bakan

David Bakan (1966) advanced a similar claim about masculinity and femininity. He argued that two fundamental modalities characterize all living beings: agency and communion. Agency is the masculine modality; communion is the feminine. Agency refers to the characteristics of living beings as individuals and is manifested in self-protection, self-assertion, and self-expansion. Communion refers to the characteristics of living beings as they exist in some larger organism of which they are a part and manifests itself in being at one with other organisms. Bakan also had a developmental perspective: the fundamental goal of human existence was to try "to mitigate agency with communion" (1966, p. 236). For Bakan, unmitigated agency represented evil; viability required the successful integration of agency and communion.

Jeanne H. Block

Jeanne H. Block (1984) provides some evidence in favor of Bakan's (1966) theory. She asked university students in Norway, Sweden, Denmark, Finland, England, and the United States to describe the "kind of person I would most like to be." Then she compared the ideal selves of males and females across the six countries. Ideals were similar across the six cultures with males more often affirming characteristics consistent with agency and females affirming characteristics consistent with communion.

Block (1984) proposes that individuals at higher stages of ego and moral development will have integrated aspects of both agency and communion into their identities. Individuals with more primitive levels of ego and moral development identify themselves in terms of sex-typed characteristics (agency for males, communion for females). She provides data from two studies, which are consistent with her proposal. At more advanced levels of ego development, females not only identify themselves in terms of characteristics reflecting commmunion, but also those reflecting agency. Extrapolating from the Bakan/Block argument to aging, one could propose that among the elderly, it would be those women who have integrated agency and communion who would be better equipped to cope with the challenges and threats of aging. On the one hand, agency would ensure self-confidence and feelings of efficacy; on the other hand, communion would ensure a sense of belonging in family, community, and culture.

PHYSICAL AND SOCIAL CHALLENGES

Physical Challenges

Numerous physical changes are associated with the aging process. Among these changes are a decline in the functioning of the immune system, diminished lung capacity, a decrease in cardiac output, a decline in carbohydrate metabolism, and marked changes in the central nervous system (Hooyman & Cohen, 1986; Trofatter, 1986). There appears to be a decrease in levels of the neurotransmitter dopamine, even among those elderly for whom there is no diagnosis of Parkinson's or other neurological disorders (Busse, 1986). There is also evidence for cortical atrophy and ventricular enlargement in the normal aging process (Busse, 1986).

Although physical changes affect both women and men, there are also aspects of the physical aging process that selectively or exclusively affect women: for example, menopause and the concomitant decrease in estrogen and progesterone production. In the age range of 65 to 79, women are more likely than men to suffer from a variety of chronic diseases: hypertension, hypertensive heart disease, elevated serum cholesterol, osteoarthritis, rheumatoid arthritis, loss of vision (Verbrugge, 1983).

Despite the fairly negative portrayal of the physical health of elderly women, professionals (e.g., Ostrow, 1980) have argued that some deteriorations in physical health are due more to abuse or disuse than to the aging process. Consequently, some of the negative physical changes of aging women are probably not inevitable, though frequently both the elderly and medical practitioners continue to regard them as such (Riley & Bond, 1983).

Among developmental theorists discussed previously, Thomae (1970, 1983; Thomae & Simons, 1967) emphasizes that changes or stresses have a psychological impact only when they are perceived and of concern to the person experiencing them. Consequently, if the physical challenges listed in this section were of no concern to

aging women, they would have no impact. That such is not the case
is underscored by numerous studies. Although elderly adults generally report fewer sources of stress than younger adults, they consistently report physical health as a source of greater stress than younger adults (Folkman & Lazarus, 1980; Gurin, Veroff, & Feld,
1960; House & Robbins, 1983; Riddick, 1982). Folkman, Lazarus,
Pimley, and Novacek (1987) report the results of a study of 66 men
and 75 women between the ages of 65 and 74. Compared with a
younger group of adults (35 to 45 years), these older adults were
significantly more likely to report health-related issues as a source
of stress. Furthermore, physical health was of equal concern to both
aging men and aging women. Changes in physical health are perceived by elderly women and are of concern to them.

Socioemotional Challenges

Retirement

Research on the adjustment of women to retirement has surfaced
since 1980 (Szinovacz, 1982). Prior to this decade, such research
focused on males. Keith (1982) compared predictors of life satisfaction among retired elderly women and elderly women who had been
homemakers (72 to 97 years). There were some important demographic differences between these two groups of women: retired
women had more education than homemakers; homemakers were
more likely to be married; homemakers had more children who
were still living. Different variables predicted life satisfaction for
these two groups of elderly women. Among the retirees, the variables that significantly predicted life satisfaction were, in order of
importance, perceived improvement in health status over the past
seven years, loneliness (negatively related to life satisfaction), involvement in civic organizations, increased church involvement,
greater numbers of contacts with acquaintances (i.e., not confidants
or family members). Among the homemakers, the variables that
significantly predicted life satisfaction were, in order of importance, loneliness (negatively related), more education, perception
of current health as good, increase in number of acquaintances over
the past seven years.

The major difference between sources of satisfaction for elderly retired women and elderly homemakers was the positive correlation between satisfaction and greater involvement in civic and religious organizations among the retirees and the positive correlation between satisfaction and education among the homemakers. Contrary to what might be expected, involvement with family members was not a significant predictor of satisfaction for the elderly home-makers.

Stereotyping

Schonfield (1982) questioned adults ranging from college age to the elderly about aging stereotypes. Their agreement with traditional stereotypes (e.g, "old people tend to be inflexible") ranged from a high of 77% to a low of 20%. Furthermore, most of these adults agreed that there were many elderly individuals who did not fit these stereotypes. In fact, fewer than 20% of the adults surveyed thought that the stereotypes they were evaluating described as many as 80% of the elderly. Schonfield (1982) concludes that negative stereotyping of the elderly is limited.

Schonfield (1982) did not question his subjects about stereotypes of aging women versus aging men. However, Walsh and Connor (1979) did. They asked undergraduates to rate articles written by applicants for the position of art columnist on a local newspaper. When the article (always the same) was described as one written by a 64-year-old man, they were unwilling to publish it or to ask the writer's advice about art. When the article was portrayed as one written by a 64-year-old woman, the students were both willing to publish it and to consult the writer's advice about art.

Older women do not fare as well in portrayals by the major television networks. Aronoff (1974) analyzed prime-time network dramas for the years 1969 to 1971. He reported that for females increasing age was associated with decreased chances of achieving goals. Across both genders and all age groups, it was only the group of female elderly who were portrayed as more likely to fail than to succeed at achieving their goals. Signorelli (1983) replicated Aronoff's (1974) findings in an analysis of prime-time dramas that appeared on television from 1969 to 1981. Among older adults, 37% of the males were portrayed as successful, whereas 23% were portrayed as unsuccessful. In contrast, only 17% of elderly women were portrayed as successful, whereas 35% were portrayed as unsuccessful. At no other age were there gender differences in the portrayal of success by television characters.

The results of these studies of stereotyping of elderly women are far from consistent. To the extent that negative stereotypes are held by individuals who form the support system for elderly women, they are clearly detrimental (Riley & Bond, 1983). The full impact of negative stereotypes on the lives of aging women is still unknown. Riley and Bond (1983) suggest that some of the stereotypes of the biological process of aging do have a negative effect on the delivery of medical services to the elderly.

In line with Thomae's theory (1970, 1983), researchers need to address an unanswered question: to what extent are stereotypes perceived by and of concern to elderly women? Assuming that stereotypes of aging (medical, social, emotional) are perceived by and of concern to elderly women, they constitute a stress factor with which aging women have to cope. It may be less the physical problems of aging than the stereotyping of these problems as inevitable and immutable that is the source of the stress associated with the health concerns of the elderly. Being told "Well, what do you expect at your age?" is simultaneously demeaning and unhelpful.

Living Alone

The challenge of living alone is one faced by many elderly women. Even among elderly women who do not live alone, many are widowed and thus perceive themselves as alone or lonely (Lopata, 1980).

Henderson, Scott, and Kay (1986), report the results of a study of 268 community-dwelling residents of Hobart, Australia, all of whom were 70 years of age or older. They found significant sociodemographic differences between the elderly living alone and those living with relatives. Those living alone were more likely to be older, female, unmarried, widowed, more likely not to have siblings in the same town, and more educated. Nonetheless, there were very few differences in social relationships and mental health between those elderly who lived by themselves and those who lived with others. Those living alone rated themselves as more lonely and as having significantly fewer affectionately close relationships. Even so, those who lived alone did not differ from those who lived with others in their perceptions of the adequacy of these relationships, nor in perceptions of the availability and adequacy of social integration means. There were no differences between the groups in DSM-III diagnoses of major depression. However, those living alone did score higher on items assessing complaints about physical health, sleeping difficulties, loneliness, unhappiness, and recent crying.

Essentially the same pattern of results is revealed when only the data for elderly women are considered. Thus, among elderly women living alone, there is a higher frequency of symptoms of depression but no evidence for diagnoses of depressive disorder nor for isolation from social relationships.

A longitudinal study by Lund, Caserta, and Dimond (1986) qualifies the above picture somewhat. They investigated the adjustment of widows and widowers aged 50 or older from three weeks following the death of their spouse to two years later. They found no adjustment differences between widows and widowers. From three weeks post-bereavement to two years later, widows and widowers had significant improvements in life satisfaction scores and significant decreases in scores for emotional shock, helplessness/avoidance, anger/guilt/confusion, grief resolution behaviors and depression. Thus, the passage of time following bereavement does alleviate some symptoms of depression.

There are variables other than the passage of time that appear to mitigate the loneliness of widowhood and/or living alone. Heller and Mansbach (1984) interviewed 43 women aged 60 to 97 who were patrons of two city nutrition sites for low-income individuals. They found that, after they had controlled for age, three variables significantly and independently predicted life satisfaction for these elderly women: frequency of church attendance, social network size, and proportion of network members considered as intimates or confidantes.

Similarly, Lowenthal and Haven (1968) emphasize the importance of having a confidante. They investigated elderly community residents who had been widowed. They found that a widow with a confidante was better adjusted than a married woman without a confidante! In line with Heller and Mansbach (1984), Gallagher, Thompson, and Peterson (1981-1982) report the results of several studies that support the importance of church attendance and/or religious beliefs in the adaptation of widows to the death of their husbands.

Generally, research suggests that the bereaved elderly and those living alone are more unhappy than those who are married and/or living with others. This conclusion may need to be qualified by the results of several recent investigations.

Fooken (1985) reports the results of an investigation of the psychosocial status of four subsamples of women from the Bonn Longitudinal Study of Aging. All of the women were born between 1890 and 1905. Fooken's description of these women suggests that when they were in their 70s, the never-married women and the recently widowed were better adjusted. The women who were still married in their mid to late 70s were more preoccupied with health and physical impairment and were more concerned about perceived restrictions of social activities. They appeared to have more psychosomatic symptoms than the other groups. Never-married women in their 70s spent their time with relatives (siblings and nieces/nephews), maintained social contacts, entertained guests, and read books. Recently widowed women in their 70s were more identified with the maternal role and were more involved with their children than women in the other groups. They did not feel restricted by health problems. Long-time widowed women (usually since World War II) in their 70s had high tendencies toward psychosomatic complaints and neuroticism and reacted to health problems with depression.

West and Simons (1983) report that for elderly women being married may be a mixed blessing. In a sample of 167 women aged 65 and over living in the midwestern United States, they found that the relationship of life events to illness was much higher for married women than for those who were unmarried (single, widowed, or divorced). That is, having elevated scores on a life events schedule was much more likely to be related to experiencing illness for married elderly women than it was for unmarried elderly women.

Similarly, Morgan (1976) reports greater life satisfaction among elderly widows (after the passage of some time since bereavement) than among elderly married women. However, with statistical controls for income or occupational status, Morgan (1976) reported no relationship between marital status and life satisfaction. In Fooken's (1985) study, no such statistical controls were carried out. Since the never-married women had more education and better health than the other three groups and since the financial problems of the widows had been great in the past, such controls appear to have been needed. Similarly, in the West and Simons (1983) study, income moderated the relationship between life events and illness.

This review of the literature suggests that being widowed or living alone may be challenges or stresses with which women must cope and may lead to symptoms of depression. More tightly designed studies that control for income and occupation are necessary. Longitudinal studies that include married, divorced, and ever-single women are also necessary. Finally and most important, with rare exception (e.g., Lopata, 1969) no one has asked the bereaved woman what kind of relationship she had with her late spouse. If the relationship was poor, death may well bring relief. Differences in perceptions of the marital relationship both before and after bereavement may well account for whether widowhood and living alone constitute a stress with which elderly women must cope. Future longitudinal studies need to include questions about the availability and adequacy of intimate relations prior to as well as after the deaths of spouses, friends, relatives, and other sources of intimate relationships.

RESEARCH ON THE COPING OF AGING WOMEN

Is There an Increase in Active Coping After Midlife?

Gutmann (1985a, 1985b, Neugarten & Gutmann, 1958) proposed that active coping or active mastery increases as women who have children move into the postparental period. Cooper and Gutmann (1987) used a masculinity/femininity measure, a self-report measure of gender identity, and a measure of ego mastery based on the Thematic Apperception Test to assess Gutmann's hypothesis.

There were differences consistent with the hypothesis on the self-report measure of gender identity.

Women with children at home described themselves as more submissive and less aggressive than did women whose children had already moved away from home. These latter women described themselves as having more self-confidence, independence, assertiveness, problem-solving skills and creativity than did women with children still at home. There were no differences between the two groups of women in their descriptions of themselves as nurturant or concerned about relationships with others. Women with children no longer living at home were also more likely to be classified as expressing active mastery than were the women with children still at home.

However, Cooper and Gutmann's (1987) results were not consistent across all measures. In particular, the masculinity/femininity scale did not discriminate between the two groups of women. There are problems with using masculinity/femininity scales to study developmental changes; increased scores on some items from a scale may be offset by decreased scores on other items from the same scale. An additional problem with the Cooper and Gutmann (1987) study is the fact that the authors do not clearly discriminate the identity or role of parent from the responsibilities of parenting. If it is the diminishing of caregiving responsibilities that is related to an increase in active coping, then it is not the role of "mother" or the fact of aging that would account for differences in active and passive mastery. Instead, any person with primary responsibility for caring for another individual would be more nurturant and less aggressive than other persons not having the primary responsibility of caring for another individual.

Unfortunately, much of the research that could lead to conclusions about increases or decreases in the active coping of women in later years is distorted by the use of "masculinity" and "femininity" scales to measure specific attributes that are neither inherently "masculine" or "feminine." The use of such terms obscures the nature of the items contained, confuses the contribution of specific items to developmental differences, and conceals the reasons for age-related changes.

Spence and Helmreich (1978, 1981) prefer to use "instrumentality" or "agency" instead of "masculinity" to refer to such attributes as independence, activity, competitiveness, self-confidence, ambition, and assertiveness. Rather than by "femininity," emotional expressivity or communion are assessed by means of such characteristics as kindness, gentleness, being helpful to others, awareness of the feelings of others, affection, and compassion. However, specific and divergent attributes still remain hidden within the broader categories of instrumentality and expressivity or agency and communion. It is the individual attributes that must be assessed and studies on women who have never had children must be included in order to answer the question, "Is there an increase in active coping after midlife?"

Are Aging Women Who Integrate Agency and Communion Better Adjusted?

Bakan's (1966) proposal that the goal of life is to integrate agency and communion has been interpreted to mean that those individuals who do manage to integrate the two will be better adjusted than those who do not. Block (1984) suggested that, for women, having only the characteristics of emotional expressivity and communion is associated with being unhappy. She evaluated the "femininity" scores of 68 female subjects from the Oakland Growth Study and the Berkeley Guidance Study when they were 30 to 40 years of age. Those women who were highest on femininity and also were highly socialized were also dissatisfied, indecisive, vulnerable, and lacking in spontaneity.

Livson (1981, 1983) analyzed the data on some of these same women when they were between 40 and 50 years old. She compared those women whose adjustment to middle age was healthy with those whose adjustment was not. She found that androgynous women (i.e., having both agency and communion) were more likely to fall into the healthy category than were feminine women (communion only). Women in the latter category were more likely to be classified as having an unhealthy adjustment to midlife.

Is this pattern maintained into the older years? The participants in the Oakland Growth Study are now in their late 60s; those in the Berkeley Guidance study will turn 60 within the next several years.

Data on these women can help answer this question. In the meantime, several other studies suggest that this pattern may well endure past midlife. Holahan (1984) followed up some of the participants in Terman's study of gifted children, who were reevaluated when they were in their 30s. Holahan (1984) assessed these same individuals when they were in their 70s and found that for career-oriented women, there was a positive relationship between life satisfaction at age 70 and feelings of having attained earlier life goals by age 70. For non-career-oriented women, life satisfaction and happiness were negatively related to the attainment of earlier life goals. These women were all born around 1912. Possibly, those who were career oriented in the 1940s when they were in their 30s were fairly high on agency. The extent to which these career-oriented women also embodied attributes of femininity or communion is unknown.

There is some additional evidence that among elderly women, the integration of agency and communion is consistent with better adjustment. Frank, Towell, and Huyck (1985) found that androgynous women aged 47 to 68 scored higher on mastery and self-esteem than feminine women in the same age range. Other researchers have suggested that better adjustment is associated with more effective coping patterns (McCrae & Costa, 1986). Nonetheless, there are also several results that are not completely consistent with this interpretation.

Androgynous women (high on both masculinity and femininity) actually score lower than masculine women on measures of mastery and self-esteem (Frank, Towell, & Huyck, 1985). Part of the problem with relating masculinity, femininity, and androgyny to mastery and esteem is that items assessing mastery and esteem are included on masculinity scales. Thus, the high correlations between masculinity and these adjustment scales may be an artifact of the similarity of the items on the scales. Other measures of adjustment such as life satisfaction or the balance between positive and negative affect (McCrae & Costa, 1986) need to be used in future research.

Although our culture values masculinity and androgyny more than femininity, ample evidence exists that seeking social support is a very effective coping mechanism (Roos & Cohen, 1987). Women seek more social support than men (Butler, Giordano, & Neren,

1985) and profit more from the receipt of it than men (Holahan & Moos, 1986). Future research on aging women can seek to determine whether social support is beneficial for all elderly women and what the differences are among the following groups of women: those who cope by providing social support, those who cope by receiving social support, those who cope by integrating the provision and receipt of social support (Black, 1985). It may be that agency and communion have different relationships not only to adjustment issues but also to the efficacy of such coping mechanisms as seeking, receiving, and providing social support.

Is There an Increase in Integrity as Women Age?

Recall that for Erikson integrity involves the acceptance of one's own life and the lives of others. It also includes a detached yet active concern with life as one prepares for the end of one's own life. Does current research on coping support the Eriksonian prediction that in normal-functioning elderly women integrity predominates? In longitudinal studies, does integrity increase with age?

Folkman et al. (1987) present evidence that supports the assumption that in normal-functioning older people, coping patterns associated with integrity predominate. Analyses comparing the coping patterns of older and younger adults revealed several significant age differences. With the exception of coping responses to health-related stressors, there were no significant age-by-gender interactions. The age-by-gender interaction that occurred for coping patterns in response to health-related stressors was caused by differences in coping patterns between younger men and women with these differences evening out among the elderly. That is, in this study, the coping patterns of elderly men and women were virtually the same.

Older adults coped with stressors by accepting more responsibility for the stresses in their lives and by using more positive reappraisal than younger adults, but also by using more distancing. This latter mechanism seems to be consistent with Erikson's concept of the development of some detachment. Nonetheless, in the area of health-related stressors, older adults used more confrontive coping than younger adults. That is, for the stressor that was of most concern to them, elderly women and men used the most active coping mechanism.

McCrae (1982) provides evidence that also is consistent with Erikson's assumptions about aging. He reports significant decreases with age in six coping patterns: hostile reaction, escapist fantasy, sedation, assessing blame, wishful thinking, and indecisiveness. There was also a significant increase with age in one coping mechanism: faith.

McCrae and Costa (1986) evaluated the effectiveness of all these coping mechanisms by asking 151 adults ranging in age from 21 to 90 to indicate whether each coping technique helped solve a problem or made them feel better. Of those six coping patterns found by McCrae (1982) to decrease significantly with age, four were in the top seven least-effective coping mechanisms reported by McCrae and Costa (1986): hostile reaction, escapist fantasy, wishful thinking, indecisiveness. The one coping mechanism, faith, that increased significantly with age in McCrae's (1982) investigation was ranked as the most successful coping mechanism in McCrae and Costa's (1986) investigation. These two studies provide striking evidence that for elderly adults, coping effectiveness increases. The use of ineffective coping declines with age; the use of effective coping increases.

A problem with the Folkman et al. (1987) and McCrae (1982) studies is that the age comparisons are cross-sectional. It may be that the older subjects in their studies have always had more effective coping mechanisms or have always had more of the characteristics associated with integrity.

Mussen (1985) studied the parents of the participants in the Berkeley Guidance Study from 1968 to 1970. The average age of the women in the study was 69. Mussen found that several personality characteristics of these women when they had been in their 30s were significantly predictive of their life satisfaction in their late 60s and early 70s. In particular, self-assurance, cheerfulness, not being fatigued, satisfaction with one's lot, and mental alertness at age 30 were all significantly positively correlated with life satisfaction in the older years. Worrisomeness (a measure of anxiety) was significantly negatively correlated with life satisfaction. Thus, Mussen's (1985) study does provide some evidence that early adjustment is predictive of later adjustment. Erikson (1963) has long argued that such is the case.

Nonetheless, Olbrich (1985) presents some data from the Bonn Longitudinal Study of Aging supporting positive advances in coping patterns during the older years. In dealing with health problems, Olbrich's (1985) subjects most frequently used very active, effective coping mechanisms. Furthermore, over a ten-year period, there were significant decreases in preferred usage of two dysfunctional techniques: hope for change and active resistance. The former involves nothing other than wishful thinking. The latter is self-defeating as it includes acting in direct opposition to medical advice.

Ryff and Heincke (1983) investigated adult's self-perceptions of integrity as well as other personality characteristics at different points in the life cycle. They asked young adults, middle-aged adults, and elderly adults to rate themselves on 16 items that reflected Erikson's concept of integrity. All three groups were asked to rate themselves on the integrity items for three time points in their lives: young adulthood, middle adulthood, and older adulthood.

Adults in all three age groups rated themselves as higher on integrity in older adulthood than at any of the other three time points. Older adults thought they had more integrity at the present time than when they were 25 or 45 years old. Middle-aged adults thought that they would have more integrity in their older years than they had currently or than they had had at the age of 25. Young adults thought that they would have more integrity as older adults than they had currently or than they would have at the age of 45. Thus, adults perceive that their acceptance of their own lives is or will be higher in their elderly years.

Although recent research on coping is certainly consistent with Erikson's assumption that integrity is both related to adjustment during the younger years and also predominates among the elderly, there is one serious source of error for this conclusion. Much recent medical research (e.g., Barefoot, Dahlstrom, & Williams, 1983; Julius, Harburg, & Cottington et al., 1986; Siegman, Dembroski, & Ringel, 1987) suggests that individuals with seriously maladaptive coping mechanisms may well die prior to the older years, in part because of cardiovascular disease. Thus, age-related declines in dysfunctional coping mechanisms and increases in functional ones may be due to the fact that individuals without functional coping mechanisms and with dysfunctional ones simply do not live long enough to reach old age.

This subject is of great importance to future research on the coping of aging women because almost without exception the research on coping and early death has focused on men. Since premenopausal and postmenopausal women fall into different risk groups for cardiovascular problems and death due to myocardial infarction, it is the coping mechanisms of the higher-risk postmenopausal group that require the most urgent research attention.

Is the Perception of Stress Related to Coping in the Elderly?

Thomae's (1970, 1983) theory of aging includes the assumption that perceptions of change or stressors are more related to behavior than are objective measures of stressors or change. Olbrich and Thomae (1978) found that among elderly West Germans, objective health scores were less predictive of health-related coping behaviors than were perceptions of health-related stressors. In their study, perceptions of economic stress were better predictors of life satisfaction than were actual measures of income.

Olbrich (1985) also presents evidence that as perceived stress increased during the 1966-1976 decade for the Bonn Longitudinal subjects, so did their intensity of coping. Thus, there is ample evidence in support of the assumption that it is the perception of stresses among the elderly that predicts coping with those stresses.

SUMMARY AND CONCLUSIONS

At the beginning of this article, several questions were raised about coping patterns of aging women. The literature reviewed suggests that women's integrity and coping effectiveness increase with age. The question of whether instrumentality and agency change after midlife cannot yet be answered.

The source of, or reason for, the increase in coping effectiveness is still a matter of speculation; research to specify the sources of change needs to be conducted. Age-related coping changes in women may be related to role changes (e.g., worker to retiree, wife to widow), to responsibility changes (caregiver to noncaregiver), to changes in age-related tasks (e.g., facing death), or to younger age at death of those individuals with dysfunctional coping mechanisms.

Increases with age in coping effectiveness and integrity seem to be true for most women. These changes are not nomothetic or universal: in all studies *average* coping effectiveness or integrity increases. There are also clearly identified idiographic coping patterns among aging women; that is, there are individual differences in coping. These different coping patterns are associated with other variables: coping patterns at earlier points in the life cycle, demographic characteristics (e.g., retired versus homemaker), the integration of agency and communion.

The theories of Erik Erikson and Hans Thomae have received substantial empirical support. Integrity and coping effectiveness do increase with age. Furthermore, perceptions of stress or change do appears to be more relevant to coping efforts than objective measures of stress or change. There is also some support for the Bakan/Block proposal that the integration of agency and communion is associated with better adjustment than agency or communion alone. The evidence for Gutmann's hypothesis that active mastery increases as women age beyond midlife is less convincing.

Much research remains to be done on the coping patterns of aging women, although a fairly coherent picture emerges from existing data. In general, elderly women accept their lives as having been well spent; cope effectively; use varied coping patterns that are associated with demographic differences, personal past history, and degree of integration of agency and communion; and use coping patterns that are related to their perceptions of stress and change.

As the next several generations of women age, can we anticipate any changes in this picture of the coping patterns of aging women? It is highly unlikely that coping effectiveness or integrity will diminish among elderly women. Recall that Ryff and Heincke (1983) found that the 45-year-olds and 25-year-olds of the 1980s look forward to high integrity in their elderly years. The major difference we can anticipate in the next 30 to 50 years appears to be some shifts in the demographic variables that characterize elderly women. Consequently, we may see changes in the variables that are associated with successful aging for the average elderly woman.

Recall that Keith (1982) found differences in the variables that predicted successful aging according to whether elderly women were retirees or homemakers. As the proportion of retirees to homemakers increases among elderly women, we can anticipate a need to increase opportunities for elderly women to participate in civic and religious organizations.

What does the picture of aging women's coping patterns imply for practitioners who offer social or medical services to aging women? Thomae's (1970, 1983) theory and the data that support it suggest that in assessing the stresses faced by an elderly client, the practitioner should ask the client what she perceives the stresses in her life to be and how severe she thinks they are. Furthermore, the practitioner should ask the client how adequate she perceives her close relationships to be. It is her perception of the adequacy of these relationships that will predict future psychological adjustment, not an objective measure of adequacy.

Erikson's theory (1963, 1968, 1978) and the data that support it suggest that elderly women in general accept their lives as having been well spent. This implies that elderly women are comfortable with the way they have done things in the past. If so, then a practitioner working with an elderly client may find that the best way to help her cope with whatever problem she is facing is to ask her what she did to solve related problems in the past and whether these coping methods worked for her. If they did and there are no physical or mental changes that will impede her repeating the same coping methods, then she should be encouraged to use them again: she does know best.

REFERENCES

Aronoff, C. (1974). Old age in prime time. *Journal of Communication*, 24(4), 86-87.

Bakan, D. (1966). *The duality of human existence*. Boston: Beacon Press.

Baltes, P. B., & Nesselroade, J. R. (1973). The developmental analysis of individual differences on multiple measures. In J. R. Nesselroade & H. W. Reese (Eds.), *Life-span developmental psychology: Methodological issues* (pp. 219-251). New York: Academic Press.

Baltes, P. B., Reese, H. W., & Nesselroade, J. R. (1977). *Life-span developmental psychology: Introduction to research methods*. Monterey, CA: Brooks/ Cole.

Barefoot, J. C., Dahlstrom, W. G., & Williams, R. B., Jr. (1983). Hostility, CHD, incidence, and total mortality: A 25-year follow-up study of 255 physicians. *Psychosomatic Medicine, 45*, 59-63.

de Beauvoir, S. (1977). *Old age*. Middlesex, England: Penguin Books.

Black, M. (1985). Health and social support of older adults in the community. *Canadian Journal of Aging, 4*(4), 213-226.

Block, J. H. (1984). *Sex role identity and ego development*. San Francisco: Jossey-Bass.

Bühler, C. (1933). *Der menschliche Lebenslauf als psychologisches Problem*. Leipzig: Hirzel.

Busse, E. W. (1986). The brain and aging. *Clinical Obstetrics and Gynecology, 29*, 374-383.

Butler, T., Giordano, G., & Neren, S. (1985). Gender and sex-role attributes as predictors of utilization of natural support systems during personal stress events. *Sex Roles, 13*, 515-524.

Cooper, K. L., & Gutmann, D. L. (1987). Gender identity and ego mastery style in middle-aged, pre- and post-empty nest women. *Gerontologist, 27*, 347-352.

Erikson, E. (1963). *Childhood and society* (2nd ed.). New York: Norton.

Erikson, E. (1968). *Identity: Youth and crisis*. New York: Norton.

Erikson, E. (Ed.). (1978). *Adulthood*. New York: Norton.

Folkman, S., & Lazarus, R. S. (1980). An analysis of coping in a middle-aged community sample. *Journal of Health and Social Behavior, 21*, 219-239.

Folkman, S., Lazarus, R. S., Pimley, S., & Novacek, J. (1987). Age differences in stress and coping processes. *Psychology and Aging, 2*(2), 171-184.

Fooken, I. (1985). Old and female: Psychosocial concomitants of the aging process in a group of older women. In J. M. A. Munnichs, P. Mussen, E. Olbrich, & P. G. Coleman (Eds.), *Life-span and change in a gerontological perspective* (pp. 77-101). Orlando, FL: Academic Press.

Frank, S. J., Towell, P. A., & Huyck, M. (1985). The effects of sex-role traits on three aspects of psychological well-being in a sample of middle-aged women. *Sex Roles, 12*, 1073-1087.

Gallagher, D. E., Thompson, L. W., & Peterson, J. A. (1981-1982). Psychosocial factors affecting adaptation to bereavement in the elderly. *International Journal of Aging and Human Development, 14*(2), 79-95.

Gilligan, C. (1982). *In a different voice*. Cambridge, MA: Harvard University Press.

Gurin G., Veroff, J., & Feld, S. (1960). *Americans view their mental health*. New York: Basic Books.

Gutmann, D. L. (1985a). Beyond nurture: Developmental perspectives on the vital older woman. In J. K. Brown & V. Kerns (Eds.), *In her prime: A new view of middle-aged women* (pp. 198-211). South Hadley, MA: Bergin & Garvey.

Gutmann, D. L. (1985b). The parental imperative revisited. In J. Meacham (Ed.), *Family and individual development* (pp. 31-60). Basel: Karger.

Haan, N. (1977). *Coping and defending*. New York: Academic Press.

Heller, K., & Mansbach, W. E. (1984). The multifaceted nature of social support in a community sample of elderly women. *Journal of Social Issues*, *40*(4), 99-112.

Henderson, A. S., Scott, R., & Kay, D. W. (1986). The elderly who live alone: Their mental health and social relationships. *Australian and New Zealand Journal of Psychiatry*, *20*, 202-209.

Holahan, C. J., & Moos, R. H. (1986). Personality, coping, and family resources in stress resistance: A longitudinal analysis. *Journal of Personality and Social Psychology*, *51*, 389-395.

Holahan, C. K. (1984). Work and family goal orientations in early adulthood and satisfaction in aging: The Terman men and women. *Gerontologist*, *24*, 301.

Hooyman, N., & Cohen, H. J. (1986). Medical problems associated with aging. *Clinical Obstetrics and Gynecology*, *29*, 353-373.

House, J. S., & Robbins, C. (1983). Age, psychosocial stress, and health. In M. W. Riley, B. B. Hess, & K. Bond (Eds.), *Aging in society: Selected reviews of recent research* (pp. 175-197). Hillsdale, NJ: Erlbaum.

Julius, M., Harburg, E., Cottington, E. M., Johnson, E. H. (1986). Anger-coping types, blood pressure, and all-cause mortality: A follow-up in Tecumseh, Michigan (1971-1983). *American Journal of Epidemiology*, *124*, 220-233.

Keith, P. M. (1982). Working women versus homemakers: Retirement resources and correlates of well-being. In M. Szinovacz (Ed.), *Women's retirement: Policy implications of recent research* (pp. 77-91). Beverly Hills, CA: Sage.

Lazarus, R. S., & Folkman, S. (1984). *Stress, appraisal, and coping*. New York: Springer.

Livson, F. B. (1981). Paths to psychological health in the middle years: Sex differences. In D. Eichorn, J. Claussen, N. Haan, M. Honzick, & P. Mussen (Eds.), *Present and past in middle life* (pp. 47-98). New York: Academic Press.

Livson, F. B. (1983). Gender identity: A life span view of sex role development. In R. Weg (Ed.), *Aging: An international annual (Vol 1). Sexuality in the later years: Roles and behavior* (pp. 105-124). Menlo Park, CA: Addison-Wesley.

Livson, N. (1973). Developmental dimensions of personality: A life-span formulation. In P. B. Baltes & K. W. Schaie (Eds.), *Life-span developmental psychology: Personality and socialization* (pp. 97-122). New York: Academic Press.

Lopata, H. Z. (1969). Loneliness: Forms and components. *Social Problems*, *17*, 248-262.

Lopata, H. Z. (1980). The widowed family member. In N. Datan & N. Lohmann (Eds.), *Transitions of aging* (pp. 93-118). New York: Academic Press.

Lowenthal, M. F., & Haven, C. (1968). Interaction and adaption: Intimacy as a critical variable. *American Sociological Review*, *33*, 20-30.

Lund, D. A., Caserta, M. S., & Dimond, M. F. (1986). Gender differences through two years of bereavement among the elderly. *Gerontologist*, *26*, 314-320.

McCrae, R. R. (1982). Age differences in the use of coping mechanisms. *Journal of Gerontology*, *37*, 454-460.

McCrae, R. R. , & Costa, P. (1986). Personality, coping, and coping effectiveness in an adult sample. *Journal of Personality, 54*, 385-405.

Morgan, L. A. (1976). A reexamination of widowhood and morale. *Journal of Gerontology, 31*, 687-695.

Munnichs, J. M. A., & Olbrich, E. (1985). Life-span and change in a gerontological perspective: An outline. In J. M. A. Munnichs, P. Mussen, E. Olbrich, & P. G. Coleman (Eds.), *Life-span and change in a gerontological perspective* (pp. 3-11). Orlando, FL: Academic Press.

Mussen, P. (1985). Early adult antecedents of life satisfaction at age 70. In J. M. A. Munnichs, P. Mussen, E. Olbrich, P. G. Coleman (Eds.), *Life-span and change in a gerontological perspective* (pp. 45-61). Orlando, FL: Academic Press.

Neugarten, B. L., & Gutmann, D. L. (1958). Age-sex roles and personality in middle age: A thematic apperception study. *Psychological Monographs, 72* (No. 470).

Olbrich, E. (1985). Coping and development in the later years: A process-oriented approach to personality development. In J. M. A. Munnichs, P. Mussen, E. Olbrich, P. G. Coleman (Eds.), *Life-span and change in a gerontological perspective* (pp. 133-159). Orlando, FL: Academic Press.

Olbrich, E., & Thomae, H. (1978). Empirical findings to a cognitive theory of aging. *International Journal of Behavioral Development, 1*, 67-84.

Ostrow, A. C. (1980). Physical activity as it relates to the health of the aged. In N. Datan & N. Lohmann (Eds.), *Transitions of aging* (pp. 41-56). New York: Academic Press.

Riddick, C. C. (1982). Life satisfaction among aging women: A causal model. In M. Szinovacz (Ed.), *Women's retirement: Policy implications of recent research* (pp. 45-59). Beverly Hills, CA: Sage.

Riley, M. W., & Bond, K. (1983). Beyond ageism: Postponing the onset of disability. In M. W. Riley, B. B. Hess, & K. Bond (Eds.), *Aging in society: Selected reviews of recent research* (pp. 243-252). Hillsdale, NJ: Erlbaum.

Roos, P. E., & Cohen, L. H. (1987). Sex roles and social support as moderators of life stress adjustment. *Journal of Personality and Social Psychology, 52*, 576-585.

Ryff, C. D., & Heincke, S. G. (1983). Subjective organization of personality in adulthood and aging. *Journal of Personality and Social Psychology, 44*, 807-816.

Schonfield, D. (1982). Who is stereotyping whom and why? *Gerontologist, 22*, 267-272.

Siegman, A. W., Dembroski, T. M., Ringel, N. (1987). Components of hostility and the severity of coronary artery disease. *Psychosomatic Medicine, 49*, 127-135.

Signorelli, N. (1983). Health, prevention and television: Images of the elderly and perceptions of social reality. In S. Simson, L. B. Wilson, J. Hermalin, & R. Hess (Eds.), *Aging and prevention: New approaches for preventing health and mental health problems in older adults* (pp. 97-117) New York: Haworth Press.

Smith, T. W., & Anderson, N. B. (1986). Models of personality and disease: An interactional approach to Type A behavior and cardiovascular risk. *Journal of Personality and Social Psychology, 50,* 1166-1173.

Spence, J. T., & Helmreich, R. (1978). *Masculinity and femininity: Their psychological dimensions, correlates and antecedents.* Austin: University of Texas Press.

Spence, J. T., & Helmreich, R. L. (1981). Androgyny versus gender schema: A comment on Bem's gender schema theory. *Psychological Review, 88,* 365-368.

Szinovacz, M. (1982). Introduction: Research on women's retirement. In M. Szinovacz (Ed.), *Women's retirement: Policy implications of recent research* (pp. 13-21). Beverly Hills, CA: Sage.

Thomae, H. (1959). Entwicklungsbegriff und Entwicklungstheorie. In H. Thomae (Ed.), *Handbuch der Psychologie, B. 3, Entwicklungspsychologie* (2nd ed.). Gottingen: Verlag fur Psychologie.

Thomae, H. (1970). Theory of aging and cognitive theory of personality. *Human Development, 13,* 1-16.

Thomae, H. (1983). *Alternsstile und Altersschicksale: Ein Beitrag zur Differentiellen Gerontologie.* Bern: Huber.

Thomae, H., & Simons, H. (1967). Formen der Reaktion auf Belastungssituationen im Alter. *Zeitschrift fur experimentelle und angewandte Psychologie, 4,* 290-312.

Trofatter, K. F. (1986). Immune responses and aging. *Clinical Obstetrics and Gynecology, 29,* 384-396.

Verbrugge, L. M. (1983). Women and men: Mortality and health of older people. In M. W. Riley, B. B. Hess, & K. Bond (Eds.), *Aging in society: Selected reviews of recent research* (pp. 139-174). Hillsdale, NJ: Erlbaum.

Walsh, R. P., & Connor, C. L. (1979). Old men and young women: How objectively are their skills assessed? *Journal of Gerontology, 34,* 561-568.

West, G. E., & Simons, R. L. (1983). Sex differences in stress, coping resources, and illness among the elderly. *Research on Aging, 5,* 235-268.

Women and Aging:
A Clinical Social Work Perspective

Toba Schwaber Kerson, DSW, PhD

Clinical social workers most often help older women because the autonomy of the women or those whom they care for has been threatened through poverty, physical or mental frailty, crushing social responsibility, or loss. The high value that social work places on self-worth, self-determination, and individual entitlement to dignity and security, clinical social work's focus on social role and the relationship of the individual to society, and the fact that the majority of clinical social workers are women who are aging place aging women high on the clinical social work agenda (Monk, 1981).

"The world of the aged is increasingly a society of old women" (Hess, 1980, p. 42). Elderly women are poorer than men. The poverty rate among elderly women living alone is approximately 30% (Lewis, 1987). Unfortunately, "although the vast majority of clients seen by social workers are women, research rarely addresses issues unique to female clients" (Quam & Austin, 1984, p. 360). In articles about women's issues published in eight social work journals from 1970 to 1981, only 1.7% focused on aging and widowhood (Quam & Austin, 1984). Because of the dearth of materials dealing exclusively with issues of women and aging, the sources for this article were clinical informants, books, and articles describing programs, and studies that included women and aging.

In general, clinical social work helps aging women to manage the physical and psychological realities of aging. Dual overarching goals, therefore, are women's sense of empowerment and acceptance of limitations (Milinsky, 1987). Although only a small por-

Toba Schwaber Kerson is Professor, Graduate School of Social Work and Social Research, Bryn Mawr College, 300 Airdale Road, Bryn Mawr, PA 19010.

123

tion of social work and aging programming, research, and literature focuses purely on women, the overwhelming majority of aging clients are women. Women live longer and are more likely to require social work intervention as a result of poverty, social, or physical need. For example, in 1984, 15% of women 65 and over were living in poverty as opposed to 8.7% of men of the same age. Almost one-fourth of women of Spanish origin and more than one-third of black women 65 and over lived in poverty (U.S. Bureau of the Census, 1985).

In terms of physical need, the incidence of many devasting chronic illnesses increases dramatically in the elderly (Kerson, 1985). Almost half of people 65 and over experienced some limitation of activity because of a chronic condition. The percentage rises for those 85 and over. In addition, it is thought that between 18% and 25% of older people have significant mental health symptoms (Cohen, 1980).

> The vulnerability of older women to mental health problems results not from longevity per se but from the fact that longevity can cause a woman to outlast her personal financial resources and to overwhelm current prevention, treatment and rehabilitation capabilities in the community. (Lewis, 1987, p. 11)

In addition, possibly because it is sex linked and certainly because incidence increases with longevity, Alzheimer's disease is more frequently found in women. Also, women are more susceptible to drug-induced dementia (Lewis, 1987).

Clinical social work for aging women focuses on two different stages in the life span of women: middle age and old age. The problems of each group are distinctive but hardly discrete. In middle age, women often seek the help of social workers because they are widows, displaced homemakers, or caregivers to elderly parents as well as children. Sometimes, they wish to understand the effects of menopause or redefine their relationship with parents (Shaw, 1987). In old age, problems worsen if women's economic situations become perilous and as physical and/or mental deterioration increase. Role transitions and losses that may occur in middle age through death or divorce of a spouse often escalate dramatically in old age.

Basically, clinical social work programs can be categorized as oriented towards well or frail elders. The goal of the first group is to support and restore the well in order to maintain independence. Examples are activities designed to foster employability and crisis intervention programs that help the recently widowed or divorced to confront their losses and, with support, move forward in their lives. The goal of the second category is to help the physically and/or mentally debilitated to avoid institutionalization if possible, to retain maximal independence, and to redefine autonomy in ways that reflect an adult status that may be dependent but is not diminished. Examples are programs to maintain the frail elderly at home or autonomy-enhancing activities in nursing homes. Such programs hope to maintain people at their present level of functioning as long as possible to forestall a more dependent or sequestered state.

Specific clinical services to aging women are available in a broad range of agencies and institutions from large public departments of health and human services offering public assistance, Medicaid, and protective services to small private family agencies providing individual crisis intervention, support services, mutual aid groups, and socialization activities. Many programs are designed to reach as many of the elderly as possible. Others are designed specifically for women, or minority populations such as gay and lesbian elderly, or the disabled elderly. Clinical social work services are available to aging women throughout the spectrum of long-term care in projects to maintain the frail elderly at home, hospitals, rehabilitation centers, home care agencies, nursing homes, and hospices (Kerson, 1988). In these organizations, clinical social workers act as program planners and managers, outreach workers and marketers, brokers of concrete services, counselors, psychotherapists, case managers, family surrogates, and advocates.

A BRIEF HISTORY OF CLINICAL SOCIAL WORK IN AGING

The spectrum of services available to aging women has increased since the birth of social work around the beginning of the twentieth century. Primarily, before the Great Depression, there was some attempt to address the economic insecurity of the elderly (Achenbaum, 1983). In the 1920s, because of the manner in which their problems were defined, the needs of the elderly were largely ignored by social caseworkers who embraced psychoanalytic theory. "The elderly were not seen as capable of this new view of self-mastery perpetuated by the social work profession. The spirit of charity still remained the root of social service for the elderly" (Dunkle, 1983, p. 11). The Great Depression and the Social Security Act of 1935 accelerated federal funding for the elderly. At that time, assistance to the needy was redefined as a public obligation. The elderly were most typically clients of the new public agencies that managed income problems rather than the older voluntary agencies that addressed psychological troubles (Dunkle, 1983).

The most dramatic increase in social welfare programs for the elderly occurred in the 60s and early 70s with the passage of the Older American's Act (1965), Medicare (1966), and Supplemental Security income (1972). Each piece of legislation has expanded opportunities for social programs and clinical social work services for the elderly. Basically, "community services are seen as ways to enhance the independent living of the elderly, in turn preventing or delaying institutionalization" (Stone, 1986, p. 1). In 1984, 26 million people over 65 in the United States were living outside institutions. Only 22% had used community services (primarily senior centers) during the preceding year; 1% used homemakers; 3% visiting nurses; and 2% home health aides. All services were utilized to a greater extent by women than men. Use tends to increase with age, functional limitation, and for those who live alone (Stone, 1986).

Perhaps partly in response to increased public interest in problems of the elderly and opportunities for clinical social work, in 1980, the Council on Social Work Education identified "Services to the Aged" as a practicum field of practice. "Social workers may not have designed the social policy that has so dramatically improved the economic plight of some elderly, but they have been the agents responsible for implementing these services" (Dunkle, 1983). Thus, gerontological social work has become an important area of concentration for social work practitioners.

CLINICAL SOCIAL WORK WITH WOMEN IN MIDDLE YEARS

Services to women in middle years, the years from 45 to 65, focus primarily on widows, displaced homemakers, and caregivers. Actually, in the middle years, role transition rather than age is the meaningful marker. Life events that characterize the middle part of the life span are having children leave home, reaching an occupational plateau, menopause, grandparenthood, retirement, the onset of chronic illness, having to care for aged parents and widowhood. Clinical interventions range from employment strategies to individual counseling to mutual-aid groups. It is thought that interventions that promote independence for women in middle years will prevent or reduce dependency in later years (Blau, Rogers, & Stephens, 1979).

The authors of *Clinical Practice with Women in Their Middle Years* say that the goal of clinical practice with middle-aged women is to help them resolve developmental conflicts. "The aims of clinical practice are accomplished by increasing the clients' awareness of such issues, helping them integrate these conflicting urges, encouraging behavior change, and helping women cope with the consequences of these changes" (Sands & Richardson, 1983, p. 40). In middle age, women reassess interpersonal relationships with spouse, children, parents, and other significant people in their lives. Because particular signs of aging escalate during middle age, women take particular note of gray hair, wrinkles, and weight gain. They anticipate then experience menopause, reassess and, perhaps, redefine sexuality, work, and achievement (Kobosa-Munro, 1977). Also, "during midlife, many women struggle to realize a long-standing ambition" (Sands & Richardson, 1986, p. 39).

Sometimes, the importance of work in a woman's life is reaffirmed. In many situations, women who have stayed out of the workforce return to school or to the workplace. In other situations, women leave the workforce shifting their orientation toward intimacy and affiliation. One study of female retirees reports that women fare better who want to retire despite physical capacity (Levy, 1980-81). Another reports that women who continue to work beyond the usual retirement age do so out of the need to support themselves or others, because they are more highly educated and because of a continued need in the workplace (Kaplan & Cabral, 1980).

Clinical Practice with Employed Women describes ways to focus on work-related problems of women by screening for increased stress due to multiple role responsibilities (Freeman, Logan, & McCoy, 1987, p. 415). The following four overlapping high-risk status profiles are described:

1. single women (divorced, widowed, never married) living alone or with few external supports whose children have not been taught age-appropriate personal and household skills and who do not have models for handling multiple roles including work
2. married women whose husbands do not want them to work, who have difficulty delegating responsibilities, whose family do not share responsibilities, and who do not have models or external supports for handling multiple roles
3. women who do not have job skills, training, or experience, with low-paying, unrewarding and difficult jobs, who are vulnerable to sexual and racial harassment and discrimination, and who do not have support at work or elsewhere for coping with these work conditions
4. women who have recently returned to work after an absence of five or more years (especially middle-aged women who must shift to an inner-directed frame of reference), whose husbands are unemployed, who are beginning new training or educational experience, and who do not have role models or external supports for coping with transitions.

Citing role and problem-solving theory, the article advocates use of a social worker-client contract that emphasizes the client's active participation in the process and the use of small groups for normalizing role transitions and teaching problem-solving techniques. Interventions include problem-focused exercises, discussions, role playing, and homework assignments. Often, too, workers serve as role models. One ongoing exercise, the Situations-Options-Consequences-Solutions exercise (SOCS), uses concrete examples to teach problem-solving techniques. As a group, members also often decide to attend self-help activities such as weight-reduction programs for additional mutual support.

In *A Social Work Response to the Middle-Aged Housewife,* Klass and Redfern (1977) describe "Three-To-Get Ready" classes whose goal was affirmation and positive self-worth for the middle-aged housewife. Using educational-group experiences, the classes provided an opportunity for women to take psychological tests, develop self-awareness, receive help with resume preparation, analyze specific job skills, and utilize information about vocational, educational, and volunteer opportunities. Classes helped women to be more self-confident and aware of themselves and options available for work, volunteer, and leisure activities. Of the 110 women interviewed after participating in the program, 51% were employed, 60% were involved in some sort of educational experience, a few women began a new volunteer commitment and many discontinued serving in a voluntary capacity.

Another study of clinical social work for middle-aged women "explores the dynamic link between parental decline and the emergence of disturbing symptoms in adult children" (Shaw, 1987). Here, several clinical interventions help clients with the separation issues that are activated by parental decline by restructuring the relationship between adult child and parent. The first recommends abolishing the hierarchical boundaries between parent and child. Thus, adult children learn to relate to parents as if they are equals rather than as child to parent. In the second, the goal is the attainment of filial maturity sot hat in middle age the adult can perceive the parent as the person she was before the child was born. Emphasis is on the interactional process, and here, in the interaction between parent and adult child, development continues. Thus, treatment can be confined to the adult child but can also involve parents and siblings.

The third approach attempts to bridge the gap between parent and child by attacking old rules that no longer apply and establishing a mutually positive atmosphere. The fourth uses family-of-origin work to help adult children discontinue viewing their parents as they did when they were small children. Quoting Framo, the article notes, "When it comes to dealing with parents, the residuals of those early affects of love, hate, shame, and awe almost never disappear" (Shaw, 1987, p. 412).

WIDOWS AND DISPLACED HOMEMAKERS

Widowhood involves many kinds of losses that are addressed by clinical social work. Widowhood itself substantially increases the risk of being poor (Burkhauser, Holden, & Myers, 1985). Limited economic resources are thought to be a key factor in the decline of well-being in widowhood (Arens, 1982-83). It has also been demonstrated that widowhood results in an immediate decrease in perceived health, but that long-term consequences to health are minimal (Ferraro, 1985-86).

Social isolation often does not increase immediately after the death of a spouse but it does increase five or more years later (Ferraro, 1984). Although more women than ever work, they continue to see the man as the prime breadwinner, and the family obligation of caring for home and small children perpetuates the dependency (Lopata & Brehm, 1986). Most women who did not work before widowhood do not work after widowhood (Morgan, 1980).

Widows can be seen as part of a larger group of middle-aged women referred to as displaced homemakers. The term "displaced homemaker" refers to any individual between 35 and 64 years of age who (1) has worked in the home for a substantial number of years providing unpaid household services for family members; (2) is not gainfully employed; (3) has had, or would have, difficulty in securing employment; and (4) has been dependent on the income of another family member but is no longer supported by such income because of separation, death, or divorce (Benokraitis, 1987, p. 76). Such women are usually ineligible for other assistance programs because they have never worked, are too young for old-age benefits, and do not qualify for AFDC because their children are grown.

Many educational programs like the Three-To-Get-Ready program have been established to help women who find themselves without support. One article, "Older Women and Reentry Problems: The Case for Displaced Homemakers," examines what happens to displaced homemakers after they have been identified, counseled, trained, and sent out into the employment world (Benokraitis, 1987). The article describes the employment processes and problems of displaced homemakers and why they exist. It reports three employment problems for displaced homemakers: low self-esteem and lack of confidence, health problems, and unrealistic job aspirations.

Often, program have prepared women for jobs without being sure that there were jobs available in the area. Many women continue to be afraid of testing and interviews. Once they have been out in the work world, many women feel they need training in specific skills like assertiveness and stress management. Basically, the author suggests that training centers know the current needs of the job market before training and that there be more emphasis on how general job training and specific skills can be applied to a variety of jobs. Overall, she says that overcoming employment problems on a system level is considerably more difficult than at the individual or group level. All women must "continue to lobby, sue if necessary and seek positions through which women can enforce existing anti-discrimination laws" (Benokraitis, 1987, p. 91).

CAREGIVERS

Caregiving elderly parents and spouse is usually a family function frought with conflict (Brody, 1981, 1985; Brody et al., 1984). "Family, is in most cases a euphemism for closest female relative" (Simmons, 1985, p. 10). Adult children of the aged are the "sandwich generation," squeezed and stressed by the needs of both children and parents (Brody, 1983). At this point in the life span, the giving of resources and service for outweighs receiving or exchanging them (Miller, 1981). "Wives, daughters, daughter-in-laws and other female relatives make up 72% of the caregivers of the frail elderly" (Glasse, 1987, p. 14). Many women derive satisfaction and legitimacy from the role but pay a high price (Simon, 1986). Often, women forfeit other activities including paid, outside work and are subject to increased stress and health problems (Lewis, 1987, p. 10; Simon, 1987, p. 180; Simon, 1986). Although their average age is 57, many caregivers are old and/or chronically ill themselves.

The goal of many caregiving programs and studies is to prevent institutionalization of the elderly client. Often, the conclusions describe the great toll taken by the caregivers in achieving the goal of keeping a relative at home (Enright & Friss, 1987; Tobin & Kulys, 1981). Much of the clinical work reported in this section on middle age can be summerized by saying that middle age is a time spent in preparing for old age. If middle age is the time for women to prepare for old age, is care for elderly relatives reasonable preparation? (Naysmith, 1981) This question is not only individual or clinical but societal. What are "the rights and obligations of family and informal support systems compared with the obligations of government and voluntary agencies?" (Morris, 1980)

In one study, elderly wives of elderly severely chronically ill or disabled men reported problems of isolation, loneliness, economic hardship, and role overload (Fengler & Goodrich, 1979). Those with low morale as compared with the rest of the group were poorer, could rely less on their husbands for companionship, and had less social supports.

Another report of family caregivers and dementia demonstrated that the presence of a family caregiver was a major factor in preventing institutionalization but that the caregiver felt a greater burden when the patient's mental status was poor as a result of the disease progression or when the emotional relationship between the caregiver and the patient had not been close (Pratt, Schmall, & Wright, 1986). Almost 80% of the caregivers felt that caregiving had negatively effected their health. Institutionalization generally meant guilt and a sense of personal failure. The authors of this paper describe several interventions that build on already-existing coping strategies: educational and other programs that would be designed to increase the caregiver's confidence in problem solving, to help caregivers redefine difficult situations, and to teach caregivers how to marshal social support (Pratt, Schmall, & Wright, 1986, p. 122).

Another article describes the Natural Supports Program of the Community Service Society of New York, which assists family members in caring for their elderly relatives through a combination of counseling and support services (Getzel, 1981, 1982). Here, using an extended task-centered approach to counseling, social workers are available to caregivers as needed. "All efforts are made to avoid the intrusion of the social worker's judgments about the caregiver's role. . . .The focus remains the support of caregiving activity by kin as a developmental task of significant personal meaning and of societal importance" (Getzel, 1981, p. 208). Awareness of the meaning of caregiving is explored, the older person is involved in all decisions, a contract and ongoing counseling activity are used if possible, and service is seen as a tool to be used by the caregiver in maintaining activities. In addition, problem-solving is used with the primary caregiver to solve family tensions (Brody et al., 1984).

In the case a marital couple in which a spouse is profoundly impaired, it becomes important to help "the caregiving spouse with the multifarious consequences of his or her obligations" (Getzel, 1982, p. 518). Assisting aging couples in crisis involves a sequence of issues: (1) the emergence of the spouse caregiving crisis, (2) the presentation of the idealized historical marital interaction, (3) confronting interactional behaviors, spousal regrets and behavioral accommodation, (4) facing human finitude and biological uncertainty, and (5) recognition and resignation. Again, the social worker recognizes and supports the caregiver.

SUPPORT AND MUTUAL AID

Many of the programs and interventions described for middle-aged and elderly women focus on support and mutual aid (Lieberman, 1985). Silverman describes sources of help for midlife women as (1) formal, reciprocal help from professionals, (2) informal help from those who have successfully coped (Silverman, 1979). The emphasis is on mutuality and interdependence. "Policy to aid mutual help groups should be directed toward facilitating the exchange of information, the key to the program's success" (Silverman, 1979, p. 15).

Obviously, supportive, primary-group relationships such as contact with relatives, friends and associates and children are vital to older women, although findings vary as to the importance of each group (Beckman, 1981; Goldberg, Kantrow, & Kramer, 1986; Longino & Lipman, 1982). One study reports that aged parents remained the most improtant support for new widows (Bankoff, 1983), and another that mother-daughter relationships in later life are characterized by mutuality, interdependence, and positive connection (Bromberg, 1983).

One successful program described in the literature is the Widow to Widow Program first begun as a research and demonstration project and now existing in many communities across the country. Run by widowed volunteers, this program helps women reach out in friendship to new widows. In using volunteers in the same predicament, this program avoids the stigma of having to receive help without being able to repay by including the opportunity to reciprocate (Silverman, 1986; Silverman & Cooperband, 1984). In a variation of this program, a social service agency serving the Jewish community in a neighborhood in transition offered help to all new widows regardless of religion. Almost all of the 93 women were working-class housewives. Basically, for this version of the program, a social worker contacted all of the widows. More than half allowed an intensive first contact. More than one-third continued contact in which the social worker helped with exploration of feelings, support and ventilation, relocation, outreach information about agency services, and referral to other agencies.

Effective outreach is vital in services such as these. Programs must be accessible, provide diverse activities to appeal to a range of interests and capacities, and employ social workers who are caring, empathic, and nonjudgmental (Foley, 1976).

ELDERLY WOMEN

Services to elderly women can be seen as part of a natural progression. As with midlife women, poverty, poor mental or physical health, and a lack of natural supports sometimes mean greater need for clinical social work intervention. For example, while midlife women may be confronting divorce, their mothers may need support because of the negative effects of the divorce for them (Johnson, 1981). Just as was stated in the secion on midlife woman, often the caregiver needs as much or more clinical social work as the identified client or patient.

Programs for elderly women focus on maintaining independence often in the face of increasing frailty. Women generally value independence and sometimes see themselves as problems when they must depend on other people (Dudley, 1983). In the next sections, a discussion of clinical practice with older women will be followed by a description of community programs including home care, foster care, long-term case management, relocation services, and nursing home services.

CLINICAL PRACTICE WITH OLDER WOMEN

Clinical services to elderly women are also based on functional ability. Innovative programs for the well elderly encompass a wide range of services. For example, the Supportive Older Women's Network (SOWN) helps older women cope with their specialized aging concerns through initiation and facilitation of support groups (SOWN, n.d.). The groups meet weekly for an hour and a half in varied locations such as apartment buildings, senior centers, and churches and synagogues to discuss topics such as myths of aging, self-image, widowhood, stress reduction, assertiveness training, coping with loss and changing relationships with family members. A SOWN staff member facilitates the first eight meetings after which many groups choose to become a permanent support entity. After the completion of the eight-week program, SOWN offers leadership training seminars and provides ongoing consultation.

Another example of innovative service to the elderly is SAGE (Senior Action in a Gay Environment), which serves more than 500 older gay men and women each month through a myriad of programs in which recipients of service and volunteers are often interchangeable. SAGE sponsors special programs for women such as "women's day at the drop-in" in which one is invited to have coffee and conversation with some of the most interesting women in town, free women's groups including an age 40-49 rap, 40 + rap, 50 + rap, and women's assertiveness training (SAGE, 1984).

One final example of creative programming is Seniors Teaching Seniors, a program that taught group leadership and teaching skills to active, well, retired elderly people (Kaye, Monk, & Stuen, 1983; Kaye, Stuen, & Monk, 1985). Three-quarters of the participants were women. The eight-week module emphasized pedagogical skills acquisition, group dynamics, the psychosocial condition of aging and special-interest instruction. The program acted as a confidence builder for beginners and a skill builder for those with some teaching experience. Some of the 150 participants successfully used these skills to teach in their local neighborhoods. Retired Faculty Linkage, a related project, contacted a group of Columbia University retirees to ask if they might be interested in consulting, advising, and lecturing at community organizations. As a result, a number of retiree-community program linkages were made (Stuen & Kaye, 1985).

"In discussing clinical practice with older women, it must be noted that, commonly, elderly people are not thought to be amenable to psychotherapy. All are considered difficult or impossible to treat" (Lewis, 1987, p. 10). Medicare pays no more than $250 a year for psychotherapy and only when it is conducted by a physician. Many clinicians and programs view the primary needs of the elderly as concrete services such as transportation, legal aid, and programs involving in-home services (Keith, 1978). This view is not universally shared. "Perhaps the most neglected late life issue is the simple loneliness that stems from many of the oldest, frailist women outliving their mates, friends, older family members and even their own children, particularly male children" (Lewis, 1987, p. 10).

Some clinical social work services have been directed specifically to psychological issues of aging. For example, using a developmental model, one group treatment program counteracted defensive behavior in depressed, isolated elderly people who were living independently. The clinician who led the group thinks that "people requesting concrete help are unaware that their unmet emotional needs are frequently the basis for these requests" (Milinsky, 1987, p. 174). Using excellent outreach skills, the social worker set the group meeting time, duration, and place. Initial themes were concerned with "differences and similarities," "not getting," and "disappointed expectations." "Members openly shared their feelings about isolation and loneliness without the usual embarrassment found in younger groups when dealing with this topic" (Milinsky, 1987, p. 176). The group encouraged members to think positively, live in the present, and make an effort. Early in the life of the group, three members purchased hearing aids to wear to the sessions. Hearing what was being said and being able to respond became very important to each member. Using the group, members developed new coping strategies and regained feelings of autonomy.

Another clinician discussed the diagnostic and therapeutic value of reminiscence. Reminiscence can be used in the service of denial and to help maintain self-esteem and allay anxiety caused by physical and intellectual deterioration. In addition, reminiscence can provide material for life review that may help in personality reorganization and life acceptance and that can further interaction. It can help someone cope with the depression and grief that accompany loss (Kaminsky, 1978). Further, writing and reminiscing can help people to reconstruct, to transmit life experiences, to fuse and integrate, to become more observant, and to communicate with others (Kaminsky, 1985).

Most important, reminiscence provides ways for women to rediscover self-worth. Thinking about times when they felt more powerful and in charge and then redefining those traits for the present can effectively empower women to substitute new roles for ones that seemed more satisfying in the past. Reminiscing allows a woman to recognize the strength and capacity she demonstrated in the past and then adapt that strength to current possibilities. Thus, oral and written reminiscence are powerful means of expression.

Such clinical work is not restricted to those living outside of institutions. In another example, a group in the Detroit Jewish Home for Aged that was composed primarily of women met weekly for 20 weeks to discuss the meaning of being old (Harris, 1988). In fact, the participants named their group the "Being Old" group. Significant outcomes included a new camaraderie and support among members that carried beyond the group, and a "Positive Aspects of Aging" bulletin board for the lobby of the home. Most important, members who were originally resistant to sharing feelings examined, worked through, and came to terms with their feelings about being old.

Social work services have also been developed for elderly victims of abuse and rape. Drawing from a series of case studies, Rathbone-McCuan (1982) lists the following characteristics of victims of abuse: female; 65 or older; functionally dependent because of inadequate resources or functional limitations; history of alcoholism, retardation or psychiatric illness for either the caregiver or elderly person; history of inter or intragenerational conflict; and previous history of related incidents.

Authors in this area suggest that following the assessment, relationship interventions must be offered to the abused person after other crisis help such as food, shelter, clothing, medical care, in-home services, and transportation have been provided. It is important to determine precipitating factors, the consequences of abusive behavior, and the abuser's level of emotional anger and self-control and, then, to focus intervention on changing the environment and/or helping the abuser control anger. Finally, the clinician must determine the association of the abusive behavior with other problems (Rathbone-McCuan, 1984). In the case of rape, the clinician must help the victim make changes in the environment of her victimization, to move beyond self-blame and inadequacy, realize she is a unique individual and has the right to help, derive assistance that goes beyond the crisis, and participate in her own problem solving. Task-centered and behavior interventions are favored (Davis & Brody, 1979; Hooyman, Rathbone-McCuan, & Klingbeil, 1982; Rathbone-McCuan & Hashimi, 1982).

Generally, clinical social work for elderly women follows a support, task-centered, or case-management model of service. For example, *Social Work with the Aged and Their Families* is concerned with the elderly person's functioning within the family system (Greene, 1986). The family is seen as a developmental unit, a social system, and a set of reciprocal roles. Here, functional rather than actual age is the marker. Functioning is, of course, the prime divider between the independent elderly with good health and enough money and the dependent elderly with declining health, dementia, and/or very limited resources. Attitude and control of life also are important.

MAINTAINING THE FRAIL ELDERLY IN THE COMMUNITY

Clinical social workers work with the frail elderly in the community and in institutions. In the community, services are provided to the frail elderly through home care, foster home care, long-term case management, and adult day care. Often, these programs have been developed in order to contain costs and prevent institutional-ization. Although the primary service of home care is nursing, so-cial workers provide consultation and direct services such as mobi-lizing support networks, expediting protective service referrals, securing financial benefits, and coordinating long-term care plans (Lotz, DuChainey, & Kerson, 1988).

Foster care programs, which are still rare, have been shown to maintain or improve mental status and activities of daily living scores of participants, to result in better nursing outcomes, and to be more likely to have clients get out of the house than nursing homes. However, in those communities without adequate transpor-tation and social activities for the elderly, social isolation can be more of a problem in foster care than in a nursing home (Oktay & Volland, 1987).

Long-term case management provides a continuum of care in-cluding health and social services over an extended period of time to functionally impaired, chronically ill persons. The social worker acting as case manager uses the relationship with her client as a conduit for implementing a continuum of services that promote the client's functional ability and enhance her quality of life (Kirwin, in press). Thus, after helping the client to regain strength through al-lowing others to contribute to her care, the social worker works toward having the client regain independence in self-care and then to retain this independence with support.

In adult daycare, use of social services, nursing, medical, and rehabilitation services by clients with psychosocial or physical limi-tations maximizes functioning and allows continued community liv-ing (Goldstein, 1983). Comprehensive adult day care includes pro-gramming for at least five or six hours a day and assistance for participants in managing their lives when the center is not open. Opportunities for socialization, mutual aid, problem solving, health and nutrition services, transportation, and family support services are part of the day care experience (Kirwin, 1986). Often, multi-impaired clients who use daycare services do not seek other support services (Kirwin, 1988).

When an individual can no longer live independently, a clinical social worker can expedite relocation. Moving, especially moving from one's own home to a nursing home, can be traumatic (Pollack,

1981). Studies recommend that each client be incorporated fully in the process, visit several homes from which she can choose, and be assisted throughout the process by an available social worker acting as relocation counselor (Kaplan & Cabral, 1980).

SERVICES IN NURSING HOMES

Clinical services in nursing homes are designed to promote independence and interaction with peers, family, and friends. Many clinical services focus on the prevention of depression and isolation. Prevention and treatment of depression fosters mastery and self-worth of the residents and a noncontrolling, supportive environment for both residents and staff (Wetzel, 1980). One study reports that an optional activity instituted during an otherwise inactive period of the day demonstrated that environmental restructuring can reestablish and maintain social behavior (Blackman, Howe, & Pinkston, 1976). Interaction was encouraged by using a small activity area in which spatial arrangements were conducive to interaction and approximating a "koffee klatch."

Obviously, the nature of the service must match the capacities of the clients. In nursing homes, services are also available for patients with Alzheimer's disease who benefit from attention, caring, and structure. For example, "Alzheimer's Disease: Intervention in a Nursing Environment," describes the use of crisis intervention and problem solving with family and staff and behavioral techniques such as modeling and reinforcement to help a woman with Alzheimer's disease reduce her anxiety and the resulting wandering, rummaging, and suspiciousness (Mercer & Robinson, 1988). Although in Alzheimer's disease, progressive deterioration is inevitable, this eight-week program resulted in more independent self-care for the client and greater understanding and support from family and staff.

SUMMARY AND RECOMMENDATIONS

As the numbers of aged women continue to grow and social work continues to develop new programs and interventions for elderly women, clinical social work will make work with elderly women a high priority. "A balance between support and dependence, autonomy and assistance, is difficult to achieve and more difficult to finance" (Weinberg, 1987). Addressing the psychological, social, physical, legal, and financial strengths and problems of their clients, clinical social workers will continue to maximize self-determination while providing the supports necessary for the client to live as independently as possible.

Social work for aging women will continue to work on the most micro level of reminiscence, self-awareness, self-worth, and empowerment and the most macro level of advocacy for policy formulation and change (Morris, 1980). With regard to advocacy, some specific alterations in public programs such as old age, survivors, and disability insurance, funding of custodial care particularly for those with Alzheimer's disease as well as in private pension systems, may help women to avoid poverty in widowhood (Root & Tropman, 1984). Clearly, to develop innovative policies advocacy groups comprised of the elderly, their families, and professionals will have to work closely with all levels of government to meet present policy and program needs of all elderly women (Muller, 1983).

In the future, clinical social work will increase services to middle-aged women that are preventive in nature, that is, services focusing on an independent old age. For example, although interpersonal networks are developed during the lifetime of a person, learning to depend again on peer relationships during middle age will help prepare women for a time when many will lose husbands and perhaps sons (Poulin, 1984; Robertson, 1978). So many of the techniques that social work has developed for children and adolescents about the value of peer relationships can be adapted in work with middle-aged women. If a person does have to live in an institution, peer relationships are critical to adjustment. In addition, clinical social work will teach women in middle age that early intervention is more effective than late intervention at a time when those involved are often depleted, alienated, isolated, and angry.

Clinical social work will be responsible for educating itself, its clientele, and those with whom it must advocate to obtain increased services. Education will include knowledge of women's aging process; the biological, social, economic, and psychological problems of aging; and skills for intervening in the care of elderly women

(Bromberg, 1983; Miller, 1981; Rathbone-McCuan, 1984). Since most social workers are women and everyone who lives will age, these problems are our own personal as well as professional future. Thus, increasingly, each social worker will examine her own attitudes, values, and experiences with aging in order to avoid responses that interfere with helping the client.

As is our tradition, clinical social work's commitment to aging women will grow as the population and program funding increases. Already, there is a fine tradition of work in this area with superb examples of clinical intervention and program planning and implementation for middle-aged and elderly women from a wide spectrum of backgrounds and experiences. No doubt, the future will bring increased problems and, along with them, heightened clinical social work commitment and skill in helping elderly women to achieve a balance between dependence and autonomy.

REFERENCES

Achenbaum, W. A. (1983). Towards the next watershed in aging America. In W. A. Achenbaum (Ed.) *Shades of gray: Old age, American values and federal politics since 1920* (pp. 137-167). New York: Little, Brown.

Arens, D. A. (1982-1983). Widowhood and well being: An examination of sex differences within a causal model. *International Journal of Aging and Human Development, 15*, 27-40.

Bankoff, E. A. (1983). Aged parents and their widowed daughters: A support relationship. *Journal of Gerontology, 38*, 226-230.

Beckman, L. J. (1981). Effects of social interaction and children's relative inputs on older women's psychological well-being. *Journal of Personality and Social Psychology, 41*, 1075-1086.

Benokraitis, N. (1987). Older women and reentry problems: The case of displaced homemakers. *Journal of Gerontological Social Work, 10*, 75-92.

Blackman, D. K., Howe, M., & Pinkston, E. M. (1976). Increasing participation in social interaction of the institutionalized elderly. *Gerontologist, 16*, 69-76.

Blau, Z. S., Rogers, P. R., & Stephens, R. C. (1979). School bells and work whistles: Sounds that echo a better life for women in later years. In *Midlife women: Policy proposals on their problems*. Committee on Aging, U.S. House of Representatives.

Brody, E. M. (1981). Women in the middle and family help to older people. *Gerontologist, 21*, 471-480.

Brody, E. M. (1983). Women's changing roles and help to elderly parents: Attitudes of three generations of women. *Journal of Gerontology, 38*, 597-607.

Brody, E. M. (1985). Parent care as a normative family stress. *Gerontologist, 25*, 19-29.

Brody, E. M., Fulcomer, M. C., Johnson, P. T. (1984). What should adult children do for elderly parents: Opinions and preferences of three generations of women. *Journal of Gerontology, 39*, 736-746.

Bromberg, E. M. (1983). Mother-daughter relationships in later life: The effect of quality of relationship upon mutual aid. *Journal of Gerontological Social Work, 6*, 75-91.

Burkhauser, R. V., Holden, K. C., & Myers, D. A. (1985). Measuring the well-being of older women: The transition from wife to widow. *IRP Discussion Paper*, 21-24.

Cohen, G. D. (1980). Prospects for mental health and aging. In J. E. Birrin & R. B. Sloane (Eds.), *Handbook of mental health and aging* (pp. 971-993). Englewood Cliffs, NJ: Prentice-Hall.

Davis, L. J., & Brody, E. M. (1979). *Rape and older women: A guide to prevention and protection*. Washington, DC: National Center for Prevention and Control of Rape.

Dudley, A. (1983). Relationships and male and female elders. *Smith College Studies in Social Work, 5*, 177-187.

Dunkle, R. E. (1983). An historical perspective on social service delivery to the elderly. *Journal of Gerontological Social Work, 7*, 5-19.

Dunkle, R. E. (1987). Protective services for the elderly. In A. Minahan (Ed.), *Encylopedia of social work* (pp. 391-396). Washington, DC: National Association of Social Workers.

Enright, R., & Friss, L. (1987). Employed care givers of brain impaired adults: An assessment of the dual role. In *Family Survival Project*. San Francisco, California.

Fengler, A. P., & Goodrich, N. (1979). Wives of elderly disabled men: The hidden patients. *The Gerontologist, 19*, 175-183.

Ferraro, K. F. (1984). Widowhood and social participation in later life: Isolation or compensation? *Research on Aging, 6*, 451-468.

Ferraro, K. F. (1985-1986). The effect of widowhood on the health status of older persons. *International Journal of Aging and Human Development, 21*, 9-25.

Foley, L. M. (1976). *Stand Close by the Door*. Sacramento, CA: School of Social Work, California State University.

Freeman, E. M., Logan, S., & McCoy, R. (1987, September). Clinical practice with employed women. *Social Casework, 68*, 413-420.

Getzel, G. S. (1982). Helping elderly couples in crisis. *Social Casework, 62*, 515-521.

Getzel, G. S. (1981). Social work with family caregivers to the aged. *Social Casework, 62*, 201-209.

Glasse, L. (1987). Public policy, personal caregiving are closely tied to each other. *Perspectives on Aging*, 14-15.

Goldberg, G. S., Kantrow, R., & Kramer, E. (1986). Spouseless, childless elderly women and their social supports. *Social Work, 31*, 104-112.

Goldstein, R. (1983). Adult day care: Expanding options for service. *Journal of Gerontological Social Work*, *5*, 157-168.

Greene, R. (1986). *Social work with the aged and their families*. New York: Aldine de Gruyter.

Harris, P. B. (1989). Group work with the institutionalized elderly: The being old group revisited. In T. S. Kerson (Ed.), *Social work in health settings*. New York: Haworth Press.

Hess, B. B. (1980). Old women: Problems, political and policy implications. In E. W. Markson & G. R. Batra (Eds.), *Public policies for an aging population* (pp. 39-59). Lexington, MA: Lexington Books.

Hooyman, N. R., Rathbone-McCuan, E., & Klingbeil, K. (1982). Serving the vulnerable elderly: The detection, intervention and prevention of familial abuse. *The Urban and Social Change Review*, *15*, 9-14.

Johnson, E. S. (1981). Older mothers' perceptions of their child's divorce. *Gerontologist*, *2*, 395-401.

Kaminsky, M. (1978). Pictures from the past: The use of reminiscence in case-work with the elderly. *Journal of Gerontological Social Work*, *1*, 9-32.

Kaminsky, M. (1985). The arts and social work: Writing and reminiscing in old age. In G. S. Getzel and M. J. Mellor (Eds.), *Gerontological social work practice in the community* (pp. 225-246). New York: Haworth Press.

Kaplan, M., & Cabral, R. M. (1980). Relocation trauma counseling for the elderly: A demonstration project. *Journal of Gerontological Social Work*, *2*, 321-329.

Kaye, L. W., Monk, A., & Stuen, C. (1983). The efficacy of a self help teacher training program for older adults. *Gerontology and Geriatrics Education*, *4*, 75-87.

Kaye, L. W., Stuen, C., & Monk, A. (1985). The learning and retention of teaching skills by older adults: A time series analysis. *Educational Gerontology*, *11*, 113-125.

Keith, P. M. (1978). Factors associated with need: Community health and social services among the elderly. *Journal of Community Development Society of America*, *9*, 70-79.

Kerson, T. S. (1985) *Understanding chronic illness: Medical and psychosocial dimensions of nine diseases*. New York: Free Press.

Kerson, T. S. (1988). *Social Work in Health Settings: Practice in Context*. New York: Haworth Press.

Kirwin, P. M. (1986). Adult day care: An integrated model. In R. Dobrof (Ed.), *Social work and Alzheimer's disease* (pp. 59-71). New York: Haworth Press.

Kirwin, P. M. (1988). The challenge of community long-term care. *Journal of Aging Studies*.

Kirwin, P. M. (in press). Correlates of service utilization among adult day care clients. *Home Health Care Services Quarterly*.

Klass, S. B., & Redfern, M. A. (1977). A social work response to the middle-aged housewife. *Social Casework*, *58*, 101-110.

Kobosa-Munro, L. (1977). Sexuality in the aging woman. *Health and Social Work*, *2*, 71-88.

Levy, S. M. (1980-1981). The adjustment of the older woman: Effects of chronic ill health and attitudes toward retirement. *International Journal of Aging and Human Development*, *12*, 93-110.

Lewis, M. (1987). Sex bias dangerous to women's mental health. *Perspective on Aging*, *16*, 9-11.

Lieberman, M. (1985). Self-help groups: An overview. *Generations*, *10*, 45-49.

Longino, C. F. Jr., & Lipman, A. (1982). The married, the formerly married and the never married: Support system differentials of older women in planned retirement communities. *International Journal of Aging and Human Development*, *15*, 285-297.

Lopata, H. Z. (1987). Widowhood. In G. L. Maddox (Ed.), *Encyclopedia on Aging* (pp. 693-696). New York: Springer.

Lopata, H. Z., & Brehm, H. P. (1986). *Widows and dependent wives; from social problem to federal program*. New York: Praeger.

Lotz, N., Duchainey, D., & Kerson, T. S. (1989). Reestablishing a coordinated care program: Home health services. In Kerson, T. S. (Ed.), *Social Work in Health Settings*. New York: Haworth Press.

Mercer, S. O, & Robinson, B. (1989). Alzhiemer's disease: Intervention in a nursing home environment. In Kerson, T. S. (Ed.), *Social work in health settings*. New York: Haworth Press.

Milinsky, T. S. (1987). Stagnation and depression in the elderly group client. *Social Casework*, *68*, 173-179.

Miller, D. A. (1981). The sandwich generation: Adult children of the aging. *Social Work*, *26*, 419-423.

Monk, A. (1981). Social work with the aged: Principles of practice. *Social Work*, *26*, 61-68.

Morgan, L. A. (1980). Work in widowhood: A viable option? *The Gerontologist*, *20*, 581-587.

Morris, R. (1980). Social welfare policy and aging: Implications for the future — between the good earth and pie in the sky. In E. W. Markson, & G. R. Batra, (Eds.), *Public policies for an aging population* (pp. 121-131). New York: Lexington Books.

Muller, C. (1983). Income supports for older women. *Social Policy*, *14*, 23-31.

Naysmith, S. M. (1981). Parental care: Another female function? *Canadian Journal of Social Work Education*, *7*(2), 55-63.

Oktay, J. S., & Volland, P. J. (1987). Foster home care for the frail elderly as an alternative to nursing home care: An experimental evaluation. *American Journal of Public Health*, *77*, 1505-1510.

Pollack, S. (1981). Places called home. *Health and Social Work*, *6*, 54-58.

Poulin, J. E. (1984). Age segregation and the interpersonal involvement and morale of the aged. *Gerontologist*, *24*, 266-269.

Pratt, C., Schmall, V., & Wright, S. (1986). Family caregivers and dementia. *Social Casework*, *67*, 119-124.

Quam, J. K., & Austin, C. D. (1984). Coverage of women's issues in eight social work journals, 1970-81. *Social Work, 29*, 360-365.

Rathbone-McCuan, E. (1984). The abused older woman: A discussion of abuses and rape. In G. Lesnoff-Caravaglia (Ed.), *The world of older women* (pp. 419-470). New York: Human Sciences.

Rathbone-McCuan, E. (1984). Older women, mental health and social work education. *Journal of Education for Social Work, 20*, 33-41.

Rathbone-McCuan, E., & Hashimi, J. (1982). *Isolated Elders*. Rockville, MD: Aspen.

Rathbone-McCuan, E., & Voyles, B. (1982). Case detection of abused elderly parents. *American Journal of Psychiatry, 139*, 189-192,

Robertson, J. F. (1978). Activity preferences of community-residing aged as a guide for practice emphases. *Journal of Gerontological Social Work, 1*, 95-109.

Root, L. S., & Topman, J. E. (1984). Income sources of the elderly. *Social Service Review, 58*, 384-403.

SAGE: Senior Action in a Gay Environment. (1984). *Practice Digest, 7*, 17-20.

Sands, R. G., & Richardson, V. (1986). Clinical practice with women in their middle years. *Social Work, 31*, 36-43.

Shaw, S. B. (1987). Parental aging: Clinical issues in adult psychotherapy. *Social Casework, 68*, 406-412.

Silverman, P. R. (1979). Mutual help: An alternative arrangement made for midlife women. In *Midlife women: Policy proposals on their problems*. Washington, DC: Committee on Aging, U.S. House of Representatives.

Silverman, P. R. (1986). *Widow to widow*. New York: Springer.

Silverman, P. R., & Cooperband, A. (1984). Widow-to-widow: The elderly widow and mutual help. In Lesnoff-Caravaglia, B. (Ed.), *The world of the older woman: Conflicts and resolutions* (pp. 144-161). New York: Human Sciences.

Simmons, T. (1985). Caregiving: A woman's issue. *Generations, 10*, 9-13.

Simon, B. L. (1986). Never married women as caregivers to elderly parents: Some costs and benefits. *AFFILIA Journal of Women and Social Work, 1*, 29-42.

Simon, B. L. (1987). Never married women. Philadelphia: Temple University.

SOWN (Supportive Older Women's Network) (n.d.). Brochure. Philadelphia: Author.

Stone, R. (1986). Aging in the eighties: Age 65 and Over—use of community services. *Advance Data, 124*, 1-15.

Stuen, C., & Kaye, L. W. (1985). Creating educational alliances between retired academics, community agencies and elderly neighborhood residents. *CATALYST, 14*, 21-24.

Tobin, S., & Kulys, R. (1981). The family in the institutionalization of the elderly. *Journal of Social Issues, 37*, 145-157.

U.S. Bureau of the Census. (1985). Money income and poverty status of families and persons living in the United States. Current Population Reports (Series P. 60, No. 149). Washington, DC: U.S. Government Printing Office.

Weinberg, J. K. (1987). Aging and dependence: Toward a redefinition of autonomy. *Social Casework, 68,* 522-532.

Wetzel, J. W. (1980). Interventions with the depressed elderly in institutions. *Social Casework, 61,* 234-239.

Physical Health of Elderly Women

Barbara P. Pearson, RN, MN
Cornelia M. Beck, PhD, RN

With the many advances of medical science in reducing mortality from major diseases in America, women are experiencing a "mixed blessing." While there is rejoicing at the prospect of a longer life, there is fear that they will experience major health problems with which they will be unable to cope. Health is a major determinant of the quality of life and is intricately connected to the social, environmental, and economic aspects of the lives of elderly women. This chapter will address the health concerns of elderly women, including a historical overview of health care advances for the elderly, physical changes normally occurring with the aging process, and future projections concerning the health and services needed to promote the highest quality of life for elderly females in our society.

HISTORICAL OVERVIEW

With the passage of the Social Security Act in 1935, the United States began its attention to the overall social welfare of the elderly. The health and health services to meet the needs of the elderly segment of the population have been an area of increasing concern, especially in the past three decades.

The focus on health and other social concerns of the rapidly growing aged members of society intensified in the 1950s, with the

Barbara P. Pearson is Professor, College of Nursing, University of Arkansas for Medical Sciences, Little Rock, AR 72205.

Cornelia M. Beck is Professor, College of Nursing, and Assistant Professor, Department of Psychiatry, College of Medicine, University of Arkansas for Medical Sciences, Little Rock, AR 72205.

First National Conference on Aging in 1950, followed by the establishment of a Federal Committee on Aging and Geriatrics in 1951. Various committees and councils on aging studied needs of the elderly and coordination of programs in the ensuing ten years.

In 1961, the First White House Conference on Aging was held, with subsequent White House Conferences in 1971 and 1981. In 1963, John F. Kennedy sent the first presidential message on elderly citizens to the Congress and an Office on Aging was established. In 1965, under President Lyndon Johnson, the Administration on Aging was established and the Social Securities Act was amended to establish the Medicare program, initiating growing government involvement in financing health care for the elderly. Since that time, a variety of governmental measures, at both the national and state levels, have focused on assistance to the aged in relation to health, housing, nutrition, age discrimination in employment, transportation, volunteer programs, and other areas of the lives of the aged. In 1974, the National Institute on Aging was established within the National Institutes of Health, further recognizing the growing national dilemma about the needs and resources of the most rapidly growing segment of the American population.

From the mid 1960s through the late 1970s, governmental involvement in programs to address the problems of the increasing number of "graying" Americans proliferated, with a growth in the political voice of the aged themselves. In the decade of the 1980s, however, the fiscal impact of the governmental commitment to programs for the elderly for health care and other assistance has become a major issue within the spiraling national debt. Beginning in 1981, proposals to reverse this trend of increasing budget deficits have precipitated changes in federal assistance to the aged, such as taxing of Social Security benefits and the institution of cost-containment measures for health care. Simultaneously, the costs of health care, especially the costs of long-term care for the disabled elderly, have rapidly accelerated. Currently, 30% of the federal budget is utilized to provide benefits to the elderly. Of the overall health care expenditures in the United States, one-third of the costs are for the care of persons who are age 65 and older (Binstock, 1985). As the nation struggles with the reduction of the national debt, programs for the elderly will undoubtedly continue to be one of the proposed targets of measures to lower federal spending.

It is elderly women who will be primarily affected by increased longevity, the concomitant risk of increased health problems, and the reduction in financial support for health care. The fastest-growing segment of the population in our country is women who are age 65 and over. Since only 5% of the elderly are currently being institutionalized, most of these women remain at home. However, they may have as many as three chronic illnesses, on the average (Abdellah, 1985).

Concern about the health care services that are provided to older women becomes a key issue in relation to the quality of life. The current health care delivery system in America focuses primarily on disease and illness. This illness orientation is reinforced by the funding provided by Medicare and Medicaid, as well as private insurances, which do not cover many preventative and disease-detection services (Older Women's League, 1987).

The attention to the health of older women in this system has also been influenced by two other major factors—a gender bias in the practice of physicians, who are predominantly males, and an age bias among health providers, who may often place less value on the care of the elderly (Older Women's League, 1987).

PHYSICAL CHANGES IN ELDERLY WOMEN

To identify and address the physical health needs of elderly women, it is essential to begin with an understanding of the physiological changes that are a part of the aging process. Although there is some understanding of the aging process as it specifically relates to the physical changes in women, this understanding is limited by two major areas of deficit in the current state of research on aging. First, very little research in aging addresses the differences between women and men; second, the research does not clearly differentiate "normal" aging changes from those that signify "pathology." These deficits are more pronounced in the physical and emotional domains; most research has addressed the social changes faced by older women. The following overview of systems summarizes the common physical changes associated with aging and, where possible, addresses what is known about the effect of aging on women.

Skin and Tissue

For women who live in the youth- and beauty-oriented culture of the western world, the early aging changes that occur in the skin, hair, and body tissues are perhaps the most noticeable and have the greatest initial influence. Two major events, the graying of the hair and wrinkling of the skin, signal the onset of aging and are usually a source of concern to females.

Changes in the elastin and collagen in the skin begin in the early to mid 40s. As the elastic characteristics of the skin are reduced and the collagen bundles become larger and stiffer, the epithelium (outer layer of the skin) becomes thinner and the subcutaneous fatty layers of the skin are reduced. These changes result in wrinkling of the skin, especially on the face, neck, and hands. The creases and folds in the skin of the face, commonly referred to as "crows feet," "laugh lines," and "worry lines," tend to reflect the facial expressions an individual has demonstrated throughout her life, as well as the effect of gravity on tissue that is less elastic. While genetic factors influence the extent of wrinkling, the exposure to sun is the most important determinant in causing earlier and more severe wrinkling. Therefore, the use of sunscreens to protect the skin from ultraviolet rays cannot be overemphasized. Research on the effects of smoking in women suggests that smoking also precipitates earlier and increased wrinkling of skin.

Other changes occur that influence the quality and characteristics of the skin of a woman as she ages. There is a decrease in melanocytes, the cells that affect skin pigmentation, resulting in lighter skin in aging white women. The blood vessels of the skin become more fragile and are easily damaged by bumping or pressure, which results in small hemorrhages called purpura. In addition, there is a decrease in the size, number, and function of the sweat glands that contributes to dryness and itchiness of the skin, especially during the winter. These multiple skin changes also cause healing to be slower in aging skin.

Changes in the hair of women are also of major concern in relation to their appearance. The decrease in melanocytes that can cause changes in pigmentation in the skin also causes decreased melanin production in the hair follicles, which results in the loss of color, or graying, of the hair. In addition, because there is a progressive loss of the deep dermal blood vessels in the scalp, hair tends to grow less, and the new hairs are lighter and thinner. After age sixty, virtually all women experience hair loss. This loss of hair occurs on the legs, arms, and in the axillary and pubic areas as well, especially in advanced age, when the individual's body may seem to have virtually no body hair. In white women, the growth of facial hair, known as hirsutism, may be an additional nuisance, resulting from changes in hormones as the female ages.

The changes of subcutaneous fat in body tissues accounts for many of the other observable characteristics of aging, especially noticed in peripheral body parts. In general, the fatty tissue of the body tends to shift from the extremities to the trunk of the body, with increasing amounts of fat in the abdomen, hips, and, at times, the ankles of the older woman. As these redistributions occur, the arms and legs appear thin, breasts tend to sag, eyes may appear sunken because the fat layer around the orbit of the eye disappears, areas around the armpit and clavicle may appear more hollow, and bones and muscle contours become more visible. This is especially true in the hands of the aged, in which the bones, veins, and tendons become prominent.

In addition to the changes in appearance, the alterations in distribution of body fat and the changes in the functioning of the sweat glands have implications for the tolerance of the aged to heat and cold. The loss of the insulating fat can cause the older person to feel cold more readily. The decreased function of the sweat glands can cause susceptibility to heat exhaustion, since the body does not cool itself as efficiently through perspiration.

Sensory

Changes in the senses of vision, hearing, taste, smell, and touch are of special importance in the older woman, since they are the means through which she communicates with her environment and they can significantly affect her ability to maintain independence and a sense of security.

While the rate of change is variable, the eye and acuity of vision undergo predictable changes in the process of aging. The most common visual change is presbyopia, sometimes called "old age vision." At about age 40, the lens of the eye and the muscles that control its thickening and flattening lose their elasticity, resulting in an inability to focus clearly on near objects. Few people avoid this change and the need for magnification for reading and close work; bifocal glasses or lenses are commonly used to adapt to this change in the ability of the lens to accommodate.

The pupil of the eye becomes smaller and sometimes irregular in size, causing the eye to react more slowly and not as completely to changes in light and to require more illumination to be able to see. To see objects well at age 60, it is estimated that one needs two times the light needed at age 20; three times the light is needed by age 80 (Ebersole & Hess, 1981; National Institute on Aging, 1987). This change in the pupil also causes aging individuals to be more sensitive to glare and to have poorer vision at night.

As one ages, color vision is also altered, probably because of the progressive yellowing of the lens of the eye. This change causes more difficulty in distinguishing greens, blues, and violets, while reds, yellows, and oranges are fairly easy to see. Other changes that aging precipitates are decreased ability to respond to rapidly moving objects and decreased breadth of vision, in which objects in the peripheral vision are not as clear or may not be seen.

With aging, increases in the opacity of the lens of the eye occur and the ability of the eye to reabsorb the fluid in the eyeball generally decreases. For many, these changes can result in sufficient visual difficulties to warrant medical intervention and are discussed under the overview of major health problems of aged women.

Another relatively common eye development that can begin as early as the second or third decade of life is the formation of a lipid (fatty) material on the periphery of the cornea, which can eventually evolve from a small speck to a whitish circle at the outer edge of the iris. This age-related change, known as *arcus senilis*, unlike other eye changes, does not affect vision or eye function.

While not directly related to visual difficulties, a decrease in the function of the lacrimal apparatus of the eye does cause older individuals to experience increased dryness of the eyes and sometimes itching. If excessive and not treated with lubricants (artificial tears), the dryness can cause damage to the lids and eye itself. The reduction in production of tears is more dramatic in women after menopause.

Beyond the age of 50, individuals generally experience a decrease in their ability to hear. Women are affected by this condition, presbycusis, less than men, but do usually experience some loss of hearing acuity, ability to understand speech clearly, and changes in the range of sounds that can be heard (National Institute on Aging, 1987). These deficits are commonly caused by age-related changes in the sensory mechanisms of hearing, which can be damaged from exposure to loud noises, diseases, or the use of medications. Mechanical obstruction by excessive ear wax can also cause the symptoms, but can usually be treated relatively simply through cleansing regimens.

In presbycusis, the individual loses the ability to hear high-pitched sounds, has difficulty with common consonants of speech, including *s*, *z*, *t*, *f*, *g*, *sh*, and *ch* sounds, and frequently is unable to discriminate speech that is rapid or is occurring in environments with background noises. Hearing abilities can be influenced by the individual's ability to concentrate and center attention, but whatever the cause of the decreased hearing, it can contribute to frustration, fear, and isolation.

Over 10 million American men and women suffer from chemosensory disorders involving the senses of taste and smell, most of which occur after age 60. The ability to smell declines less rapidly in women than men and can contribute to decreased taste as well (National Institute on Aging, 1987). As one ages, the number of taste buds decreases and as many as two-thirds of the taste buds may atrophy, but the ability to discriminate between the four basic tastes of salt, sweet, sour, and bitter are usually retained, although they are not generally as distinct.

While the changes in taste and smell may result from physical changes in the body, other factors that influence the sensory systems include nasal obstructions, upper dentures that obstruct the palate, medications, and allergies. Changes in the senses of taste and smell are especially important in terms of their potential to decrease appetite in aging individuals. To compensate for the changes in food taste, older persons may use increased spices and/or salt, both of which can be detrimental. Some elderly may also compensate by increased intake of carbohydrates and fats, which can, in turn, lead to increased obesity and to less efficient tissue repair. In some instances, the decrease in taste, smell, and appetite can lead to malnutrition, because of decreased dietary intake.

Musculoskeletal

The changes of aging also are reflected in deterioration of the muscles, bones, and joints of the body. Muscle fibers decrease in size, with a proportionate decrease in muscular strength. The decrease in overall muscle mass can be masked by the increase of fat and collagen in areas formerly containing muscle. The extent of muscle wasting, as aging progresses, is generally judged by the wasting of muscle on the top of the hand. The muscles also respond more slowly and are fatigued more rapidly than when the person was younger.

A similar change in bone mass occurs after the age of 45. Changes in bone mass for women are accelerated after menopause, because of the decline in estrogen. Although bone growth continues, generally into and beyond the sixth decade, the reabsorption of the interior of long and flat bones occurs at a faster rate than the growth. In this complex process, protein and minerals are lost from the bone matrix.

Both weight- and nonweight-bearing joints in the body begin undergoing changes at the age of 20 to 30, with acceleration of the changes after age 40. The cartilage gradually progresses from a smooth surface to one with deep fissures and shredding; eventually, erosion of the cartilage may take place. When this occurs, bones within the joints come in contact with each other. These events can result in pain, crepitation, and eventually the development of irregular bone growth as the body attempts to strengthen the joints where erosion has occurred. Similarly, the synovial membranes in the joints undergo shredding and the fluid becomes thicker, creating less movable joints. The overall effect of the changes in the muscles, bones, and joints is more restricted movement, both in terms of range and speed of movement.

The spine is most noticeably affected by these changes, resulting in decreased height. During the middle-age years, the discs between the vertebra (bones) in the spine suffer a loss of thickness due to a loss in water content. As aging progresses, the vertebra themselves narrow, further shortening the spine. The chest increases in diameter from front to back (sometimes called barrel chest) and the thoracic spine becomes more convex, a condition called kyphosis. All of these changes, combined with the decreased extension in the knees and hips of elderly individuals, can cause a shortened height ranging from .5 inch to 2 inches and the "bowed" posture so often depicted in pictures of the aged.

Heart and Lungs

The major organs of the body also undergo multiple changes as a part of the aging process. An in-depth discussion of the complex physiological alterations is beyond the scope of this article; therefore, the focus will be primarily on the functional decreases that result from these physiological alterations.

The heart, in general, may be reduced in size, as are other muscles of the body, except in the presence of disease for which the muscle is attempting to compensate by enlarging. In aging, the heart muscle experiences reduced efficiency and a consequent decreased output of blood as it contracts. The heart rate, at rest, remains relatively unchanged and may be slower in some individuals than the resting state at a younger age. When increased heart rate is needed to meet body demands, the heart does not respond as rapidly, nor does it return to the resting rate as quickly, once the heart rate is elevated.

Although these changes result in decreased cardiac efficiency, the cardiovascular functioning is usually sufficient to meet the needs of the body because body demands are also decreased as one ages. Difficulties can, however, be encountered when the aged individual is physically taxed or emotionally stressed, causing demands for increased blood circulation that are greater in amount or needed more rapidly than the heart can respond to.

The vessels of the cardiovascular system sustain alterations that are reflected in changes in circulation. The normal elasticity of blood vessels decreases, resulting in increasing stiffness and less distensibility. They may also fragment, split, and fray, and usually straighten and become longer. In addition, the inside diameter (lumen) of the vessels may be narrowed because of deposits of fat and calcium, thereby changing the blood flow to organs. These factors can combine to cause increases in both the systolic and diastolic blood pressure.

Whereas elevations in blood pressure tend to occur with aging, some elderly persons experience a sudden drop in blood pressure when they sit or stand. This occurrence, called orthostatic or postural hypotension, can have many causes and can create increased risks for injury among the aged.

The changes in the respiratory system in the aged include alterations in the functioning of the lungs and in the structure of the chest cavity. There is little change in the size of the lungs, but the elasticity of the lungs decreases, causing more rigidity of the tissue and less effective lung expansion. The lung expansion is also affected by changes in the ribs. The ribs become more stationary and move less freely because of increased calcium in the cartilages that support the ribs and decreased efficiency in the respiratory muscles of the chest wall.

The combined effects of kyphosis, increased diameter of the chest, and decreased strength of the muscles are evidenced in decreased effectiveness of breathing and diminished cough reflex. Therefore the individual may be less able to clear substances from the respiratory tract, further complicating ventilation.

Nervous System

In aging, the nervous system undergoes complex changes in the cells, neurotransmission mechanisms, and cerebral blood flow. The brain weight decreases gradually after age 30, with an approximate loss of 7% by age 80 (Kenny, 1982). Although millions of neurons are lost during the aging process, this loss may have little effect on the functioning of the brain if disease is not present (National Institute on Aging, 1987).

The overall effect of these nervous system changes is gradually evidenced in the slowing of response and decrease in sensory perception as one ages. Aged individuals generally react to stimuli more slowly and move less rapidly. The response to pain is often decreased, as is the sense of position and balance.

In normal aging, these changes are particularly relevant to the safety of the person, as they may precipitate falls, cause the aged not to respond quickly enough to heat and cold with resulting tissue damage, and/or decrease the ability to react fast enough in other situations of danger. To accommodate for these changes, the individual generally uses more caution and is more deliberate and tentative in movement.

The intellectual functioning is generally not altered as one ages, unless disease occurs. This is especially true for those who remain active and pursue activities requiring intellectual stimulation. The loss of memory, so often attributed to aging, may in fact be more a result of decreased attention and concentration, increased anxiety and/or slower retrieval time than from true mental or memory losses (National Institute on Aging, 1987).

Reproductive System

In women, the aging changes in the reproductive system are multiple. Breast changes begin around age 35, with fat gradually replacing the glands of the breasts and decreased size and function of the ducts of the breast. Ovaries decrease in size and become fibrotic, but continue to function. The uterus, cervix, and vagina become smaller with changes in their function, especially in terms of their secretory activity.

Menopause, commonly known as the "change of life" for women, is considered to occur one year after a woman's last menstrual period. The average age of menopause is 50, leaving nearly one-third of her life expectancy to be lived once a woman reaches the end of her ability to reproduce (National Institute on Aging, 1987).

Changes prior to the end of the menses can occur over a period of nearly five to ten years, called the climacteric. During this time, women can experience many problems, including moodiness, irritability, changes in skin, lack of energy, loss of sex drive, insomnia, vaginal atrophy, and hot flashes.

The hot flashes, although uncomfortable, are a severe problem for only an estimated 10% of women, who may require hormone therapy. Whereas estrogen replacement therapy (ERT) used to be relatively common treatment for menopausal symptoms, it is prescribed less frequently for this purpose because of its potential for causing increased risk of uterine cancer (National Institute on Aging, 1987).

The changes in the structure and function of the vagina can create discomfort, especially during sexual activity. With the thinner walls of the vagina and decreased secretions, women can experience increasing pain during sexual intercourse. Lubricants are utilized to prevent the pain and abrasion that occurs, and frequent intercourse is known to decrease the problems encountered (National Institute on Aging, 1987).

Genitourinary

With aging, the bladder decreases in size and is thus able to hold less urine; it also does not empty as completely. The sensations enabling one to know when the bladder needs to be emptied undergo changes that may cause an individual to be less aware of the fullness of the bladder.

Changes in the muscles of the urethra also occur, making it less able to control the flow of urine. As tissue quality diminishes, the mucosa of the urethra may collapse into the opening, creating a situation that can require surgical repair.

PHYSICAL HEALTH CONCERNS OF ELDERLY WOMEN

With the increasing longevity of women, the effects of the physical changes of aging are often manifest in disease processes that vary in severity for elderly women. This overview describes the major physical diseases that can result in chronic disability and/or death of women.

Cardiovascular Disease

Heart disease, generally thought of as a disease of men, is the leading cause of death in women over the age of 65, when one of every four women has some form of heart disease. Diseases of the cardiovascular system occur 10 to 20 years later in women than in men, with a dramatic increase following menopause of American women. Prior to menopause, the estrogen levels in females seem to protect them (National Institute on Aging, 1987). Black women are at greater risk for heart disease after age 45, whereas the disease risk for white women is greater after age 55 (McKeever & Martinson, 1986).

Although women develop heart disease at a later age and may have milder forms of the disease, they are more likely to die of heart attacks than men in nearly every age group (Older Women's League, 1987). Similarly, if a woman survives a first heart attack, she is two to three times as likely to suffer a second heart attack in the subsequent five years as a man is (National Institute on Aging, 1987). Women also do not benefit from the use of aspirin or bypass surgery to control/correct heart problems to the degree that men benefit from these measures (National Institute on Aging, 1987).

Hypertension is one of the primary cardiovascular diseases influencing the toll on life and productivity in women. Hypertension, a sustained elevation in the blood pressure, is the most common cause of heart and vascular disease (Older Women's League, 1987). Women with hypertension are three times more likely to have heart attacks, five times more likely to suffer from congestive heart failure, and eight times more likely to have a stroke. By age 65, 66% of white women have some degree of hypertension and 82% of black women suffer from the condition (National Institute on Aging, 1987). Called the "silent killer" because of the absence of symptoms, hypertension requires early diagnosis and treatment for improvement of the overall health status of women. Treatment for the disease consists of medications, diet, and exercise.

Cerebral vascular accidents, commonly called strokes, are the third leading cause of death in women. Strokes are caused by decreased blood supply to the brain, which can occur from blockage or occlusion of the major vessels supplying the brain or from hemorrhage from vessels that leak or rupture. The severity of stroke can vary widely from transient ischemic attacks (TIA), with little tissue damage, to paralysis, or near instant death.

The risk factors for stroke are multiple, including atherosclerosis, hypertension, stress, diabetes, and increased cholesterol levels. The incidence of stroke increases markedly after age 55, with 70% of all stroke deaths occurring in persons over age 70. Stroke-related illnesses account for a vast majority of the use of health resources and are a major cause of disability in elderly women (Gioiella & Bevil, 1985).

Cancer

Cancer is the second leading cause of death in the United States. In women, it is the leading cause of death for ages 35 to 54, the second leading cause of death for ages 56 to 74, and third leading cause of death for women over the age of 75 (Older Women's League, 1987). For over 50 years, breast cancer has caused the most deaths from cancer in women. In 1987, for the first time, the American Cancer Society estimates that lung cancer will become the leading cause of cancer deaths among women, although breast cancer still is projected to rank highest in incidence. Scientists have predicted that lung cancer deaths in women would eventually predominate because of the increase of cigarette smoking among females since World War II and the low survival rate; only 13% of lung cancer patients live five or more years after diagnosis. With early detection, the survival rate rises to 33%, but less then one-fourth of lung cancers are diagnosed in an early stage of development (American Cancer Society, 1987).

Table 1 lists the 1987 estimates for incidences and deaths of women from cancer, projected by the American Cancer Society. While statistics on current incidence and death from cancer in the elderly, by sex and race, are not readily available, it is generally recognized that cancer increases with advancing age. Currently, one of every eight deaths among women over 65 years of age is from cancer. The majority of the deaths is from cancer of the gastrointestinal tract, breast, lungs, pancreas, and uterus (National Institute on Aging, 1987; Woods, 1985).

The risk of breast cancer and cancers of the reproductive system in women is of special note. The American Cancer Society now

TABLE 1. Cancer in Women: 1987 Estimates of Incidence and Deaths.

Incidence		Deaths	
Breast	27%	Lung	20%
Colon/Rectum	16%	Breast	18%
Lung	11%	Colon/Rectum	14%
Uterus	10%	Leukemia & Lymphomas	9%
Leukemia and Lymphomas	7%	Ovary	5%
Ovary	4%	Pancreas	5%
Urinary	4%	Uterus	4%
Skin	3%	Urinary	3%
Pancreas	3%	Skin	2%
Oral	2%	Oral	1%
All other	13%	All Other	19%

Source: Cancer Facts and Figures, 1987. American Cancer Society.

estimates that one in every ten women will experience breast cancer at some point in her lifetime (American Cancer Society, 1987). Uterine cancer claims over 10,000 women over age 60 each year (Older Women's League, 1987). The incidence of endometrial (body of the uterus) cancer in white women is double that of black women, whereas the cases of cervical cancer occur twice as frequently in blacks (American Cancer Society, 1987).

As technology for detection of cancer improves, the use of mammography, PAP smears, and other types of diagnostic procedures can reduce the incidence of these cancers through early detection. Similarly, preventive measures, including diet, smoking cessation, decreased exposure to ultraviolet sun rays, and judicious use of medications known to increase female cancer risks, can reduce the toll in terms of death and disability. The American Cancer Society estimates that such prevention measures and early detection can reduce cancer by one-half (National Institute on Aging, 1987).

Incontinence

Changes in the genitourinary structure and function can cause women to experience an inability to control the passage of urine, called urinary incontinence. This condition occurs most frequently in women who have had numerous children and in obese women. The severity of the incontinence varies, with "stress incontinence" being the most common form, occurring during sneezing, coughing, or lifting. Treatment for incontinence includes exercises to increase the integrity of the muscles and in some cases surgery. Incontinence is often the precipitating factor for institutionalization of elderly women who have previously managed on their own or been cared for by family members (Abdellah, 1985; Soldo & Manton, 1985).

Musculoskeletal Disorders

Three major musculoskeletal disorders — osteoporosis, osteoarthritis, and rheumatoid arthritis — are associated with disability in aging women and represent significant threats to the mobility and maintenance of independence of women as they age.

Osteoporosis is a disorder in which the progressive loss of bone that occurs with aging is greater than normal, resulting in bones that are weak, porous, and more prone to fracture. Although bone loss is a part of the aging process, as previously described, the process in women accelerates after menopause with the change in body hormones and can cause serious health problems for many women.

Osteoporosis affects primarily the vertebra of the spine, the neck of the femur of the leg, the bones in the wrists, and other bones in the leg. Consequently, women with osteoporosis are susceptible to fractures in these areas, most notably hip fractures and "crush" or compression fractures of the spinal vertebra. Many women are not aware that they are suffering from osteoporosis and the attendant risk of fractures until they experience one of these injuries. The fractures may occur with little or no trauma, that is, spontaneously, simply due to the weakness of the bones.

The thinning of the bones, beginning after age 35, has been estimated to affect half of women over age 45 and nine in ten women over age 75. After age 40, women's bone loss is two times that of men, and following menopause may be four times as great (Older Women's League, 1987).

Currently, an estimated one out of every four women over age 65 have evidence of osteoporotic fractures. The increasing incidence of these fractures in women has been termed a "silent epidemic," resulting in accelerated health care costs, disability, and at times, death (Lindsay, 1987).

White women who are fair and slim are at higher risk for osteoporosis. Other risk factors for all women include early menopause or surgical removal of the ovaries, dietary deficiencies of calcium and vitamin D, high caffeine and alcohol intake, smoking, sedentary life style, and cortisone medications (Lindsay, 1987; National Institute on Aging, 1987).

All the physiologic mechanisms of osteoporosis are not well understood, but it is believed that women can protect themselves by developing a life style at an early age that includes sufficient calcium intake, regular exercise, and avoidance of substances that interfere with bone metabolism, including soft drinks, coffee, red meat, and cigarettes. In addition, the use of estrogen replacement to slow the progression of osteoporosis is gaining increased acceptance (Lindsay, 1987).

Osteoarthritis is the most common type of arthritis, afflicting men more before age 45, but more common in women after age 45.

Unlike rheumatoid arthritis, osteoarthritis is not a systemic condition. In the course of the development of the disease, the cartilage covering the ends of the long bones of the body is damaged and/or worn away, bone comes in contact with bone, and bony spurs may develop as the body tries to compensate for the loss of joint integrity.

The disease is usually manifest in sore, swollen joints with accompanying pain and tenderness. The joints most affected are weight-bearing joint surfaces, such as the hip, knee, and cervical and lumbar spine regions. The most noticeable involvement is that seen in the joints of the hands, where osteoarthritic nodes commonly develop. Although the disease may initially cause only pain and stiffness, it can progress to marked loss of joint mobility that is accompanied by increasing pain and incapacitation. Past the age of 60, the disease causes debilitating changes in 25% of women (Gioiella & Bevil, 1985).

In the early stages of osteoarthritis, treatment is directed to reducing the pain and stiffness, thereby maintaining joint movement. Therapy may include anti-inflammatory and pain medications and physical therapy measures such as heat, massage, and ultrasound. When these measures are not successful and the debilitation of patients increases, surgical joint replacement may be performed. The most common joint replacements are the hips, knee, elbow and finger joints.

Rheumatoid arthritis is a chronic, systemic form of arthritis in which connective tissue changes result primarily from inflammatory processes affecting the synovial lining of the joint spaces. Irreversible joint damage is progressive. The disease is two and a half to three times more common in women than men (Carter, 1986; Luckman & Sorenson, 1987). The disease may develop at any age, with the onset commonly occurring between ages 20 and 40 and the incidence increasing with aging.

In rheumatoid arthritis, the small joints of the hands, wrists, and feet are the most commonly affected, with bilateral involvement. The symptoms include pain, swelling and stiffness, similar to those of osteoarthritis, but because of the systemic nature of the disease, patients generally also experience fatigue, fever, anorexia, and weight loss. The pain and stiffness is generally of greater severity and lasts longer in the mornings than the symptoms of osteoarthritis. Persons with rheumatoid arthritis can also experience periods of remission of the disease, but these are usually followed by exacerbations in which the symptoms are much worse.

As the disease progresses, the involved joints undergo changes that can progress to union of the bones of the involved joints. Since the disease is systemic, it can also involve connective tissue of other types in the body, such as the heart, lungs, muscles, and blood vessels.

The early treatment for rheumatoid arthritis is similar to the measures described in the treatment of osteoarthritis. However, because rheumatoid arthritis is the most virulent type of arthritis, more extensive drug therapy may be used, including gold salts, antimalarials, steroids, and immunosuppressive agents (Carnevali & Patrick, 1986; Carter, 1986).

Sensory Disorders

Of the many disorders affecting the senses of the aging person, those that affect the vision and hearing have the greatest potential for disabling physical and emotional impact. Not only can these diseases cause the individual to lose their independence, but sensory distortions can lead to isolation and, at times, unnecessary paranoia and fear.

Diseases of the Eye

Cataracts. Cataracts are a clouding or opacification of the lens of the eye. The National Institute on Aging (1987) estimates that two-thirds of the population from the ages of 65 to 74 have some form of lens opacity. The clouding of the lens results from changes in the protein of the lens or from damage to the cells within the lens caused by other diseases, such as diabetes.

Cataracts, of several types, cause decreased visual acuity, eye fatigue, and blurred or multiple vision. As the cataracts progress, patients may also complain of sensitivity to light. Cataracts usually occur in both eyes, but may not appear at the same time or influence vision at the same pace.

The treatment for cataracts is surgical removal of the opaque lens, with replacement of a lens in the eye (intraocular lens implant) or through the use of contact lenses or glasses. The decision to perform surgery and the timing of the surgical removal are generally a function of the degree of influence the cataract is having on the individual's ability to perform her usual activities of daily living.

Cataract surgery is now being performed routinely in one-day surgery units, permitting the patient to be discharged early, unless other medical problems necessitate longer hospitalization. When cataract surgery is required on both eyes, each eye is operated on at different times. For 90% to 95% of cataract extraction patients, the surgery restores vision that will enable them to resume their usual activities of daily living (Luckman & Sorenson, 1987; National Institute on Aging, 1987).

Glaucoma. Glaucoma is the leading cause of blindness in the United States. Although the disease can occur at any age, it is more prevalent after age 40. It is estimated that 3% of the population over age 65 suffer from glaucoma (National Institute on Aging, 1987).

Glaucoma is caused by increased pressure of the fluid within the eye (intraocular pressure) resulting from inadequate drainage of the fluid. The pressure causes damage to the optic nerve, which is vital in transmitting visual messages to the brain. The damage is irreversible, gradually decreases the visual field, and eventually results in blindness, if untreated.

Of the two types of glaucoma, wide-angle and narrow-angle, the wide-angle (also called open-angle or chronic-simple) glaucoma is more common in the elderly and usually has no symptoms during its insidious development. Narrow-angle (also called closed-angle or acute-angle) glaucoma can cause intermittent symptoms, consisting of head and eye pain, colored halos around lights, and decreased visual acuity. Once the condition reaches the point that fluid drainage from the eye is completely occluded, the resulting rapid increase in intraocular pressure is considered a medical emergency and can cause blindness within 24 to 36 hours if aggressive therapy is not instituted. In the acute stage, the patient experiences severe eye pain, decreased vision, and nausea and vomiting. Treatment includes medications to increase fluid drainage, reduce fluid in the eye, and control the pain and nausea, followed by surgery to open the angle and achieve normal intraocular pressure.

In open-angle glaucoma, the course of the disease is much longer, but the lack of symptoms is a serious threat. If diagnosed and treated through the use of medications, the disease and destruction to the optic nerve can be arrested or slowed, thus preserving the remaining sight.

The key to diagnosis is routine testing for glaucoma past the age of 40. The tonometry test is a simple measurement of the intraocular pressure of the eye, which should be conducted at least annually for persons with a family history of glaucoma and at routine eye examinations for all others.

Age-related macular degeneration. Age-related macular degeneration, also known as senile macular degeneration, is the leading cause of blindness for persons over 65 years of age, with an 11% occurrence of the disease in this age group (National Institute on Aging, 1987; Carnevali & Patrick, 1986). The macula, the part of the retina that controls the sharpness of central vision, loses it function, possibly related to decreased blood supply. The disease generally affects both eyes and results in symptoms of darkened and/or distorted vision and loss of color vision. The individual gradually loses the ability to see clearly enough to engage in the normal daily activities that require central vision. The remaining peripheral vision can be utilized to assist the individual to maintain some independence and performance of necessary function. Medical treatment for macular degeneration is limited, but some success is being achieved with the use of laser treatments to halt or slow the course of the disease. Early diagnosis and treatment is critical as the disease can progress rapidly.

Hearing Disorders

Although the loss of hearing in women is primarily due to the age-related changes previously described, rather than specific disease processes, changes in hearing warrant medical evaluation if they become pronounced. Such evaluation should include audiology testing to determine the type and extent of loss. The normal aging losses of presbycusis can be accompanied by hearing problems such as vascular changes, tumors, effects of certain drugs on hearing, or other disease or environmental factors causing hearing damage. Medical intervention may be helpful in controlling causes other than age-related changes.

Whatever the source of the hearing loss, women should be encouraged to seek assistance through the use of hearing aids to improve their ability to hear. The powerful influence of hearing deficits on one's ability to communicate and interact with the environment should not be neglected. When hearing losses are allowed to progress, they can be the precipitating factor for a variety of psychological and social problems ranging from embarrassment, withdrawal, social isolation, fear, and paranoia to an inability to test reality. Boredom and loss of self-esteem are also serious problems, along with the high risk of loss of safety, due to inability to hear alarms or other signals warning of danger.

THE FUTURE

By 2010, the average female life expectancy is expected to be 86.1 years and the number of women over 85 will more than double (Older Women's League, 1987). In the U.S. census projections for 2010, 13.8% of the population will be over age 65; this segment of the population is expected to continue to grow to 20% by the year 2025 (National Institute on Aging, 1987). In the 15-year period between 2010 and 2025, a marked increase in the elderly will occur as the baby boom population reaches retirement age. Hewitt and Howe (1988) provide an overview of the staggering growth of the aged population between 1986 and 2040, when those aged 65 to 74 will increase by 85%, those aged 80 and over will increase by 300% to 400% and those 90 and over will increase by 500% to 700%. With this increased longevity, the average woman can expect to spend as many years caring for a dependent parent as for a dependent child (Older Women's League, 1987). The major physical health concerns of older women today will undoubtedly continue as the major causes of disability and death in the future. They should serve as the targets for the development of future health services. This picture of health concerns can be changed only through increased attention to health promotion and disease prevention as well as the needed changes in the health care of women who experience disease.

While there are some differences projected between women who are elderly now and those who will be in the future, there are general trends that can be expected to persist:

1. There is a likelihood that women will continue to be alone for a significant proportion of their later years.
2. There will be difficulty obtaining health insurance after being widowed because of existing physical health problems and the high cost of individual policy rates, since access to group health insurance generally is tied to employment.
3. If public policy changes are not made, women will continue to face economic hardships, related to costs for long-term care, preventive screening, medications, and other services not currently covered under Medicare, Medicaid, or private insurance.
4. There will be a continual growth in the need for home health care services as the number of disabled elderly increases.
5. There will be an increased drain on the physical, economic, and psychological resources and well-being of younger women (young-old), as they are required to serve as caretakers and/or providers for the increasing numbers of frail older family members.

The physical disorders occurring with aging cause women to need illness-oriented services, but many of the diseases they develop could be prevented or lessened in severity through health promotion and early detection services. Multiple conditions have been identified for which screening could achieve these outcomes: smoking, hypertension, ischemic heart disease, rheumatic heart disease, stroke, tuberculosis, hyperlipidemia, obesity, cancer of the colon and rectum, syphilis, chronic open-angle glaucoma, breast cancer, alcoholism, and cancer of the cervix.

Services to address the health needs of aging women must take social, economic and environmental variables into account and must interface with other community resources to maximize achievement of increased levels of wellness, decreased severity in illness, and more effective use of remaining capabilities when disability occurs. As women become more aware of their rights and political power, they can intensify the current demands of older women for a health care system that is free of gender and age bias and one that protects and promotes their health, rather than treating only episodic illness and disease.

For many of the physical diseases afflicting aged women, health-promotion services targeted on life-style modifications could impact both disease occurrence and progression. Areas for primary emphasis include nutrition, exercise, more effective stress management, smoking cessation, and reduction of alcohol consumption and other risk factors for many physical health concerns of women. The development of health-promotion programs should emphasize early initiation of life styles that can decrease women's risk for many chronic, acute, and fatal diseases (Abdellah, 1985). Similarly, such programs should focus on the total context of health, including the effect of social, cultural, environmental, and public policy issues, with the goal of assisting the aged to increase control over their own health.

Assessments are needed concerning the kinds of personal, social, physical, and economic support that would give older women the option to remain in the home and maintain their autonomy while still receiving the care they need. Home-care programs, such as visiting nurse, mutual help groups or congregate living arrangements, might enable the older woman to remain at home and maintain autonomy while at the same time contain health care costs.

Because of the high costs of institutionalization and of out-of-home services, financial and service incentives for families providing care to older women should be considered. As Glasse and Leonard (1988) have noted, our current systems of care and public policy are "heavily dependent on the exploitation of unpaid caregiving in the home," since female relatives provide 72% of these functions. Because many females are now working, they may be unable to continue the home care of the elderly at a time that the numbers of those needing care are growing faster than those able to provide it.

The need for future research on aging women and health is of utmost importance. Research on health-related issues has traditionally been undertaken with male subjects or has not differentiated findings in relation to gender or age. Such deficits generate difficulties in the efforts to design and implement health care programs for women that are based on scientific data and rationale.

Future research should address a wide scope of topics that can be grouped in several major categories: (1) accessibility, utilization, and economic barriers to use of health care services; (2) types of services that would yield optimal outcomes for women's health in the areas of promotion, disease prevention, early detection, treatment, and rehabilitation; (3) types of health care providers who could provide necessary health activities in the most cost-effective manner; (4) treatment and prevention of diseases that specifically increase the mortality and morbidity of aging women; and (5) increased studies of the effect of environment and life styles on the maintenance of health and progression of disease in women.

CONCLUSION

The future will see the older woman as an important consumer of health care services whose unique needs will demand consideration. It is imperative that the unique characteristics and health concerns of the older woman be addressed in the design of health care services and in the development of research priorities.

REFERENCES

Abdellah, F. G. (1985). The aged woman and the future of health care delivery. In Haug, M., Ford, E., & Sheafor, M. (Eds.), *The physical and mental health of elderly women* (pp. 254-258). New York: Springer.

Binstock, R. H. (1985). The oldest old: A fresh perspective on ageism revisited. *Milbank Memorial Fund Quarterly Health and Society, 63*, 420-451.

Carnevali, D. L., & Patrick, M. (1986). *Nursing management for the elderly* (2nd ed.). Philadelphia: Lippincott.

Carter, M. A. (1986). Rheumatic disorders. In S. Price, & L. Wilson. (Eds.), *Pathophysiology: Clinical concepts of disease processes* (3rd ed.). New York: McGraw-Hill.

Ebersole, P. & Hess, P. (1981). *Toward healthy aging*. St. Louis: Mosby.

Gioiella, E. C., & Bevil, C. W. (1985). *Nursing care of the aging client*. Norwalk, CT: Appleton-Century-Crofts.

Glasse, L., & Leonard, F. (1988). Policy from the older woman's perspective. *Generations, 12,* 57-59.

Hewitt, P., & Howe, N. (1988). Generational equity and the future of generational politics. *Generations, 12,* 10-13.

Kenney, R. A. (1982). *Physiology of aging.* Chicago: Year Book.

Lindsay, R. (1987). The aging skeleton. In Haug, M., Ford, E. & Sheafor, M. (Eds.), *The physical and mental health of elderly women.* New York: Springer.

Luckman, J., & Sorenson, K. (1987). *Medical surgical nursing: A psychophysiologic approach.* Philadelphia: W.B. Saunders.

McKeever, L., & Martinson, I. (1986). Older women's health care. In Kjervik, D., & Martinson, I. (Eds.), *Women in health & illness.* Philadelphia: W.B. Saunders.

National Institute on Aging. (1987). *The aging woman.* Washington, DC: U.S. Department of Health, Education, and Welfare.

Older Women's League. (1987). The picture of health for mid-life and older women in America. *Mother's Day Report.* Washington, DC: Author.

Soldo, B., & Manton, K. (1985). Health status and service needs of the oldest old: Current patterns and future trends. *Milbank Memorial Fund Quarterly Health and Society, 63,* 286-319.

Woods, N. F. (1985). New models for women's health care. *Health Care Women International, 6,* 193-208.

Mental Health of Elderly Women

Cornelia M. Beck, PhD, RN
Barbara P. Pearson, RN, MN

The mental health of elderly women has only recently become a focus of study and public concern, so the amount of knowledge specific to this area is limited. Therefore, much of what is presented here is an extrapolation of information from the literature on women and mental health and the literature about the aged and mental health.

A brief historical overview of mental health of aging women will be presented, followed by information on the incidence of mental illness in aged women and their utilization of mental health services. Then several factors influencing older women's mental health will be addressed. Finally, some of the major mental health problems of elderly women will be discussed.

HISTORICAL OVERVIEW

Freud, in commenting on mental health problems in the elderly, advised that psychotherapy was not useful with people over 50 years of age because of the inelasticity of their mental processes and their ineducability. It was not until 1950 that Segal published the first clinical material describing analytic sessions with an elderly client. In the 1960s, Melanie Klein published theoretical formulations on the normal psychological adaptation of the elderly. During

Cornelia M. Beck is Professor, College of Nursing, and Assistant Professor, Department of Psychiatry, College of Medicine, University of Arkansas for Medical Sciences, Little Rock, AR 72205.

Barbara P. Pearson is Professor, College of Nursing, University of Arkansas for Medical Sciences, Little Rock, AR 72205.

the 1970s the federal government began to focus more attention on the unique problems of the elderly, but little concern was given to mental health problems. Finally, at the Third White House Conference on Aging in 1981, the American Psychiatric Association and the Committee on Long-term Care recommended that mental health be an integral part of a comprehensive health and social service program. Since that time, the federal government has concentrated more on the mental health problems of the elderly.

Recently, there is evidence that attention is now being paid to the unique mental health problems of elderly women. For example, at a 1987 conference sponsored by the National Institute on Aging, it was concluded that few behavioral scientists have focused on gender differences in the aged (Holden, 1987) and that study needs to be directed to this area. Two issues that are now beginning to be addressed are the incidence of mental illness in elderly women and their utilization of mental health services.

INCIDENCE AND MENTAL HEALTH SERVICES UTILIZATION

A long-standing contention in the literature on mental health and aging is that older persons have a greater incidence of mental disorders and a greater need for mental health services than other age groups. However, this notion has recently come into question (Biliwise, McCall, & Swan, 1987) as there is increasing cumulative evidence that mental health problems are related to factors other than age. In contrast to earlier reports of a 10% to 15% incidence of psychiatric syndromes in elderly persons, recent community epidemiologic studies report the incidence to be only 4% to 5% (George, Blazer, Winfield-Laird, Leaf, & Eischback, 1987).

Because mental disorders frequently are related to low income, widowhood, and social isolation, it is a reasonable assumption that older females would be particularly vulnerable to developing psychiatric illnesses. However, despite the fact that more women than men are widowed and many elderly women have considerably lower incomes and live alone, these vulnerabilities do not appear to be manifested in an impaired psychological status relative to their impaired male counterparts.

Feinson (1987) reviewed 14 community mental studies from the years 1958 to 1985 that address psychological impairment and gender in older adults. She concluded that there is lack of consistent evidence of more psychological impairment among older females than males. She offers several explanations for the lack of gender differences in mental health in the older population. First, in the later years, female and male roles become more similar than dissimilar. Second, older women and men become more similar than different in terms of control and power. Men may feel as if they have lost control (and status) when they retire from the workforce. Thus, they may be more similar to women who have felt a sense of powerlessness because of their female roles. Third, women may accumulate more positive coping strategies than men as they age and thus have an improvement in their mental health, again making them more similar to men in the later years.

It has long been acknowledged that women of any age seek mental health care more than men (Milazzo-Sayre et al., 1987). This higher utilization by women has been linked to sex bias, disadvantaged status, and current diagnostic definitions (Carmen, Russo, & Miller, 1981). On the other hand, the underutilization of mental health services by the elderly is well supported in the literature. Causative factors in this underutilization emerge from the perspective of the provider and the consumer. Health care providers may see the older person as too old for treatment of mental health problems and frequently fail to detect psychiatric problems in the elderly. The elderly may not seek care because of their negative perceptions about mental health problems and the ability of mental health professionals to assist them in resolving their problems.

Data on the utilization of mental health services by older women is limited. Kaas' (1987) review of data from the 1985 National Ambulatory Medical Care Survey (National Center for Health Statistics, 1987) and the 1985 National Hospital Discharge survey indicates the following:

1. Only 4.6% of all psychiatric office-based visits were made by women 65 years and older.
2. Of all people who made office-based physician visits for a principal diagnosis of a mental disorder, 6.7% were made by

women 65 years of age and over as compared with older men who made 3.5% of these types of visits.

3. Older women accounted for 8% of all psychiatric drug visits (those psychiatric visits in which at least one drug was prescribed) and 8.08% of the physicians' office visits that were precipitated by psychological and mental symptoms.

Kaas (1987) used a grounded theory research approach to explore how older women defined mental health, how they determined their own mental health, and how they took care of their mental health. After analyzing interviews with 30 community-living women who were 55 to 86 years old, Kaas (1987) found that older women use a comparing process to define their mental health; that is, they compare their mental health with their own prior experiences and that of others. They then identify ways in which they can manage their mental health. In addition, the language that older women use to define their mental health is not like the terminology used by the professionals. That is, older women do not identify themselves as having a mental illness, even when they clinically exhibit symptoms of psychiatric disorder. They see themselves as "going through a bad time." Therefore, the older woman is not likely to seek mental health care because she does not define herself as having a mental health problem. Mental health professionals need to adjust the language used to describe mental health problems to terminology that is more meaningful to the older woman. For example, instead of "depression," words like "having downspells" or "going through a bad time" might be used.

Kaas (1987) also found that the older women in her study generally managed their mental health alone and did not seek professional help unless absolutely necessary. Health care providers need to assess and to encourage the mental health management practices that the older woman has developed and those that fit within her definition of mental health. Before seeking professional care, the older woman has usually talked to her family and friends about her problems and has exhausted her repertoire of strategies for managing her situation alone.

SOCIAL SUPPORT

Literature on the epidemiology of mental illness clearly indicates that there is a strong correlation between an individual's social support and the likelihood that that person will develop mental illness. Although no research was found that specifically addressed this correlation in older women, it seems reasonable to assume that this same relationship would hold true.

For many older women, their family is a major component of their social support network. In one national study, 54% of noninstitutionalized American women over 65 had seen their children on the preceding day and 79% had seen a child within the preceding week. Those women who were over 80 were more likely to see their children than those who were younger, probably because when women become very old they are more likely to move in with their children or to an apartment or nursing home near one of the children (National Institute on Aging and National Institute of Mental Health, 1979).

Rathbone-McCuan and Hashimi (1982) caution that an older woman who moves in with a child's family may become isolated if she does not strive to, or is not allowed to, attain a personally appropriate balance between independence and dependence. This means that the older woman may need to learn how to make decisions without relying on a family member to make them. She needs to select activities that broaden her social network to ensure personal growth and maintain mental health. She also needs to maintain a life style that allows her personal freedom, even at the expense of making family members uncomfortable because she is trying to be "too independent."

Since a motivating force for a large proportion of women has been what is good for other people, rather than a focus on self, the older woman may need to be resocialized to develop goals for herself instead of defining her goals only as they are linked to the goals of others. Within the limits of health and economic restrictions, older women need to be encouraged to act with a sense of self that is not totally influenced by a sense of family (Rathbone-McCuan & Hashimi, 1982) and to develop social supports outside of their family network.

ROLE TRANSITIONS

The role transitions that older women experience are often sources of stress that lead to mental health problems. Widowhood and retirement are two major role transitions. Widowhood is a predictable life event for a married woman's later years and is considered the most isolating of crisis events associated with marriage. Mortality rates are higher among the recently widowed. The bereaved have also been found to have more frequent serious physical illnesses, general malaise, including dizziness and fainting, and more mental health problems, particularly grief. The older woman's loss of a marriage partner inevitably results in grief. However, there is great individual variability among widows in the duration of grieving and in how they cope with the psychological and economic effects of widowhood.

To carry out the work of grieving, widows need permissive support from family and friends. If they are supportive in accepting the widow, in allowing her to talk about her reaction to her loss and about her relationship with her husband, she will be better able to cope with her grief. Through provision of the opportunity to express and share her thoughts and feelings, the widow will be better able to resolve her grief. If the widow is successful in coping with her loss, she will be able to make the adjustment to the challenging role changes necessitated by becoming a single person (Rathbone-McCuan & Hashimi, 1982).

However, there is some research that indicates there is a time after a woman is widowed when personal networks fail. This occurs when married friends and children go back to their daily lives and the widow is left alone to deal with her problems. More information is needed about the timing and process of such events in widowhood (National Institute on Aging and National Institute of Mental Health, 1979).

The older widow may have persistent recall of past intimacy with a spouse to the extent that it blocks her from developing effective social interactions. The unresolved grief can be manifested as an avoidance mechanism; the woman may surround herself with memories of her husband and their past life together to avoid developing new relationships. In cases where the woman lacks the ability to structure opportunities to meet and interact with both men and women, this avoidance behavior may be a form of adaptation. In such cases, the older woman would benefit from having the opportunity to learn new social skills, such as those that can be developed in social skills training programs for widows (Rathbone-McCuan & Hashimi, 1982).

A number of research studies indicate that older women find the adjustment to loss of the spouse less stressful than either younger women or men at any age (Gatz, Pearson, & Fuentes, 1984). This may be explained by the fact that the socialization of women often allows for more intimate, affectional, interpersonal behavior. This prior socialization may provide women with greater access to intimate and affectionate bonds in old age. Recent network analysis research supports this view and has found that older women meet socialization needs through friends and obtain most services from children and neighbors (National Institute on Aging and National Institute of Mental Health, 1979).

It has also been suggested that older women have had many opportunities in their lives to synthesize conflicting role demands and therefore have developed a resiliency to role change. This may allow women to view widowhood as a transition that involves a future, as well as a past, rather than simply as a loss. With this focus, the future can be envisioned as encompassing new possibilities available for the rest of one's life (Gatz, Pearson, & Fuentes, 1984).

Data on the retirement of women indicates that women may experience more distress after retirement than men and thus be more likely to develop mental illness (Atchley, 1976; Fox, 1977). Levy (1980-1981) reported that women who did not want to retire expressed discontent and depression to an extent not true for men. However, married women may adjust to retirement more easily because they are more likely to have had an impermanent work history for childrearing reasons (Robinson, 1986). The older woman who retires can also be required to adapt to her husband's retirement plans, which may have been made without consideration of her needs, creating another source of emotional stress.

Women can be negatively affected during this transition period by what the husband anticipates and experiences before and during retirement and the degree to which these elements are shared and/or change the usual pattern of their lives. If there is reduced income, the woman may be prevented from continuing her previous life style or she may develop a dread of poverty. If the wife is involved in meaningful social relationships beyond the dyad of husband and wife, these may conflict with the increasing demands the retired husband can make because of his loss of social relationships in previous work roles. Thus the wife may have to give up part or all of her social world to meet the relational needs of the retired spouse (Turner, 1979).

LONELINESS

A 1981 Harris Poll indicated that 10% of those 65 and older believed that loneliness was a very serious problem for them and the majority of these were women. Although living alone does not necessarily equate with loneliness, it should be noted that more elderly women live alone than any other subgroup of the population and the proportion of those maintaining their own households is increasing. Other examples of situations that might lead to loneliness or isolation are the older woman caring for a demented spouse who no longer calls her by name, the nursing home resident who sees many persons who no longer care or call her by her name, or the woman who has been victimized by thieves or muggers and is fearful of traveling too far from home (Harper, 1985).

Widowhood and bereavement can also lead to loneliness, isolation, and depression and the potential for isolation appears to increase with age (National Institute of Mental Health, 1987). It is important that mental health professionals recognize that the loneliness of widows is very complex and therefore sometimes not easily overcome. Lopato (1983) found in studying widows that a widow missed the man who was her love object; she missed being the love object, being important to somebody; she missed having someone who thought what she said was important; she missed her companion; her escort; someone with whom to organize time.

ANGER

Since many older women grew up in environments where it was not considered feminine to express their anger, they may tend to hide any feelings of anger. They may be unable to accept that they feel anger because they have learned to suppress it. They may talk about their anger only indirectly, for example, in complaints about food, relatives, or various world events.

However, some women may be more apt to express their anger in their later years than at other stages in their lives. They may become less inhibited with age, possibly because of hormonal changes, or their defenses may not be as effective in helping them control their anger.

DEPRESSION

A review of studies on the incidence of depression in women and more specifically in older women reveals that there are many contradictory findings. A recent document on aging women from the National Institute on Aging (1987) states that women at any age are about twice as likely as men to become depressed and older people in general are about twice as likely as younger people to become depressed. Thus depression is thought by many to be the single most pressing problem affecting the mental health of older women. However, some researchers are suggesting that rates are no higher among elderly women than among younger women (Holzer, Leaf, & Weismann, 1985; Newman, 1984). Many older women who have experienced depression at a younger age continue to experience depression later in life, a relatively small number of women experience depression for the first time after the age of 65 (Holzer, Leaf, & Weissman, 1985).

One reason that the exact prevalence of depression among elderly women is not well known is that the elderly are often excluded from many community psychiatric surveys and few studies have looked at gender differences in the aged for depressive disorders. Also, scales used to measure depression are often heavily weighted on physical symptoms that may be produced in the absence of depression by the physical changes and illness so often experienced by the aged (Blazer & Williams, 1980).

Issues related to the etiology of depression in elderly women also need increased attention. The loss and isolation of elderly women place them at psychological risk for reactive depression, and the social changes that accompany aging usually compound depressive responses. The sociocultural milieu of older women defined their major social role as reproduction and nurturance and transmission of values to the next generation. Once that work is done, they may be perceived as, and believe themselves to be, socially redundant, with few hopeful options (Gatz, Pearson, & Fuentes, 1984).

Holzer, Leaf, and Weissman (1985) presented data on the risk factors for depression from a study of 23 elderly women. They found a higher prevalence of depression for the separated or divorced than for the widowed or single woman. In examining the association between living arrangements and depression for elderly females, they found that 51% of the respondents lived alone. The lowest prevalence of depression was found for those living with a spouse.

It has been suggested that the way the elderly manifest their depression may be different from younger persons. For example, an older adult's depression is more often characterized by apathy, listlessness, memory loss and somatic complaints, such as insomnia and appetite disturbance (Gatz, Pearson, & Fuentes, 1984). Holzer, Leaf, and Weissman (1985) raised the question of whether the phenomenon of depression as experienced by elderly women is different from the depression experienced by younger women. In an effort to answer this question, they studied the symptom profiles exhibited by younger women, older women whose first depression episode was earlier in life, and older women whose first depressive episode was after age 65. They found a general similarity among the symptom profiles of these three groups. This suggests that depression for elderly females is much the same process as depression among younger women and that there is no evidence for a special set of mechanisms being operative among elderly female respondents. They suggested that depression in elderly females is very much an extension of the depressive process experienced by younger females.

It is important to distinguish symptomatology from actual mental illness. Some of what is diagnosed as mental illness may be an appropriate reaction to an unhappy situation. For older women, there may be an existential component in what is called depression and this may be a part of an adaptational process.

Depression may be misdiagnosed and mistaken for untreatable senile dementia, called "pseudo-dementia." The mental changes caused by an underlying depression may be mistaken for a true loss of mental capacity. If the depression remains undiagnosed, the mental decline, which began as something treatable, might never be improved.

Despite the notion prevalent in the past that the elderly could not benefit as much as younger persons from psychotherapy, studies of the efficacy of treatment for depression suggest that the elderly may be as responsive as younger persons to a variety of treatments (Holzer, Leaf, & Weissman, 1985).

SUICIDE

The rates for suicide in women peak in the 45-50 age range and then steadily decline, whereas men show a direct linear increase to age 75 (Stenback, 1980). Suicide rates are dramatically lower for women at all ages, but some see trends for increases among older women (Butler & Lewis, 1982). Studies have confirmed that women make more attempts at suicide than men, but men complete their attempts more often. It has also been found that the elderly are usually successful in carrying out their suicide plans. They use methods that are more likely to be fail-proof. However, it is not known whether or not elderly women are more successful than their younger counterparts in their suicidal attempts (Block, Davidson, Grambs, & Serock, 1978).

Marital problems seem to be a significant factor in the suicide rate of older women, as they are in depression. Although widowhood has been directly associated with suicide, widows and wives do not seem to differ significantly in suicidal rate. It has been suggested that women who have strong attachments to people will be less likely to commit suicide than those who have no close associations. Physical health is also directly linked to suicide in older women. Older women may choose suicide so that they die while they are still physically and mentally able to make decisions; this is especially true if they are facing a debilitating terminal illness and are alone. They may consider suicide as a way to rejoin deceased loved ones and frequently choose the anniversary date of an important loss for a suicide attempt. Even when they have been taught that suicide is wrong, their guilt feelings may be overcome by a strong belief that they have a right to choose when and how to die (Beck, 1988).

Some elderly persons are not even aware of their own tendency to injure themselves; this has been called subintentional suicide. This self-destructive behavior may be seen in the older woman who finds it impossible to deal with widowhood and dies shortly after the spouse's death. It may also occur among elderly women who are placed in a nursing home. Signs of self-destructive tendencies often seen in the elderly are injuries such as accidental falls, unusual weight problems, heavy smoking, failure to plan for and get proper medical treatment, refusing to eat, refusing medication, or not taking care of other physical needs. Drug abuse and alcoholism are also signals of the older woman's desire to destroy herself.

COGNITIVE IMPAIRMENT

Although mental decline is not a part of normal aging, deterioration in brain function, known as dementia, occurs more frequently with aging. In fact, cognitive impairment is thought to be the primary mental health problem of older people. The rate of mild cognitive impairment is 14% for both women and men; the rate for severe impairment is 3% for females and 5.6% for males (U.S. Congress, 1987).

Cognitive impairment is one of the principal reasons for institutionalization of the elderly. It is estimated that about half of the elderly living in long-term care institutions are there because they were diagnosed as senile, and the diagnosis is not always justified. Too frequently a mistaken diagnosis is made because physicians and families attribute mental decline and behavioral change caused by physical conditions to senility and fail to initiate appropriate and timely treatment. The mental confusion of aged women, often attributed to senility, can be managed if they have access to continuing, well-informed services of health care professionals and patient education (Abdellah, 1985).

Dementia can have multiple causes, some of which are reversible. The two primary causes of dementia are Alzheimer's disease and multi-infarct dementia. Alzheimer's disease accounts for approximately 54% of all cases of dementia with multi-infarct dementia or a combination of the two accounting for the rest (Weiler, 1987).

Alzheimer's disease affects more women than men, primarily because the majority of its victims are over age 80, an age at which women outnumber men by nearly two to one. Multi-infarct dementia is more commonly encountered in men than women (Kermis, 1986). The major predisposing factors associated with multi-infarct dementia seem to be arterial hypertension and emboli originating from vascular disease of the great vessels of the neck and vascular disease of the heart (American Psychiatric Association, 1987). Persons with multi-infarct dementia have many of the same symptoms as Alzheimer's patients. However, in multi-infarct dementia, there is a stepwise deteriorating course with "patchy" distribution of deficits (i.e., affecting some functions, but not others). In Alzheimer's disease there is a steady declining pattern with a multifaceted loss of abilities.

ALCOHOL AND DRUG ABUSE

About two-thirds of older alcoholics become addicted before age 50 and about one-third become alcoholics later. Women tend to become alcoholics later in life as their children leave home and the realities of old age begin to surface. The older woman who is an alcoholic receives less understanding and acceptance than the alcoholic man and is therefore more likely to be a hidden alcoholic and difficult to identify (White House Mini-Conference on Older Females, 1981). Groups of women especially vulnerable to alcohol and drug abuse are (1) isolated and depressed women who live alone; (2) women in unhappy marriages; (3) women institutionalized in nursing homes and psychiatric settings; and (4) the non-

English-speaking who are culturally isolated and those lacking the resources to enter treatment programs (Russo, 1985).

Even if they had the financial resources, some women would have difficulty entering a treatment program or facility because of their responsibilities for the care of others. Those who approach facilities as potential clients are often rejected by counselors because younger people are assumed to have better recovery potential. If women do enter treatment facilities, they find that the services provided them are generally oriented toward male clients (Russo, 1985) and the problems of younger persons.

Older women are at high risk for drug abuse. This is partially due to the fact that tranquilizers and antidepressants are promoted as the first and unfailing solution to women's depression and anxiety. Women consume 70% of prescribed tranquilizers and 72% of prescribed antidepressants (White House Mini-Conference on Older Females, 1981). White elderly woman comprise only 6% of the population, yet they receive 17% of the prescriptions for the major tranquilizer Thorazine, 17% of those for the antidepressant Elavil, and 20% of the prescriptions for sedatives written in the United States (Jones-Witters & Witters, 1983).

The physiological absorption and excretion patterns for drugs taken by women 65 and over is much slower and the effects often lead to unanticipated drug interactions (Abdellah, 1985). These drugs also tend to be prescribed at too high a dose for older people and therefore have even more potential for serious side effects. The side effects can then be mistakenly interpreted as physical or mental illnesses.

ELDER ABUSE

The phenomenon of elder abuse has received increasing attention and it is estimated that as high as 10% of the elderly nationwide are affected by abuse. Physical abuse is the most prevalent form reported, although psychological abuse may actually be the most prevalent. Many cases involve more than one type of abuse and the abuse is usually not confined to a single incident (Sengstock & Barrett, 1984).

Older women are more likely to be abused and account for 75%

of the reported cases. The victim usually has some physical impairment and is often physically and emotionally dependent on the person who abuses. The individual who abuses is most likely the victim's caretaker and usually a close relative. Since women are more frequently in the role of caretaker, the person who abuses is often a daughter or other female relative who is under a great deal of stress that is usually precipitated by long-term medical or financial problems.

THE FUTURE

If the mental health care needs of elderly women are to be met in the future, it is important that health care providers be educated about the particular needs of elderly women and that services be designed to meet these needs. Traditional mental health models of intervention place the burden of change on the older woman, while simultaneously implying that she lacks the power for constructive change (Gatz, Pearson, & Fuentes, 1984). It has been suggested that a shift in focus from direct services to self-help/support groups not only serves more people, but also decreases the economic and social costs that would accrue from serving women individually. The economic costs of developing social support networks are minimal in comparison with direct service, and the social stigma associated with becoming a patient in the mental health system is virtually nonexistent for the participant in a support group (Rickel, Gerrard, & Iscoe, 1984). Levy (1981) has argued that older women have a special need to be helped in creating social networks. Self-help is an approach particularly compatible with a feminist perspective and has the potential of improving both physical and mental health status.

Self-help groups can be organized outside the formal structure of any human service organization and directed toward dealing with a wide spectrum of problems that a number of older women encounter. The best-known examples are based on self-help for widows. Other types of groups are appearing across the country with other problem foci, including older women who are providing caregiving functions for older spouses or whose husbands are institutionalized, those who are experiencing dislocation, and those who are victims of violence and exploitation. Banding together for mutual support and sharing services has been found to be a determining factor in the mental health of those caring for disabled spouses, a problem that also results in deterioration of physical health (Crossman, London, & Barry, 1981).

The community-based voluntary association alternative is one of the major conceptual and programmatic cornerstones of the aging network and its approach to isolation (Estes, 1979). Significant numbers of older women find meaningful social connectedness through involvement in volunteer activities. There are literally thousands of volunteer programs operating throughout the United States that are staffed solely by older women. The volunteer role is one that is traditionally compatible with older women's previous socialization and is linked to family and nurturing functions. Such volunteer associations could also be utilized for health promotion, disease detection, and rehabilitation programs, in association with health professionals (Rathbone-McCuan & Hashimi, 1982).

In the promotion of social support, it is very important that we distinguish between social support and creating an overdependency and lack of autonomy. Social support must be aimed at assisting the older woman to maintain her independence and functional abilities and enhance her dignity and self-esteem (Harper, 1985). It is also important that funding for women's self-help support groups be considered because standard health insurance does not currently reimburse these services.

Some non-Western countries have been innovative in finding alternatives to the isolation and loneliness of the older woman and the issue of care once aging results in decreased physical capacities or disease. In Liberia, West Africa, the middle-aged women have organized cooperatives for their parents. Cooperatives for agriculture, health education, or literacy classes, for example, permit the older women to remain socially useful and productive. In several countries, older women with larger houses adopt a younger family who moves in and shares expenses and pledges to care for the older woman when she becomes frail. In China, several older women without children will move in with young couples. The older woman will help with the childrearing and other domestic functions. In return, the young couple pledges to care for the older woman in her frail days.

It has also been projected that the changing sex roles will have an adverse effect on the number of women who will become alcoholics in the future. Because of the high costs of institutionalization and of out-of-home services, financial and service incentives for families providing care to older women should be considered.

Research is also needed to determine whether the apparent underservice of mental health problems represents a choice by older people, lack of access, provision of inappropriate services by providers, or other factors. Studies are particularly needed to examine special service needs of elderly women with severe mental illness (National Institute of Mental Health, 1987).

REFERENCES

Abdellah, F. G. (1985). The aged woman and the future of health care delivery. In M. R. Haug, A. B. Ford, & M. Sheafor (Eds.), *The physical and mental health of elderly women* (pp. 254-258). New York: Springer.

American Psychiatric Association. (1987). *Diagnostic and statistical manual of mental disorders* (4th ed.). Washington DC: Author.

Atchley, R. C. (1976). Selected social and psychological differences between men and women in later life. *Journal of Gerontology, 31,* 204-211.

Beck, C. (1988). The aged adult. In C. Beck, R. Rawlins, & S. Williams (Eds.), *Mental health-psychiatric nursing: A holistic-life cycle approach* (pp. 840-864). St. Louis: Mosby.

Biliwise, N. G., McCall, M. E., & Swan, S. J. (1987). The epidemiology of mental illness in late life. In E. E. Larie, & J. H. Swan (Eds.), *Serving the mentally ill elderly: Problems and prospectives.* Lexington, MA: Lexington Books.

Blazer, D., & Williams, C. D. (1980). Epidemiology of dysphoria and depression in an elderly population. *American Journal of Psychiatry, 137,* 439-444.

Block, M. R., Davidson, J. L., Grambs, J. D., & Serock, K. E. (1978). Unchartered territory: Issues and concerns of women over 40. Baltimore, MD: University of Maryland Press.

Butler, R. N., & Lewis, M. I. (1982). *Aging & mental health: Positive psychosocial and biomedical approaches* (3rd ed.). St. Louis: Mosby.

Carmen, E., Russo, N., & Miller, J. (1981). Inequality and women's mental health: An overview. *American Journal of Psychiatry, 138*(10), 1319-1330.

Crossman, L., London, C., & Barry, C. (1981). Older women caring for disabled spouses: A model for supportive services. *Gerontologist, 21,* 464-470.

Estes, C. R. (1979). *The aging enterprise.* San Francisco: Jossey-Bass.

Feinson, M. C. (1987). Mental health and aging: Are there gender differences? *Gerontologist, 27*(6), 703-711.

Fox, J. H. (1977). Effects of retirement and former work life on women's adaptation in old age. *Journal of Gerontology, 32,* 196-202.

Gatz, M., Pearson, C., & Fuentes, M. (1984). Older women and mental health. In A. U. Rickel, M. Gerrard, & I. Iscoe (Eds.), *Social and psychological problems of women: Prevention and crisis intervention.* Washington, DC: Hemisphere.

George, L. K., Blazer, D. G., Winfield-Laird, I., Leaf, P. G., & Eischbac, R. (1987). Psychiatric disorders and mental health service use in later life: Evidence from the Epidemiologic Catchment Area Program. In J. Brody & G. Maddox (Eds.), *Epidemiology in late life.* New York: Springer.

Harper, M. S. (1985). Older women: Family and community supports. Issues: The older woman alone — mental health of older women. *Kenya Nursing Journal, 13,* 15-24.

Holden, C. (1987). Why do women live longer than men? *Science, 238;* 158-160.

Holzer, C. E., Leaf, P. J., and Weissman, M. M. (1985). Living with depression. In M. R. Haug, A. B. Ford, & M. Sheafor (Eds.), *The physical and mental health of aged women* (pp. 101-116). New York: Springer.

Jones-Witters, P., & Witters, W. L. (1983). *Drugs and society: A biological perspective.* Monterey, CA: Woodsworth Health Sciences.

Kaas, M. J. (1987). Emotional referencing: The definition and management of mental health by older women, (University Microfilms) San Francisco: University of California (ADG87-23874).

Kermis, M. D. (1986). *Mental health in late life.* Boston, MA: Jones & Bartlett.

Levy, S. M. (1980-1981). The adjustment of older women: Effects of chronic ill health and attitudes toward retirement. *International Journal of Aging and Human Development, 12,* 93-110.

Levy, S. M. (1981). The aging woman: Developmental issues and mental health needs. *Professional Psychology, 12,* 92-100.

Lopato, H. Z. (1983, April). *Social change and older women's roles.* Paper presented at the Minnesota Gerontological Society Spring Conference, Brooklyn Park, MI.

Milazzo-Sayre, L. J., Benson, P. R., Rosenstein, M. J., & Manderscheld, R. W. (1987). *Use of inpatient psychiatric services by the elderly aged 65 and over, United States, 1980* (Mental health statistical note, No. 181). Hyattsville, MD: U.S. Department of Health and Human Services, National Institutes of Mental Health, Division of Biometry and Applied Sciences, Survey and Reports Branch.

National Center for Health Statistics (1987a). *1985 Summary: National Hospital Discharge Survey.* Unpublished data. Hyattsville, MD: U.S. Department of Health and Human Services, Public Health Service.

National Center for Health Statistics (1987b). *Utilization of short-stay hospitals: 1985 National Health Survey.* Unpublished data. Hyattsville, MD: U.S. Department of Health and Human Services, Public Health Service.

National Institute of Mental Health (1987). *Women's mental health: Agenda for research.* Washington, DC: U.S. Department of Health and Human Services.

National Institute on Aging. (1987). *Answers about the aging woman.* Washington, DC: U.S. Department of Health and Human Services.

National Institute on Aging and National Institute of Mental Health. (1979). *The older woman: Continuities and discontinuities*. Washington, DC: U.S. Department of Health, Education and Welfare.

Newman, J. P. (1984). Sex differences in symptoms of depression: Clinical disorder or normal distress? *Journal of Health and Social Behavior*, *25*, 136-159.

Rathbone-McCuan, E., & Hashimi, J. (1982). *Isolated elders*. Rockville, MD: Aspen.

Rickel, A. U., Gerrard, M., & Iscoe, I. (1984) *Social and psychological problems of women: Prevention and crisis intervention*. Washington, DC: Hemisphere.

Robinson, K. (1986). Older women: A literature review. *Journal of Advanced Nursing*, *11*, 153-160.

Russo, N. F. (Ed). (1985). *A women's mental health agenda*. Washington DC: American Psychological Association.

Sengstock M. C., & Barrett, S. (1984). Domestic abuse of the elderly. In J. Campbell & J. Humphreys (Eds.), *Nursing care of victims of family violence*. Englewood Cliffs, NJ: Prentice-Hall.

Stenback, A. (1980). Depression and suicidal behavior in old age. In J. E. Birren & R. B. Sloane (Eds.), *Handbook of mental health and aging*. Englewood Cliffs, NJ: Prentice-Hall.

Turner, B. (1979). The self-concepts of older women. *Research on Aging*, *1*, 218-243.

U.S. Congress, Office of Technology Assessment. (1987). *Losing a million minds: Confronting the tragedy of Alzheimer's disease and other dementias*, (OTA Publication No. OTA-BA-323). Washington, DC: U.S. Government Printing Office.

Weiler, P. G. (1987). The public health impact of Alzheimer's disease. *American Journal of Public Health*, *77*(9), 1157-1158.

White House Mini-Conference on Older Females (1981). (Report 720-019/6913). Washington DC: U.S. Government Printing Office.

A Minority-Feminist Perspective on Women and Aging

Ketayun H. Gould, PhD

In recent years, the elderly population in this country has been growing faster among minorities[1] than among whites. In 1980, 2.6 million persons, or 10% of the population 65 and over were non-white (Lowy, 1985, p. 28). By 2050, 19.7% of the elderly population are projected to be minorities (U.S. Bureau of the Census, 1984, pp. 41-94). Despite gains in civil rights, it is still true that many nonwhite elderly in this cohort will experience old age as the culmination of a lifetime of inequality and discrimination ("Symposium: Civil Rights," 1986).

Although these claims have increasingly affected our current interest in studying the minority aged, it is fair to state that up into the 1960s, most gerontological publications ignored racial and cultural variations in aging. In fact, "for many years prior to the mid-1960s,

Ketayun H. Gould is Professor, School of Social Work, University of Illinois at Urbana-Champaign, Champaign, IL 61820.

1. In this article, the terms *minority, ethnic minority,* and *nonwhite* refer to the following groups: black, Hispanic, Native American, and Asian and Pacific Islander.

195

most social gerontologists in the United States limited their research to white subjects'' (Jackson, 1985, p. 265). Since that time, a small but growing number of publications have begun to focus on the social status of aged minorities (e.g., Jackson, 1967; National Urban League, 1964). The trend, however, has fallen far short of covering the status of elderly minority women. In fact, in the early 1970s, the issues affecting *all* older women were essentially ignored in the two areas that should have revealed this concern – the literature on women and the literature on the elderly (Conable, 1986). Women's groups were addressing issues pertinent to young and middle-aged females – day care centers, abortion reform, discrimination in employment, and so forth. Lewis and Butler (1972) hit the nail on the head when they asked the following question: ''Why is a socially sensitive movement like women's liberation neglecting its older 'sisters,' leaving them to fend for themselves?''

Today, primarily as a result of consciousness raising by groups such as the Older Women's League and the National Coalition on Older Women's Issues, aging has now emerged as a major feminist issue. The burgeoning literature on elderly females reflects the fact that the scholarly world has paralleled the developments in society. But again (as demonstrated before in the literature on minority aged), elderly minority women seem to be the neglected research category. Thus, the literature on minority elderly does not provide breakdowns of data by sex, and the literature on older women does not included cross-classification of data by minority status. Somehow, because of the exclusivity of interests on the part of professionals, women and minority issues seem to be separated out for special consideration. As a result, the concerns of older ethnic-minority women are rarely addressed from a perspective that recognizes that racism and sexism interact to produce ''gender-specific race effects and race-specific gender effects''' (Smith & Stewart, 1983, p. 6). Moreover, ageism complicates the situation further by creating a particular kind of ''multiple jeopardy'' (Butler, 1975).

In view of these facts, this article proposes the development of a minority-feminist perspective (Gould, 1985) as an appropriate strategy to comprehend the social reality facing older nonwhite women. This perspective recognizes that racism, sexism, and ageism have to be viewed in an *interactive* framework to analyze the person-environment interaction of the older minority woman. The use of this model does not exclude the possibility of studying the independent effects of each of these "isms." It only asserts that part of the professional search to understand the oppressive features of society for older nonwhite females will be incomplete if an interactional framework is not recognized as a viable model for professional practice with this group.

Specifically, the article will first outline the available minority demographics related to elderly women to demonstrate the current state of the art—the database that can be used to assess the extent and parameters of specific problems. The background information will provide a framework to evaluate the physical and mental health status of older nonwhite females in its own context to avoid teaching about this group exclusively from a victimization perspective. This will be followed by an analysis of the discrepancy between needs and use of services, particularly the variables that might be related to delivery of services. Finally, this article will present a futuristic vision of what a minority-feminist perspective might contribute to this area of study.

MINORITY DEMOGRAPHICS: PROBLEMS

Before presenting the background information on nonwhite women, it might be instructive to outline some of the research problems that are evident in conducting a review of this literature. First, it is important to recognize that although there are many similarities in the various groups' experiences of discrimination because of minority status and sex, they are still members of distinctive subcultures that exhibit wide variations in strengths in adapting to old age. Often, the exclusive reliance on minority demographics has failed to clarify the bigger picture by taking account of minority differences and strengths. Of course, the same point can be made regarding the treatment of the "white" category (used for comparison with nonwhites) as if all white ethnics share similar characteristics regardless of class, culture, and generational factors (Cohler, 1982).

Second, the use of demographics in this area seems to be closely tied to answering the following question: Do the disadvantages of members of minority female groups increase with aging or is aging a great leveler of racial and sexual differences in this country? (National Institute on Aging, 1981). Jackson (1985) demonstrates that the answer to this question of "social aging" (investigation of age changes in statuses and roles) is elusive because of the general absence of ethnic minorities in longitudinal studies. Cross-sectional surveys, comparing minority and majority populations, might provide answers to whether older nonwhite females experience multiple jeopardies, but they do not permit a careful analysis of factors related to social aging. Jackson illustrates the point by showing that the differentials in income between elderly white and nonwhite women is not simply a function of race, but also of marital stability and wage histories. Thus, the interaction effects of race with period and cohort effects need to be taken into account in evaluating the question of social aging.

Furthermore, most research on on older ethnic minorities is not directed toward investigating sex differences within the population. The majority of these studies seem to present findings that document the major demographic differences between elderly blacks and whites, or between the dominant and minority populations. Therefore, the data on various groups of elderly nonwhite women that are presented in this paper are gleaned mainly from studies that use data from the 1980 United States Census of Population, or other primary or secondary sources that provide general information on ethnic minorities. The review of the literature further demonstrates that even when the information is available for older minority females, the studies focus solely on demographic differences between blacks, Hispanics, and whites. Data on Asian and Pacific Islanders and Native American elderly women are generally lacking, or are lumped into the category of "other" in the statistical analyses. Moreover, when data do exist, the information is largely inadequate. For example, Block (1979) describes the general problems of relying completely on census information on Native Americans. It seems that various agencies use different criteria to determine who is an Indian. Inaccuracies and undercounts are perennial problems when most data collection is done by non-Indians who do not speak the language and are unfamiliar with the location of Indian house-holds. Because of these gaps in information, at times the author had to resort to presenting general information on minorities and then try to extrapolate to the situation facing older nonwhite females.

POPULATION SIZES AND SEX RATIO

Among the 65 and older age category (almost 26 million persons in 1980), the white percentage (89.8%) was significantly higher than any of the minority groups: blacks (8.2%), Hispanics (2.8%), Asians and Pacific Islander (0.6%), and Native Americans (0.3%). Differences in age distribution of these groups reflect variations in their patterns of fertility, mortality, and immigration rates. Within each of the ethnic groups, the percentage of females age 65 and older as a proportion of the total number of females of all ages was as follows: blacks (8.9%), Hispanics (5.5%), Asian and Pacific Islander (6.0%), and Native Americans (5.8%). The only minority group where the numbers of the 65 and older population were higher for males than females (when the elderly were examined as a proportion of total number of males and females) was the Asian and Pacific Islander category: The numbers were 6.0% for females and 6.1% for males. This pattern reflects the influence of the excessive male immigration for this minority population during the early part of this century (Jackson, 1985, p. 272). In this context, it is interesting to note a societal stereotype. Although many authors (e.g., Kim, 1978; U.S. Commission on Civil Rights, 1980; Lee, 1985) have shown concern about the fact that the older Asian and Pacific Islander males are often isolated due to their early immigration patterns, the same concern has not been directed to examining the plight of spouseless, childless, elderly women (Goldberg, Kantrow, Kremen, & Lauter, 1986). Somehow, the societal assumption that females are more capable than males in managing their daily lives has affected professional judgment in determining which groups among the minority elderly are so disadvantaged that they need preferrential treatment (Gould, 1988).

The 1980 sex ratios (the number of males for every 100 females) for those over 65 years reveals a distinct female advantage throughout the analysis, by ethnicity. Moreover, the female advantage increases by age within each ethnic category. Thus, for blacks, the 1980 census figures show that there were 73.4 males for every 100 females aged 65 to 69, whereas for the Hispanics, Asian and Pacific Islanders, and Native Americans, the figures were 78.4, 96.6, and 82.6, respectively (Manuel & Reid, 1982, p. 36). Jackson (1971) has demonstrated that a major difference between blacks' and whites' sex ratio (80.4 for whites) is the greater presence of females compared to males for black persons under 70 years of age. For the advanced old-aged (over 85 years of age according to the 1980 census figures), a sex ratio crossover occurs between blacks and whites. Thus, the sex ratio for this age group was 42.9 among the whites and 50.0 among blacks (Manual & Reid, 1982, p 36). The "mortality selection thesis" of the crossover effect (Manton, 1982) explains the phenomenon by suggesting that the robust population of blacks who survive into advanced old age consist of a "survivor" population of both males and females. Therefore, the female advantage for this age group among blacks is pronounced but is not as substantial as among whites. The same pattern is revealed among Hispanics, Asian and Pacific Islanders, and Native Americans: Compared to the white sex ratio of 42.9 for the 85 and over age category, the figures for these three minority groups were 60.1, 61.3, and 64.5, respectively (Manuel & Reid, 1982, p. 36). This emphasis on the "survivor" factor among the minority advanced old aged should not, however, minimize the importance of recognizing that, reflective of the poor health of minorities, nonwhite females at birth can expect to live roughly three years less than white females. Even then, the general pattern changes by age 85, when minority females are expected to outlive nonminority women (National Center for Health Statistics, 1980).

At this point, it is worth reiterating that the variations among the older minority women (such as the sex ratios between the different minority groups among the 65-69 age category) should not be minimized. For example, the sex ratio among Asian and Pacific Islanders was 96.6 compared with the 73.4 ratio among blacks. As stated before, the higher ratio of Asian and Pacific Islanders can be explained by their particular immigration history, whereas the lower ratio of blacks reflects the greater mortality risks incurred by black males during the younger and middle years (Manuel & Reid, 1982, p. 37).

EDUCATIONAL AND ECONOMIC LEVELS

The 1980 census figures for the median number of years of formal education for each sex for the 65 and over age category reveal that minority women were typically slightly better educated than minority men (Jackson, 1985, p. 275). In order to put this finding in perspective, it is important, however, to examine whether the *general* educational level of each minority elderly group is significantly different than whites. For example, 6% of black elderly had no formal education in 1980, and only 17% had completed high school compared to 2% of whites who had no formal schooling and 41% who had completed 12 years of education (Agree, 1985). Thus, the educational level of today's black elderly reflect a history of discrimination in educational opportunities, and it is meaningless to put too much weight on the fact that minority females are slightly better educated than minority males. Moreover, it is important to remember that whereas nonwhite women may show a general trend of being slightly better educated than nonwhite men, their "better" educational preparation is not likely to overcome the multiple jeopardies that might prevent them from earning an income that is commensurate with their education. For example, Jackson (1985, p. 276) demonstrates that although the positive relationship between education and income that show up for white aged males is duplicated for black elderly men, poverty is almost as high among black elderly women with less than six years of schooling as among those who attended high school.

Agree (1985) also presents some data on educational levels for the other three minorities of color. Of all minority elderly, Hispanics reveal the least number of years of education. Of this group 16% have no formal education. In this respect, it is also interesting to examine the educational levels of Asian and Pacific Islander elderly, since the societal stereotypes of this minority group include a picture of high educational attainment that is not borne out by the data. In reality, 13% of this minority elderly group have no formal education compared to 1.6% of whites. For the Native Americans, although 12% of the elderly have no formal education, the quality of the education, both on and off reservations, is poor. Moreover, Manuel and Reid (1982, p. 39) have calculated that although the educational level of both the minority and nonminority elderly has improved since 1970, the gulf between the minority (for example, black) and nonminority aged has actually widened (1970-1979) by almost five percentage points among those with less than a high school education. It seems to this writer that with the preponderance of females among the nonwhite elderly (with a median educational level of less than nine years), the effects of differential accessibility to educational opportunities is not going to disappear in the next few decades (Jackson, 1985, p. 275).

Still, the most pronounced findings that demonstrate how racism, sexism, and ageism affect choices throughout the life cycle, are those related to the poverty status of nonwhite females. Older minority women constitute the poorest segment of American society. Agree (1985) provides data on median income for all races for the 65 and over age group, by sex. The median income of black elderly women ($2,825) is almost half the income of black aged males ($4,113). Comparable data are presented for the other three minorities of color: Hispanics ($2,873 for females versus $4,592 for males); Asian and Pacific Islanders ($3,476 for women compared with $5,551 for men); and Native Americans ($3,033 for females versus $4,257 for males). Lowry (1985, p. 35) provides another perspective on poverty among the current cohort of minority elderly women by showing that four out of five elderly minority women live with incomes below $2,000 per year. What this number translates to is the fact that in 1980, 44% of aged black women fell officially into the poverty category, and, if one added to the poor those in the near-poor category (persons living below 125% of the poverty level), the figure reaches a high of 82% (Minklen & Stone, 1985, p. 353).

These authors also present data on the poverty rate among elderly Hispanic women. The Hispanic rate of 31.4% is lower than the black rate, but it is still more than double the poverty rate for all women in the 65 and over age category (Minkler & Stone, 1985, p. 353). Moreover, Agree (1985) reveals that the poverty rate for rural Hispanic elderly women is higher than the total rate for the population: 38% of rural women have an income below the poverty line.

More current data on poverty status are available for black elderly women — the poorest category amongst all of the elderly groups. A report by the National Caucus and Center on Black Aged (1987, p. 2) reveals that five out of eight (64.9%) aged black females had an annual income below $5,000 in 1985, and one out of six (17.0%) had less than $3,000. Moreover, the situation is especially precarious for single, unrelated, black women or those who live with nonrelatives. About seven out of eight or 87.9% of the group are either poor or economically vulnerable (i.e., persons with income between the poverty line and twice the poverty line).

In using these data (useful as they may be), it is important to recognize that there are certain problems in using summary statistics when they are presented as being representative of the economic picture for various ethnic communities that might be grouped under one minority category. This is particularly true for such a diverse group as Asian and Pacific Islanders (more than 20 Asian populations and five Pacific Islander groups), although it is just as true for Hispanics and Native Americans. For example, Agree (1985) makes the statement that the proportion of Asian and Pacific Islander elderly living below the poverty level compares to that of the white elderly population. She cites the median income for elderly Asian and Pacific Islander women ($3,476) as being comparable to that of white aged women ($3,894). Gould (1988) has demonstrated that these summary statistics do not convey the significant differences in poverty status that exist between the various groups who make up the Asian and Pacific Islander category. This fact can be illustrated easily by pointing out that poverty level among elderly "Other Asians" is 28.6%, whereas it is 2.5% among aged Japanese (Koh, 1985, p. 4). In addition, within each of the Asian and Pacific Islander groups, the foreign-born members, particularly the most recent immigrants, have relatively low incomes (Gardner, Robey, & Smith, 1985, p. 34).

In this respect, the inherent research problems of having no data broken down by ethnic status on Asian and Pacific Islander elderly women are self-evident. What is surprising though, is the fact that, generally, even Asian and Pacific Islander professionals (who have contributed significantly to the literature on the community), have not recognized the importance of presenting their data analysis by sex — again pointing out the urgency of developing a minority-feminist perspective (Gould, 1988). Block (1979, p. 187) makes a similar case about the difficulties of using summary statistics to generalize about 266 Indian tribes spanning a 30-state geographic area. Thus, any general remarks about the *total* minority community have to be approached with caution.

In analyzing the sources of income for older nonwhite women, the available data on black elderly women reveal that in general, they receive lower Social Security benefits than white older women and are only half as likely as their white counterparts to receive a private pension. In 1984, only 5% of elderly black women received income from a private pension (National Caucus and Center on Black Aged, 1987, p. 12). That such telling information (which can promote a clearer understanding of the effects of a lifetime of sex and race discrimination on economic well-being in old age) is simply not available for older women for all minorities of color only speaks to the lack of awareness of a minority-feminist perspective. Moreover, the data on black women reveal that even after age 65 their poverty status contributes to their high representation in household and service employment: 41% of all black women employed as private household workers were 65 and over and 28% of all black women employed as service workers fell in the 65 and older age category. Furthermore, their median weekly earnings for full-time work were typically less than the wages of elderly white females ($243.15 versus $285.71, respectively; National Caucus and Center on Black Aged, 1987, pp. 13-14.). These findings on the high rates of poverty among aged minority women leave little room for optimism regarding the economic status of future elderly cohorts.

MARITAL STATUS

The data on marital statuses of older minority women reveal that in each group, women are much less likely to be married than men and much more likely to be widowed or divorced. Older black women had the lowest percentage of marrieds and the highest percentage of widows. All of the minority groups had significantly higher divorce and separation rates for females than older white women (a four-to-six percentage point difference), whereas only the Hispanic group included a higher percentage of never married females than older white women (7.1% versus 6.8%, respectively; Agree, 1985). The differences in marital status by sex are linked to sex differences in mortality because women generally outlive men and marry men older than themselves. The higher male remarriage rate is also a contributing factor in older minority men registering a higher marriage rate than aged minority females. The differences in marital status between older women by ethnicity seem to reflect a combination of biological factors (higher mortality of black males in the 65 and below age category), as well as societal pressures that might have differential impacts on the lives of white and nonwhite females from various groups. For example, "multiple jeopardies" can certainly explain part of the variance in divorce and separation statistics between older minority and nonminority females. Jackson (1985, p. 279) states that given the current patterns of marital statuses in the 65 and below age group, she sees widening gaps in the years ahead, especially in the marital statuses of aged blacks and whites.

LIVING ARRANGEMENTS

The variations in marital statuses have implications for the living arrangements of older minority females. For example, only 59.9% of 65- to 74-year-old black females continue to live in a primary family setting, compared to 71.3% of black males. Moreover, elderly black females are much more likely to maintain families (primary family head, 19.0%) than their white counterparts (7.4%; Manuel & Reid, 1982, pp. 42-43). Furthermore, the likelihood of a related child under 18 living in the same household is increased when the household is headed by a poor, aged female who is black (Jackson, 1985, p. 280). This factor is particularly interesting because Taylor (1982) has shown that elderly black women can have a kin and friendship network that becomes part of their coping strategies with aging. Still, it is important to also keep in mind the general statistics, which reveal that living alone occurs more often among the widowed or divorced aged — a category proportionately higher among minority rather than nonminority females (Jackson, 1985, p. 280). This factor would temper the stereotype that racial minorities always have a supportive and caring family network to fall back on for living arrangements. In fact, Manuel and Reid (1982, p. 41) report on a study by Manuel of a large, random sample of elderly respondents in Southern California, which revealed that less than half (40%) of the black and Mexican American respondents lived in extended families.

There are variations among the ethnic groups on how elderly females arrange their housing. For example, unlike the aged black women, roughly equal proportions of Hispanic males and females above 75 years of age live in families (Manuel & Reid, 1982, pp. 42-43). Agree (1985) also presents statistics to show that generally, a greater percentage of whites live in nursing homes compared to ethnic minorities of color. Available data on females above age 85 reveal that 26.4% of white females are in homes for the aged (refers essentially to nursing homes), compared to 13.5% of black females (National Caucus and Center on Black Aged, 1987, p. 29). These data suggest that besides the factor of available family networks, one has to consider the possibility of discrimination and poverty as possible variables in the skewed distribution of whites and nonwhites among the aged nursing home population.

One final point that needs to be stressed in this section (that is indirectly related to living arrangements) is the state of housing available to minority aged populations. Although specific data are not available regarding the condition of housing units occupied by elderly minority females, the Report of the National Caucus and Center on Black Aged (1987) stresses that fact that housing is possibly the most visible sign of deprivation among elderly blacks. The Report quotes a 1981 Louis Harris Poll, which revealed that one out of three elderly blacks found their housing to be unsuitable (National Caucus and Center on Black Aged, 1987, p. 4). The same point has been consistently stressed regarding the substandard housing occupied by many elderly Asian and Pacific Islanders, especially in crowded, urban surroundings such as Chinatowns and Little Tokyos (Fujii, 1976; Jung, 1976; Homma-True, 1976). Similarly, Block (1979, p. 184) describes the substandard housing conditions of Native American aged, stressing the fact that data on this segment of the population are lacking because its members are a "statistically insignificant minority group."

HEALTH STATUS

Minority demographics related to elderly women can serve as background information to understand the totality for their physical and mental health status in old age. In examining these findings, it is worthwhile to keep in mind that there are differences in opinion between researchers regarding the validity and reliability of the data on this topic. For example, Manuel and Reid (1982, pp. 45-46) present statistics (not broken down by sex) to show that minority elderly are more likely to assess their health as being poor than nonminority aged. Moreover, the subjective assessment of poor health is correlated to the fact that poor, elderly nonwhites experience a higher number of activity-restricted days than their white counterparts. For bed-restricted days, the disparities between minority and nonminority elderly persist for the low-income category, whereas it almost disappears for the higher income category.

Unlike Manuel and Reid, Jackson (1985) tends to believe that the higher likelihood of minority elderlys' self-assessment of their health as being poor might be related to the fact that low-income people tend to judge their health status differently from high-income people. Jackson does not support Manuel and Reid's categorical conclusion that the health status of aged minorities is inferior to elderly nonminorities. Other reports (National Institute on Aging, 1981; "Minority Elderly Facing Special Problems," 1986) point out that whereas differences in such statistics are rates of hypertension, chronic diseases, cerebrovascular diseases, and functional impairments show higher incidence among blacks relative to whites, the health disadvantage of blacks relative to whites is greater in middle age than in old age. The National Institute on Aging Report (1981) suggests that the leveling trend in old age might be due to the fact that blacks' health is so much poorer than whites' in middle age that unhealthy blacks die before reaching old age.

Specific data on health status of older black women National Caucus and Center on Black Aged, 1987, pp. 30-31) indicate that whereas coronary heart disease mortality rates are similar in white and black men, they are much higher among black women than their white counterparts. Also, the number of new cases of coronary heart disease may be increasing in black females as compared to whites. In terms of other diseases, the average size of a breast tumor at diagnosis is greater in black women than whites, suggesting that elderly black women with breast cancer are diagnosed later than are white women. Similarly, the incidence rates for cervical, colon, and lung cancer are also higher among black females than white females. The Report reveals that, unfortunately, studies show that elderly black women are less likely than older white females to have had a cervical cancer examination.

In contrast to the findings on physical health, the results of some studies on mental health reveal that, among black women, survival has fostered the development of coping strategies that allow them to solve problems as they arise (Taylor, 1982). Aging is not viewed as a problem. In fact, growing old is accepted as a natural part of life. Taylor (1982) attributes this attitude to the development of coping strategies that are fostered by a supportive kin and friendship network that includes neighbors and service providers. However, Taylor (1982, p. 97) also states that "other strategies fell categorically within the realm of the mind set of the individual as part of a cognitive process of adaptation initiated in response to situational factors." Values and beliefs that are seen as major coping resources are religious beliefs, perception of the extended family as the most dependable source of aid, and belief in the ethic of hard work, self-help, and independence. Carter (1982, p. 106) stresses the significance of religion in reporting on a study of rural elderly blacks. In presenting the anlalysis by sex, the author concludes that the black females' sustaining relationship with the church might be due to the fact that women valued church organizations more than did elderly males. The latter group felt that these church organizations did not provide a forum for meaningful involvement of men.

The previous discussion is not meant to minimize the incidence of mental health problems among older, nonwhite females. In fact, Thein (1980, p. 156) reports that depression is a major problem among elderly Asian and Pacific Islander women, with isolation playing a significant role in increased mental health problems. Factors that contribute to an increased level of stress include loss of family, loss of friends, loss of income, lack of knowledge of resources, loss of mental stimulation, loss of self-value, and inability to communicate with their younger kin because of lack of knowledge of the English language.

USE/DELIVERY OF SERVICES

Inasmuch as elderly minorities have been identified as facing special problems, it might be assumed that they use services relatively more often than nonminorities. The figures from the Administration on Aging, however, show that there has been a three-year decline in program participation by minority elderly ("Minority Elderly Facing Special Problems," 1986, p. 3). Critics have charged that the reason for the lack of utilization of services by minorities is due to the fact that the present service delivery system is geared to a white middle-class population ("Minority Elderly Facing Special Problems." 1986, p. 3). As a way to correct this situation, many ethnic-minority professionals have suggested that services to older nonwhite populations should be minority -specific, and delivery of services should be done by staff familiar with the language and culture of the recipients (Browne & Onzuka-Anderson, 1988; Downing & Copeland, 1980; Lee, Balgopal, & Patchner, 1988).

Much of the ethnogerontologic literature seems to favor the matching of staff and clients by ethnic-minority status as a way of remedying serious deficits in traditional methods of service delivery and as a political response to movements for minority rights (e.g., Jenkins, 1981). However, there have been some concerns about the conditions under which the use of bilingual-bicultural workers might be a hindrance in clients' comfort in working on personal problems (Jansen, 1987; Sue, 1981). Although specific data about elderly nonwhite womens' use of services are not available, Jansen (1987) has addressed the question of possible problems that might arise when bilingual-bicultural female workers from the same ethnic group work with Southeast Asian refugees. Because Thein (1980, p. 160) also cites various studies to show that the utilization rate of most outpatient agencies by Asian and Pacific Islander women is higher than the rate for men, the question regarding the structure and delivery of formal services is highly significant for this minority population.

The previous discussion of formal services is not meant to minimize the importance of considering the value of informal services and social networks in the total planning and delivery of services to aged minorities (Browne & Onzuka-Anderson, 1988; Colen, 1982). At the same time, it needs to be kept in mind that there is an increasing recognition that informal social networks that support aged minorities might not be available in all cases, or these networks might not have the necessary resources to fulfill the growing needs of frail elderly groups. Thus, the current literature on this topic (Downing & Copeland, 1980; Jackson, 1985; Lee, Balgopal, & Patchner, 1988) emphasizes the point that social network theory should not be used as a shield to limit the development of needed formal services for elderly minorities. In this context, Jenkins' 1981 study provides valuable data to stress that *balance* between integration and separation of services between traditional social work agencies, ethnic agencies, and social networks needs to be maintained to plan effective service delivery to minority populations. In addition, the literature stresses the fact that generally, in-home services have not been offered to aged minorities as an available alternative to long-term institutional care (National Caucus and Center on Black Aged, 1987; Zambrana, Merino, & Santana, 1979). This modality has been shown to result in an overall reduction in health care expenditures (Taylor & Chatters, 1986). In view of these findings, the lack of attention to provision of homemaker and other home care services to older minority women again suggests that professionals might be overestimating the viability of informal networks to provide assistant to this population.

RECOMMENDATIONS/FUTURISTIC VISIONS

Currently, our society is being made aware of the plight of older Americans. Gradually, this awareness has been expanded to recognize the fact that elderly women and older nonwhites might face special problems not covered under the general rubric of "older Americans" (Downing & Copeland, 1980; Graham, 1988; Hooyman, 1987; Lee, 1985; Lee, Balgopal, & Patcher, 1988; Rode-heaver, 1987). But what about the needs of older minority women? In fact, as Hooks (1981, p. 7) has pointed out in the context of black women, the professional literature has socialized out of existence the identity of nonwhite women: "The word men in fact refers only to *white* men, the word Negroes refers only to black *men*, and the word women refers only to *white* women" [italics in original]. A minority-feminist perspective in the theoretical analysis has to be the first order of business in a futuristic vision to bring some conceptual clarity to the research on this topic. The paucity of literature on this subject, and more important, the lack of consciousness of the need for data on this issue, perpetuates the invisibility of the special needs of older nonwhite females. The question that still remains to be answered, however, is why the "minority communities" as well as "women" have not advocated the adoption of a minority-feminist perspective.

Part of the reason for this lack is the fact that there is a marked separation in the discussions of feminist and ethnic-minority questions, despite the exhortations of some scholars that professionals should grasp the common core in the operation of sexism and racism in society (Gould, 1987a). Furthermore, many professionals believe that either racism or sexism, as a form of inequality, transcend each other, and these authors see the two "isms" in dichotomous terms (e.g., Hopkins, 1979). It seems that adoption of such a framework might force older nonwhite women to identify the discrimination they face as primarily racism or sexism (within their own and the dominant group), leading to the false hope that elimination of one of these types of oppression will end their status as victims in society (Gould, 1987a).

The adoption of a minority-feminist perspective may be seen as a futuristic vision because the model requires professionals to go an extra step beyond the practice framework currently advocated: developing cultural sensitivity to the needs of older minority women. The minority-feminist perspective requires that professionals recognize that a valid explanation of reality facing elderly nonwhite females can only be found in the relationship of the community to the larger macroscopic structure of society. In other words, cultural differences and minority group structure need to be examined jointly, but *within* the context of the female experience, to understand the primary stressors of elderly nonwhite females' lives.

One way to clarify the futuristic aspects of a minority-feminist perspective for older nonwhite women is to spell out its implications for education, practice, and policy. It is natural that variations in nationality and cultural origins of the various elderly minority female groups from the dominant society might encourage a tendency to teach curriculum content in this area from a strictly ethnocultural perspective (as described by Lister, 1987, in a general article dealing with curriculum content on minorities). Teaching about ethnicity and cultural pluralism is a basic ingredient in curriculum building on elderly nonwhite women since they function in at least two environments: their own culture and that of the mainstream society. However, to understand the socialization of the older minority woman, the conceptual scheme has to be extended to frame a quadruple model, which incorporates the idea that an elderly nonwhite woman has to learn the race-sex roles of both the majority and her own culture (Gould, 1985). In other words, teaching about cultural differences and minority group structure cannot ignore the fact that elderly minority women are distinct from the men in their minority culture and separate from the larger group of older women in the dominant culture.

Similarly, the literature on practice and policy with older nonwhite women necessarily has focuses on informing the professionals about cultural backgrounds and coping strategies of various groups to encourage sensitive service delivery (e.g., Block, Davidson, & Grambs, 1981, Chap. 8; Devore & Schlesinger, 1987). A missing perspective is a recognition of the ideological assumptions, values, imperatives, and prescriptions underlying practice models that prevent moving from a person-in-environment approach to a person-in-society approach. This line of reasoning argues for a framework that does not minimize the fact that a realistic comprehension of the elderly nonwhite woman's world as an operating social system involves recognition of both race and sex as inherent facets of her destiny. A person-in-environment approach does not capture the larger macroscopic structure of society within which the older nonwhite woman has to function. The approach also fails to evaluate realistically the potential of the system to respond positively to elderly minority woman's needs and the ability of professionals to produce a positive response. To put it in another way, the theoretical contribution of a person-in-society model is the fact that it does not *avoid* the conclusion that under certain conditions, striving to achieve an adaptive balance between the person and the environment is not always desirable for groups such as older minority women, especially when the basic goal of the striving is transformation of institutions to ensure a just society (Gould, 1987b).

Non of these strategies, by themselves, is a guarantee that the professionals will be able to achieve a clear enough understanding of older minority women's lives to determine whether this group's invisibility in the ethnogerontologic and women's literature needs remedy. Recent legislation in Congress to reauthorize the Older Americans Act (OAA) includes a number of items designed to make the OAA more responsive to the needs of minority elderly. There are provisions "to fund centers of gerontology to improve, enhance and expand minority personnel and training programs, as well as require service providers to specify how the service needs of low-income minority individuals will be served" ("Older Americans Act Reauthorization," 1987, p. 1). Yet, it is interesting to note that the American Association of Retired Persons (AARP) Report that describes this legislation ("Older Americans Act Reauthorization," 1987) meticulously separates out the coverage on this topic to include only "minority affairs," with no mention whatsoever about elderly nonwhite women. This point is all the more significant since AARP has used this forum to announce that its Minority Affairs Initiative has convened a National Ad Hoc Task Force on Minority Affairs—which again makes no reference to older nonwhite females.

REFERENCES

Agree, E. M. (1985). *A portrait of older Americans*. Washington, DC: American Association of Retired Persons, Minority Affairs Initiative.

Block, M. R. (1979). Exiled Americans: The plight of the Indian aged in the United States. In D. E. Gilfand & A. J. Kutzik (Eds.), *Ethnicity and aging: theory, research and policy* (pp. 184-192). New York: Springer.

Block, M. R., Davidson, J. L., & Grambs, J. D. (1981). *Women over forty: Provisions and realities.* New York: Springer.

Browne, C., & Onzuka-Anderson, R. (1988). Community support systems for the elderly in Hawaii. In D. S. Sanders & J. L. Fischer (Eds.), *Visions for the future: Social work and Pacific-Asian perspectives* (pp. 95-112). Honolulu: University of Hawaii School of Social Work.

Butler, R. N. (1975). *Why survive? Being old in America.* New York: Harper & Row.

Carter, A. C. (1982). Religion and the black elderly: The historical basis of social and psychological concerns. In R. C. Manuel (Ed.), *Minority aging: Sociological and social psychological issues* (pp. 103-107). Westport, CT: Greenwood Press.

Cohler, B. J. (1982). Stress or support: Relations between older women from three European ethnic groups and their relatives. In R. C. Manuel (Ed.) *Minority aging: Sociological and social psychological issues* (pp. 115-120). Westport, CT: Greenwood Press.

Colen, J. N. (1982). Using natural helping networks in social service delivery systems. In R. C. Manuel (Ed.), *Minority aging: Sociological and social psychological issues* (pp. 179-183). Westport, CT: Greenwood Press.

Conable, C. W. (1988). Aging and the global agenda for women: Conversations in Nairobi. Washington, DC: American Association for International Aging.

Devore, W., & Schlesinger, E. G. (1987). *Ethnic-sensitive social work practice* (2nd ed.). Columbus, OH: Merrill.

Downing, R. A., & Copeland, E. J. (1980). Services for the black elderly: National or local problems? *Journal of Gerontological Social Work, 2*, 289-303.

Fujii, S. (1976), Elderly Asian Americans and users of public services. *Social Casework, 57*, 202-207.

Gardner, R. W., Robey, B., & Smith, P. G. (1985). Asian Americans: Growth, change and diversity. *Population Bulletin, 40*, 1-44.

Goldberg, G., Kantrow, R., Kremen, E., & Lauter, L. (1986). Spouseless, childless elderly women and their social supports. *Social Work, 31*, 104-112.

Gould, K. H. (1985). A minority-feminist perspective on child welfare issues. *Child Welfare, 64*, 346-351.

Gould, K. H (1987a). Feminist principles and minority concerns: Contributions, problems, and solutions. *AFFILIA Journal of Women and Social Work, 2*, 6-19.

Gould, K. H. (1987b). Life model versus conflict model: A feminist perspective. *Social Work, 32*, 346-351.

Gould, K. H. (1988). Asian and Pacific Islanders: Myth and reality. *Social Work, 33*, 142-147.

Graham, V. (1988). I chose life! *Modern Maturity: Publication of American Association of Retired Persons, 31*, 30-37.

Homma-True, R. (1976). Characteristics of contrasting Chinatowns. *Social Casework, 57*, 155-159.

Hooks, B. (1981). *Ain't I a woman: Black women and feminism*. Boston, MA: South End Press.

Hooyman, N. R. (1987). Older women and social work curricula. In D. S. Burden & N. Gottlieb (Eds.), *The woman client: Providing human services in a changing world* (pp. 263-279). New York: Tavistock.

Hopkins, T. J. (1979). Another conflict (Letters). *Social Work, 24*, 259-260.

Jackson, J. L. (1967). Social gerontology and the Negro: A review. *The Gerontologist, 7*, 168-178.

Jackson, J. L. (1971). Sex and social class variations in Negro older parent-adult child relationships. *Aging and Human Development, 2*, 96-107.

Jackson, J. L. (1985). Race, national origin, ethnicity, and aging. In R. H. Binstock & E. Shane (Eds.), *Handbook of aging and the social sciences* (2nd ed., pp. 264-303). New York: Van Nostrand Reinhold.

Jansen, G. (1987). Empowerment of refugee women: An interpretive study of a socio-cultural adjustment approach. Unpublished manuscript.

Jenkins, S. (1981). *The ethnic dilemma in social services*. New York: Free Press.

Jung, M. (1976). Characteristics of contrasting Chinatowns. *Social Casework, 57*, 149-154.

Kim, B. C. (1978). *The Asian-Americans: Changing patterns, changing needs*. Montclair, NJ: Association of Korean Christian Scholars in North America.

Koh, J. Y. K. (1985, February 17). *Working with Asian-Americans: Strategies, roles of social work and implications for social work education session at the 1985 Asian-American social work educators/practitioners symposium*. Annual Program Meeting of the Council on Social Work Education. Washington, DC.

Lee, J. J. (1985). Asian American elderly: A neglected minority group. Unpublished manuscript.

Lee, J. J., Balgopal, P. R., & Patchner, M. A. (1988). Citizen participation: An effective dimension for serving the Asian American elderly. In D. S. Sanders & J. L. Fischer (Eds.), *Visions for the future: Social work and Pacific-Asian perspective* (pp. 113-124). Honolulu: University of Hawaii School of Social Work.

Lewis, M. I., & Butler, R. N. (1972). Why is women's lib ignoring old women? *International Journal of Aging and Human Development, 3*, 223-231.

Lister, L. (1987). Ethnocultural content in social work education. *Journal of Education for Social Work, 23*, 31-39.

Lowy, L. (1985). *Social work with the aging*. New York: Longman.

Manton, K. G. (1982). Differential life expectancy: Possible explanations during the later ages. In R. C. Manuel (Ed.), *Minority aging: Sociological and social psychological issues* (pp. 63-68). Westport, CT: Greenwood Press.

Manuel, R. C., & Reid, J. (1982). A comparative demographic profile of the minority and nonminority aged. In R. C. Manuel (Ed.), *Minority aging: Sociological and social psychological issues* (pp. 31-52). Westport, CT: Greenwood Press.

Minkler, M., & Stone R. (1985). The feminization of poverty and older women. *The Gerontologist, 25*, 351-357.

"Minority elderly facing special problems." (1986). *NASW News, 31,* 3.

National Caucus and Center on Black Aged. (1987). *The status of the black elderly in the United States.* Washington, DC: U.S. Government Printing Office.

National Center for Health Statistics. (1980). *Vital statistics of the United States, 1978: Life tables* (Vol. 2, section 5). Washington, DC: U.S. Government Printing Office.

National Institute on Aging. (1981). *Aging and minorities.* Washington, DC: U.S. Department of Health and Human Services.

National Urban League. (1964). *Double jeopardy—the older Negro in America today.* New York: Author.

Older Americans Act Reauthorization Focuses on Minority Elderly. (1987). *AARP Highlights, 5,* 1, 9.

Rodeheaver, D. (1987). When old age became a social problems, women were left behind. *The Gerontologist, 27,* 741-746.

Smith, A., & Stewart, A. J. (1983). Approaches to studying racism and sexism in black women's lives. *Journal of Social Issues, 39,* 1-15.

Sue, D. W. (1981). *Counseling the culturally different: Theory and practice.* New York: Wiley.

Symposium: Civil rights, affirmative action, and the aged of the future: Will life chances be different for blacks, Hispanics and women? (1986). *The Gerontologist, 26*(2).

Taylor, R. J.. & Chatters, L. M. (1986). Patterns of informal support to elderly black adults: Family, friends and church members. *Social Work, 31,* 432-438.

Taylor, S. (1982). Mental health and successful coping among aged black women. In R. C. Manuel (Ed.), *Minority aging: Sociological and social psychological issues* (pp. 95-100). Westport, CT: Greenwood Press.

Thein, T. M. (1980). Health issues affecting Asian/Pacific American women. In U.S. Commission on Civil Rights (Ed.), *Civil rights issues of Asian and Pacific Americans* (pp. 153-164). Washington, DC: U.S. Government Printing Office.

U.S. Bureau of the Census. (1984). Projections of the population of the United States by age, sex, and race: 1983 to 2080. *Current Population Reports* (series P-25). Washington, DC: U.S. Government Printing Office.

U.S. Commission on Civil Rights (Ed.). (1980). *Civil rights issues of Asian and Pacific Americans.* Washington, DC: U.S. Government Printing Office.

Zambrana, R. E. & Merino, R., & Santana, S. (1979). Health services and the Puerto Rican elderly. In D. E. Gelfand & A. J. Kutzik (Eds.), *Ethnicity and aging: Theory, research, and policy.* New York: Springer.

Families, Work, and the Lives of Older Women

Naomi Gottlieb, DSW

Three strands of understandings about older women inform this discussion. The first is the impact on all women of the socialization messages received from early infancy on about the appropriate roles of women in this society. Related to this is the close connection between the enactment of those roles by younger adult women, the impact of public policies and societal programs based on these expectations of women, and the ensuing consequences for women in their later years. The roles women play and, more important, the influence of political and economic policies on their work and their family life have a compelling impact on what the latter part of their lives will look like.

The second theme is the close connection between women's roles in the family and their activities in the paid workplace. We know a great deal about the similarities of these home and workplace experiences in terms of tasks, rewards, and valuation for younger adult women, and we need to be clear about the specific effects of these forces on the lives of older women. Workplace and family work have interactive consequences for each other and, in turn, are predictive of how women will fare in their older years.

The third theme is the fairly recent and sorely needed attention to adult development. Until the last few decades, social science has been unduly influenced by the psychodynamic overemphasis on the early years as deterministic and all-important in future adult experience. We now have a burgeoning literature on changes that individuals make throughout their lifetimes. The pessimistic view implied

Naomi Gottlieb is Professor, School of Social Work, University of Washington, Seattle, WA 98195.

in the first two themes is counterbalanced by the prospect that women of all ages can change and grow.

This discussion will show full regard for the overwhelming influence of this society's views of and behavior toward women, as played out in the home and at the workplace and for the inevitable result for women as they age. However, it will also argue for the potential of older women and some of the possible changes that the future may bring, both for individual women and for the society of women as a whole.

THE LATER CONSEQUENCES
OF LIFETIME MESSAGES

The subject of socialization and development of women, particularly from different perspectives, appears in several selections in this volume, but it may be important to summarize briefly here the essential characteristics of how most women are raised so that the fuller exposition of the consequences for their later years is clear.

The pivotal message for women is that their family role is the most important one they will fulfill and that all others will be secondary. The two corollary imperatives are the centrality of relationships and affiliative activities and the obligation to nurture others and be responsible for their emotional and social well-being (Kline, 1980; Steitz, 1981; Weitzman, 1984). Women have been primarily relegated to the personal and home sphere. Much has been documented both in this volume and elsewhere about the consequences of these expectations for the development and behaviors of younger adult women and for their activities (Bart, 1980; Burden & Gottlieb, 1987). Particularly important are the power differentials between women and men, which affect all personal and political transactions (Lipman-Blumen, 1984). Women are given lip-service and Mother's Day credit for the work they do for their families in the home, and they are paid poorly for the work they do outside the home, which mirrors their family roles and is done in addition to that family work (Briar, Hoff, & Seck, 1987; England, 1984; Hooyman, 1987). Although women have made some advances in public spheres (e.g., the anchorwomen on television news programs, and the increasing numbers of women elected to local and state positions), the world at large is still clearly dominated by men, and women are reminded of that fact every day. Women continue to be held responsible for the family home, to both supply it with children and to care for both children and adults (husband, parents and grandparents, and, in some blended families, ex-parents-in-law as well). When women do work outside the home (more than half of married women do so now), their outside work is predominately in sex-segregated occupations (Baron & Bielby, 1985).

The consequences of these factors for the older woman are overwhelming. As the specifics of these consequences are considered now, the focus will be on women now in their 60s and older. This cohort of women is less likely to have been affected by the impact of the women's movement than were their younger counterparts. The older woman's growing-up years were clearly pervaded by traditional role expectations for women and were not relieved to any extent, as is true of younger women, by alternative messages of what a woman's life might be. They also have had fewer opportunities to enact other than traditional roles. They were even less likely than adult women now to other than "women's work" in the paid workforce (less likely, for example, to be admitted to professional schools and less likely to at least view other women in alternative roles). The pressure on women of color to maintain their expected roles is of a special quality. Almquist (1984) describes the "defensive strengthening" of traditional families by the mothers in ethnic-minority groups in order to maintain their cultures in the face of racist onslaughts.

A catalog of the consequences of these experiences for older women begins with the issue of power. The vast majority of women now in their 60s and older never exercised real public power nor expected to do so. They probably heard many pious statements throughout their lifetime about the crucial role women played in raising the future generation and providing a "haven" for the working man. They knew, however, that men were the ones who made the central decisions affecting their lives. Those decisions were of most importance in the public arena and had direct economic and political consequences for their families (e.g., the individual consequences of economic programs—minimum wage laws, unemployment compensation-health care policies, decisions about peace and war). With the exceptions of individuals such as Frances Perkins in Franklin Roosevelt's cabinet, these women saw few women who advocated for their concerns and who could alter their sense of powerlessness in the public sphere. Questioning this status quo presents a particular dilemma for many Black older women for whom the church, albeit a patriarchal one, forms a very important part of their lives (Terrelonge, 1984).

On a personal level, many older women also knew that their economic dependence on their husbands made it equally difficult to question his decisions and his greater power in the home. Their lack of power is thus evident in both public and private spheres (Cancian, 1985; Lipman-Blumen, 1984; Piven, 1985).

Against this backdrop of little power throughout her adult years, the older woman is rendered obsolete when the role for which she had at least some value to society is ended (Beckman & Houser, 1982). Even if she could not advocate publicly for herself and other women or even if she saw few women in positions of power who represented her, she could believe the rhetoric that praised her for her home contributions. When she is no longer nurturing and rearing children, she isn't even a candidate for that hollow applause. Grandmothers are nice to have around, but they are not considered central to the rearing of the next generation. What little real recognition women received for their family role is now gone, and even a sense of power from private accomplishments is lost.

Another consequence of the prescribed role for women is the lack of preparation for the period of their lives when the central imperative is achieved. In view of the present life expectancy of 78 years for women (Markson, 1983), most older women now will live at least a third of their lives past their childrearing years. For women who have not worked in the paid workforce, few will have developed talents or interests separate from their family role. Even for those who have been in the workforce, the restrictions of their work experiences to "women's work" will have limited the encouragement of a range of work roles or interests. The ironic feature of this situation is that the medical and public health advances that have resulted in the greater life expectancy has meant that older women will be increasingly healthy in their later years (White-Riley, 1981). The term *compressed morbidity* is now used to describe the expectations of a long period of good health in older persons followed by a fairly short last illness (Fries, 1983). Older women will thus have the physical capacity for much activity but little previous preparation in their lives to visualize their potential in roles other than family ones (Keating & Cole, 1980). Accounts of counseling services to displaced homemakers or widows are replete with examples of women who accepted their husbands' protection of them, ranging from keeping from her basic financial knowledge (e.g., his salary and their debt situation) or the essentials of house or car repair. When that "protection" ends, the woman must begin to develop these essential skills of living (Greenwood-Audant, 1984). Women who have lived such a sheltered life will have difficulty thinking about wider roles they might assume.

The irony is that although most women will spend a good part of their later years as single women (Gallagher, 1983), they have not been prepared for an independent life. For married women, the average age of widowhood is 56. Only a third of women remarry after being widowed, and by age 65, 52% of women are widowed, compared to 14% of men (Hooyman, 1987). Women of color are widowed earlier than is true for white women and so their proportion in the population of older women of color is greater (Block, Davidson, & Grambs, 1981).

Add to this the women who never marry, older lesbians, and divorced women and it becomes evident that the clear majority of older women are single. The expectation of women as they mature is that they will be partnered during their lifetime and that they will depend on their partner to take care of them financially. Even when they work outside the home, they know their husband will earn considerably more than they do and that they are not in a position to support themselves or their family to the extent he can. The actuality is that most women will have to manage on their own for a substantial part of their later years, and many will not have the practical or social resources to do so (Gottlieb, 1980).

An additional consequence of earlier socialization for many older women is that the nurturing role may never end and therefore may not even allow for possible other dreams. The older woman has been trained to care for others through the earliest role model of her mother and has been encouraged to show caregiving traits, even as a child. However, until modern health advances lengthened most lives, women could expect that if and when they reached the age of grandmotherhood, the essential caregiving tasks would be over. At the turn of the century when life expectancy was 47 years (Markson, 1983), few could conceive of four- or five-generation families. Now it is not at all unusual for a 50-year-old woman, herself in the work force, to still have an adolescent or young adult child at home and also to be responsible for the care of a 70-year-old mother *and* a 90-year-old grandmother. The naming of her as the primary caregiver here is purposeful and is based on much empirical study, which finds the woman giving most of the essential individual care, although her husband or brother may help with financial or practical support (Archbold, 1982; Brody et al., 1983). In Hispanic culture, where the norms of reciprocity among family members are clearly understood, the cultural imperatives of machismo and marianismo compel rigid gender-specific roles, and daughters are particularly expected to care for the elderly (Anson, 1984). Although the traditions of filial piety and respect for elders are strongly ingrained through many centuries among many Asian groups, that imperative comes into conflict with American culture. As has been true of many immigrant groups, newer generations of younger Asians find themselves caught between the two cultures, the bonds of intergenerational duty soften (Almquist, 1984), and so caregiving by the adult daughter creates dilemmas for the younger generation.

The impact on the daily life of the woman caregiver is considerable. The woman not in the workforce may have her life completely taken up with the hour-by-hour care of a frail, elderly relative. (In this age of blended families, the relative might be an ex-mother-in-law to whom she is still emotionally attached.) For her counterpart who also holds an outside job, the juggling of the multiple responsibilities can be overwhelming (Crossman, London, & Barry, 1981; Fengler & Goodrich, 1979; Simon, 1986). Added to the weight of the actual tasks is the decided difference between her earlier experience of caregiving of the young child and that of the older ill or frail person. In the first instance, the heavy emotional and physical investment is balanced by the excitement of a developing individual who will mature and within a reasonable and expected time period, become independent. The care of the ill elderly is quite the opposite. The end of caregiving is both indefinite and negative. The caregiving woman never knows how long the need will exist but does know that the end will be not a mature adult, eventually on his or her own, but the death of this family member, the person for whom she has given countless hours of physical and emotional attention. The lifelong imperative to be a caregiver may literally be played out for a lifetime.

Related to each of these consequences of restricted roles for women is the concomitant expectation that women will not be assertive about their own needs. It seems to be a necessary trait to fill the role. If one is to devote all of one's time and energy to the care and nurturing of other people, it is almost essential that one not give time and energy to oneself. Facilitators of assertion training classes for women report that the necessary skills are the least problematic aspect of such training. Far more important is the permission women require in order to attend to or even be aware of their own needs (Gottlieb et al., 1983). The importance of this issue to this discussion is that many older women — both those who have time and physical capabilities as well as the overwhelmed caregivers — do not have the skills nor, more essential, the self-enhancing attitudes to think of and be assertive about their needs. This makes it very difficult then to consider other roles and activities when time and health in later years permit a range of options, or even with the restriction of caregiving responsibilities, when women need to advocate for their own needs of respite care or other ways to ease their burden. Hess (1985) predicts that the sheer number of future recipients of care and the need of middle-aged women to be in the workforce will lead to a refusal by these women to continue to be the primary caregivers. However, at present, the lifelong expectation that women will place the needs of others before their own has created a barrier to their vision of themselves cast in other roles in their later years.

Society's restricted views of women affects the older woman in other personal ways. Women are disparaged for signs of old age in great contrast to our acceptance of the graying and distinguished older man (Sontag, 1972). A recent cosmetic advertisement has a young woman saying, "I do not intend to grow old gracefully. I will fight it every step of the way!'' (with the aid of the cosmetic, of course). Society's negative images of the older woman, personified by the portrait of the "old crone" plague women as they age (Payne & Whittington, 1980). Many older women seek relationships with men but are faced with the smaller numbers of older men available for partners and the men's preferences for younger women. A lifetime of sexual unassertiveness also hampers their search. When their childrearing tasks are over and women might be free to form new relationships should they be widowed or divorced, they then meet the further barrier of society's view that they are no longer acceptable as sexual beings.

Important qualifications need to be made in this general discussion of the effects of socialization messages on older women. First, there are important variations on these central themes among ethnic women of color (Almquist, 1984; Brinson-Pineda, 1984; Jackson, 1980; Nydegger, 1983). For example, the combination of work and family roles for the black women has been of a very different order. By and large, black women have been expected to work. Indeed, the work role was needed for the family's survival long before this became a necessity for many white families. Thus, the work role for black women can have salience equal to the home role (Fox & Hesse-Biber, 1984). As another example, some Asian communities expect women to achieve professionally and to experience a sense of self-worth from that as well as from the family role (Chow, 1984). Other cultural variations and effects of racism are cautions that generalizations about white women must not be assumed to be true for ethnic women of color.

Second, there is a positive side to the expectations of caring and responsibility. Women have far greater skills than men have for making and keeping rich friendships, and this can serve them well in their later years, when women predominate among elderly populations (Bernard, 1976). With these skills and with the encouragement to value women and to counteract previously held views of competition with women for men, older women can be nourished by the friendships of other older women (Candy, 1977; Kohen, 1983; Powers & Bultena, 1980). About a third of lesbians come out to family and friends after the age of 50 (Raphael & Robinson, 1980), and this phenomenon may reflect, among other factors, the need and willingness to see in other women the prospects of intimacy and nourishment. Indeed, the positive view of affiliation and responsibility for others has become a cornerstone in the consideration of new theories about women's development, which are needed to correct longstanding theories based on men's experiences of competition and autonomy and on men's views of women's worlds (Barnett & Baruch, 1978; Ehrenreich & English, 1979; Surrey, 1985).

Third, much of the description of women's socialization centers on heterosexual women who marry and have children. It is important to keep in mind that there are many older women, heterosexual and homosexual, who have never married or never have had children. The issues for them may overlap or even exaggerate the experiences of other women, but some issues are different. For example, Simon (1986) found that when family caregiving was needed, single women were expected, even more so than their married sisters, to provide that caregiving, even at the cost of their own careers. As another example, never-married women, both lesbian and heterosexual, usually have developed skills in independent living and in developing viable support systems that serve them well in their later years. They have also coped with stigmatization through their earlier years and are more able to deal with the effects of ageism as they grow older (Weitz, 1984). Lesbians also have the special issues of institutional unwillingness to accept their long-term relationships (e.g., refusal of hospital for visits by next-of-kin), and they are also denied the recognized status of widow when their partner has died (Mayer, 1985). At the same time that we need to pay due attention to the majority of heterosexual women who have families, those who do not meet those prescriptions need to be understood. In fact, all women may learn important skills from those who do not follow society's expectations.

To summarize this first theme, most women have been seen by society and by themselves as essentially the caregivers in the home and the rearers of children. They are left roleless when those obligations are done; therefore it becomes difficult for them to conceive of using their older years in self-enhancing ways. The expectations and behaviors of a lifetime form severe restrictions for many older women.

FAMILY, THE WORKPLACE,
AND THE OLDER WOMAN

For most of the present cohort of older women, family roles have clearly taken precedence over workforce participation. In considering now the realities of each of those aspects of older women's lives, the focus first will be on women's family roles. The description of older women in relation to families will provide overviews of what we know about their current life circumstances and, wherever appropriate, the connection will be made between those circumstances and the discussion above of societal imperatives. For example, the fact that more older men are married than is true of older women is not just a matter of chance. The portrayal of circumstances will not be restricted to white heterosexual women who have married and had children, although these are the majority, but will consider all women. It will also indicate how diverse women live out their later years alone and with families and friends.

Most older women are not part of a married couple. Although 77% of men over 65 are married, this is true of only 33% of women. In fact, that percentage decreases to 25% for women over 75 (Rix, 1984). More than 40% of older women will live about two-thirds of their adult lives alone (U.S. Senate Special Committee on Aging, 1986).

The explanations for this situation are varied. First, because life expectancy for men is less than for women, many older women are widowed before they reach the age of 65. As noted earlier, for women over 65, the proportion of widowhood is 52%, contrasted with a rate of 14% of men (Hooyman, 1987). The life expectancy of men is related to issues of biology and life styles, but the fact that fewer widows than widowers remarry is related to societal factors mentioned above. At age 65 and over, only 2 in a group of 1,000 women will remarry, compared with 17 men in 1,000 (U.S. Senate Special Committee on Aging, 1986). Because of the devaluation of women as they age and the emphasis, especially for women, on youth in this society, many older widows find that available men in their age range choose younger women and that there is a stigma against older women marrying younger men. Because women are socialized to be unassertive in interactions with men, many older women will not take the intiative is establishing new relationships. Also, many adult children of widows object to their mother's re-marriage and, influenced by obligations to her family role, a woman may place her own needs for a personal relationships secondary to her children's wishes. The number of single older women is also explained by women who have been divorced (this rate is now 16% for women over 45 and is increasing, Lesnoff-Caravaglia, 1984) and by never-married women, including lesbians.

The consequences for previously married women of being alone are considerable. First, their economic situation is negatively affected. Married women have been financially dependent on their husbands and when, by death or divorce, his earnings or retirement income are not available to her, her resources are drastically reduced. The proportion of older women living in poverty is 16% compared with 8.5% of men (Older Women's League Observer, 1983). The comparable rate for nonwhite women is even more severe. For example, about 55% of black women who are over 65 and who live alone are in poverty (U.S. Bureau of Census, 1986).

Retirement income for women is directly related to societal views of women. Women have been relegated to lower paying jobs, and their own retirement income is thus very low. The Social Security System was devised on the basis of traditional views of women in marriage, and most private pension systems were negotiated by strong unions in industries peopled mainly by men. Often the working older woman feels compelled by marital obligations to join her husband at the time he retires, even though her retirement income would be increased if she waited until she was older.

Second, women as a group have not been prepared to live an independent life. As noted above, many were treated in a protective way by their husbands and have not developed the necessary skills for autonomous living. Traditional socialization, which has made the family role paramount, leads to widows' feeling lost and out of control. Stillion (1984) comments on the confusion many widows feel even about what to call themselves: "Housekeeper? Home-maker?. . . . 'making a home' just for oneself is often considered a useless and self-centered vocation by our society" (p. 288). In addition, many adult children continue to assume that their mothers are inept in worldly or everyday affairs (Lesnoff-Caravaglia, 1984).

Counselors for widows frequently report that adult children take over the paternalistic role with their widowed mothers (Gottlieb, 1980).

With full awareness of the trauma for a woman of losing her husband, especially if this has been a long-term relationship, widowhood can have some beneficial effects. If the wife has been caring for an ailing husband, the end can bring relief to her. His death may also being to an end a long-term unhappy marriage. Widowhood also may provide new opportunities, in contrast to what may have been a constricting marriage — opportunities for work, new social roles, autonomy, and the development of independent skills. Services for widows that incorporate a feminist perspective and try to counteract traditional socialization find many women quite responsive to the new approach (Gottlieb, 1980).

In general, the relationship of older women with their children is a mixed picture. In looking at families across generations, it is important to note at the outset that we have more living generations than ever before in history. The four-generation family is commonplace today, and five living generations are becoming more frequent. The older people of these generations are apt to be primarily women. For many of these women, their children and grandchildren (including great-grandchildren) can be a source of pleasure and support (Timberlake, 1980). The other side of the coin is that families as they age will carry along with them longstanding tensions between the generations. As an extreme example, the incidence of neglect and abuse of the elderly by their adult children can be affected by the history of family tensions, as well as by the strains of current caregiving (Quinn & Tomita, 1986). Even in less difficult circumstances, interpersonal relationships across generations will not be "de novo" experiences but, in their diverse manifestations, will reflect the family in its younger days as well. The Native American situation is a sad example of the way in which governmental policies, causing the obliteration of cultures, resulted in the estrangement of families and the devaluation of women and the older generation (Almquist, 1984).

Even with fortunate circumstances and good intergenerational relationships, older women without partners prefer to maintain their own households. Johnson and Bursk (1980) report that family relationships seem on a better footing with separate households. In many situations, even with a relative nearby (Shanas, 1979), adult children, mobile with their own families, maintain "intimacy at a distance" (Hess & Waring, 1983). Frequent telephone and mail contact is maintained by the adult child in the far-flung community. In fact, new services are being developed to enable the distant son or daughter to engage social services in the mother's home community to provide the advocacy and coordinating role that the adult children cannot play on the spot (Richards, personal communication, 1987).

Not all older women will have had children, however, and the emphasis on the primacy of the family role for women is poignantly seen with married couples who have remained childless. Studies indicate that these marital dyads "turn inward" and often have few associations separate from their own household (Johnson & Catalano, 1981). When one of the couple dies (and this is more frequently the husband), the woman has few associations to use for support and few skills to use for her own welfare.

The situation may be very different for heterosexual women who have never married or for lesbian women. As noted earlier, these groups of women have had to manage on their own most of their lives and so have had to develop their coping skills and the practical management of their affairs through many years. Many are financially better off than their previously married counterparts through their own work history and their subsequent own retirement income, and have developed and used their own support systems. Braito and Anderson (1983) comment on the need for different measures of life satisfaction applicable to this group of women, measures not grounded in marriage and family alone, for these women appear to have many strengths separate from the family role. Although never-married elderly women represent only 7% of the population of older women, and studies of them have only begun, what is known about them is instructive, for it suggests the need for some balance in the life circumstances for many other older women. Compared with her married counterpart, the ever-single older women is better educated, in better health, places considerable importance on her workforce life, is less apt to be depressed and commit suicide, has close connections with siblings

and other interpersonal supports, and values her freedom and autonomy (Braito & Anderson, 1983). Although these attributes do suggest some important strengths missing for many older women who
have lived by societal imperatives, there is also the negative side for
the unmarried older women. She is less apt to have a caregiver for
herself when this is needed, and as a consequence, is more apt to be
institutionalized (Treas, 1977).

Being without a partner for most elderly women does not mean
that most of these women have no family and friends to turn to. The
work of Shanas (1979) indicating the close connection between the
elderly and their families has not been refuted by subsequent inquiries, although the myth of the abandonment of the elderly dies hard.
The vast majority of elderly women who are note partnered have
frequent contacts with family members. Shanas (1979) found that
most older people live within an hour's travel time of at least one
relative and have personal contact at least once a week with someone in their family. Also, for many, those contacts are a two-way
street, with the older woman giving services and material resources
to her adult children.

Siblings of the older woman often play a crucial role in both
ongoing social support and in personal caregiving (Johnson & Catalano, 1981). The sibling is apt to be a sister who, like the older
woman herself, has been widowed or is along for another reason
and who provides companionship and care (Hess & Waring, 1983).
The brothers in the family are more likely to be married still or
deceased. In any event, they are not personally available for caregiving, nor are they attuned to emotional needs, as is true for the
women members of the older family.

Other studies indicate that even when family contact is available
and used, women turn to friends even more than family members
(Hess & Waring, 1983). Many women have maintained friendships
throughout their lives (far more than is true of men) and often prefer
them to family ties, which may be emotionally complicated (Hess
& Waring, 1983). Families are more apt to be used for personal
caregiving (Hooyman & Lustbader, 1986), but the bonds with
friends are an essential and viable part of most older women's lives
(Bernard, 1976). It is an irony, in view of the portion of their lives
that women will spend alone (often one-third of their adult lives)

that same-sex, long-term friendships (often very valuable) are often thought to interfere with the marital bond and the home role (Lopata, 1977). Even after the death of friends, women can make diverse and rich new relationships, involving mutual exchange of affection and material resources (Powers & Bultena, 1980).

Older women's use of outside supports in the years when they are alone are also affected by additional factors. Inquiries have established that both health and economics affect the degree to which older persons will be available for involvements in support systems (Arling, 1976). We know that, although women live longer than men, they experience more chronic illnesses (Verbrugge, 1983). This is compounded for many women — often women of color — whose circumstances have not allowed for the basic necessities for good health or for accessibility to medical care. Furthermore, the depressed economic conditions of many older women — the result of economic dependency in prescribed social roles — do not allow them the resources to pursue outside activities and interpersonal relationships. Hooyman and Kiyak (1988) observe that "low-income women have fewer options to interact with others, fewer affordable and safe accommodations, and fewer resources to purchase in-home support services" (p. 511). Each of these precludes independent living and interaction with others when health problems arise. Thus, health and economic conditions form constraints on needed supports for the older woman alone, and these factors are in turn related to the special circumstances of women in this society.

The intent of this discussion of older women in the context of their families has been to draw the clear connection between the circumstances in which many older women find themselves and the societal expectations that have influenced them throughout their lives. Most older women, as the societal rules have prescribed, have invested most of their energies in their families, have been subordinated in that role, and have not been prepared, either financially or psychologically, for the many years they will be on their own. The condition of many older women of color has reflected the particular impact of racism as well as ageism. The personal and material resources of the never-married, including the lesbian woman, provide an interesting contrast of the experiences of women who have not met social expectations.

The discussion now of the world of work as it affects the lives of older women continues the basic argument of the import of social roles. The subject of work and the older women is treated more completely elsewhere in this volume, but a brief review of the older woman's experience in work outside the home can help us understand those connections and to see why so many older women struggle financially. Those connective themes include the secondary nature of women's paid work outside the home (secondary to her family and secondary in position in the labor force), the pigeonholing of women into jobs that mirror their family roles and low wages paid for that work, the discontinuous nature of women workforce participation, again dictated by family expectations, and the culmination of all of these experiences in low income in later years.

For most older women, labor force participation has meant a job, not a career, because family life took precedence. The woman may have gone to work to help her husband through his education or as he started his employment career. She then may have gone in and out of the workforce between child rearing and other caregiving responsibilities, and even when her earnings were essential to the family's well-being, she rarely thought of her job as requiring the same long-term investment as that of her husband (Fox & Hesse-Biber, 1984). She was clearly apt to be in "women's work" and in the secondary labor market, meaning low wages, fewer benefits (specifically the lack of a private pension), and vulnerability to being laid off (Baron & Bielby, 1985; Campbell, 1979; Lloyd & Niemi, 1979; Ozawa, 1982; Rix, 1984; Szinovacz, 1982; Trieman, Hartman, & Roos, 1984). Many older women, continuing to put their family role before their work role, assumed that their husband's pension and/or social security benefits would assure an adequate retirement. The need to worry about their economic security based on their own earnings seemed remote. Divorce and widowhood force a different picture, and the proportions of elderly women living below the poverty line—28.7% for all unmarried older women, 82% for black women—is testimony to that (Rix, 1984; U.S. Bureau of Census, 1980). The consequence of placing a woman in a dependent economic role throughout her lifetime has dire consequences for her later years (Forman, 1983; Warlick, 1985). In the following discussion, an alternative view of the interaction of work and home for women will be presented to suggest a more promising set of circumstances for later cohorts of women.

THE POTENTIAL OF OLDER WOMEN AND THE FUTURE

Another view of the future for later cohorts of older women is influenced by what we now are learning about the adult developmental process on the individual level, as well as by the impact of social movements and political changes, some already in the making and others projections for the future. This discussion suggests a more optimistic perspective on today's older woman and posits a clear connection between changed social and economic policies and the circumstances of future generations of elderly women (Giele, 1978, 1982a, 1982b; Rossi, 1986).

First, the recent adult development literature offers a refreshing orientation to the possibilities of individual growth throughout life (Fiske, 1980; George, 1982; Gilligan, 1982a). Stability has previously been emphasized as a characteristic of middle age, but there is now a growing interest in change, influenced by such social factors as "a longer postparental period, changing views of work, increasing divorce and increasing attention to the quality of life" (Knox, 1979, p. 2). It is known that women do become more assertive as they age (Gutmann, 1980; Neugarten, 1975), but now women, in particular, are seen as having the potential for other changes during their middle and later years (Rossi, 1986). Livson (1983) comments that "the parts of their personalities that were suppressed because they were not congruent with the roles of mother and young adult may now surface to add new dimensions" (p. 108). With the demands of nurturing ending for many women when children are grown, women are free to invest in other roles (Erdwins, Tyler, & Mellinger, 1980). In one exploratory study of women who made significant changes in their lives after the age of 50, women were found to be capable of and enriched by beginning entirely new careers in later life, both in employment and community activity spheres (Hooyman & Gottlieb, 1987).

Lowenthal et al. (1975) and Neugarten (1975) found that some women view growing older as a time of expansion and development of talents in self-fulfilling directions. Recent work by Giele (1982b) and Gilligan (1982b) suggest that women's involvement in caring relationships throughout their lives provides them with the social skills and social support networks necessary to use help when they need it. Similarly, Kline (1980) asserts that women's often discontinuous employment patterns provide them with a flexibility that contributes to their resolution of problems associated with aging. This faculty may also contribute to the assumption of a range of new roles (Uhlenberg, 1979).

New theories are being proposed about women's development that acknowledge the value of both their affiliative, caregiving traits and their search for autonomy while maintaining connectedness to others. These theories also imply growth throughout life (Surrey, 1985). These new understandings contain the seeds for placing appropriate worth on the nurturing tasks women perform and for correcting the second-class psychological status women have been given (Ehrenreich & English, 1979). These theoretical developments also have the potential of altering our society's view of women and changing the stance that professionals assume when troubled women seek help. They might prevent the Catch-22 dilemma faced by many women who meet society's expectations of the passive, nurturing women and then are not considered mentally healthy because they don't have valued traits usually associated with men (Broverman et al., 1970).

There is a parallel political movement, which has the considerable potential of altering that traditional view of women more dramatically and at the same time improving women's economic situation. The principle of comparable worth in the workplace appears to be accumulating political strength. As of 1985, a total of 45 states were in some stage of study or were using task forces to consider comparable worth implementation, and 9 states had assigned monies to correct inequities (Atcherson, 1987). This appears to be a new principle of economic life whose time is rapidly coming.

The increasing implementation of comparable worth principles can affect older women in two positive ways. First, if women are paid more for the work they do, their lifelong earnings will increase, and this will of course increase their retirement benefits. The financial plight of older women is such a crucial part of their general well-being that these economic changes hold great promise for the future cohort of older women.

Second, when women are paid more for the work they traditionally do — as secretaries, as nurses and nurses aides, as teachers, and the whole list of nurturing and service tasks needed by our society — those tasks, those extensions of women's roles, will be valued more in a general way. Comparable worth is, in principle, considerably different from equal pay for equal work (Remick, 1984). Comparable worth declares that different work tasks can be evaluated on the basis of overall categories, such as required training or degree of responsibility. This makes it possible for a secretary of a large corporation to be rated similarly and receive pay equal to the corporation's plumber or truck driver. At present, those salaries may have wide gaps to the detriment of women. The enactment of comparable worth says that the vitally necessary work that women do, not accorded high value because it is an extension of women's work in the home, is now worth a good deal to our society. The double effect of this economic change — more money for women both in their working and retirement years, and the enhanced esteem for the work they do — can both alter the practical resources older women will have and can lead to a changed view of themselves in society. Comparable worth is currently taking on some general reality with great potential for future older women.

There are other ways to look at the connection between women's role at home and their work in the labor force, which are more speculative but which are offered here for futuristic perspectives. All indications are that women will increasingly participate in the work place. The scenario presented now builds on that reality and suggests the reframing the question about the connection between outside work and home roles can affect women in positive ways throughout their lives.

When women were entering the workforce in increasing numbers in the 1960s, the widespread concern about the effect of their doing so on their families led to a series of studies to investigate possible harmful effects on children (Hofferth & Moore, 1979; Hoffman, 1974). The assumption was that women's partial renunication of their traditional role was a potentially dangerous development. The proposal for the future offered here takes the opposite stance and suggests that the preparation of women for a range of jobs in which, with the help of comparable-worth progress, they are paid salaries adequate to support themselves and their families, can lead to more stable family lives and better circumstances for these women in their later years.

Arguments can be made (although they will not be pursued here in view of the central focus on older women) that when women are trained and expect to be paid well for the work they do they will (1) have greater self-esteem and develop skills for independent living; (2) be less likely to want to take the chance of interfering with a future worthwhile career by risking pregnancy in adolescence, a condition that we know leads to lifelong poor earnings and serious implications for the older years (studies of risk-taking behavior and pregnancy appears to support this hypothesis, Luker, 1975); (3) enter marriage on an equal economic footing with their husbands, thereby not marrying solely for support (perhaps favorably affecting the rate of divorce), and will more likely demand an egalitarian sharing of household tasks, including caregiving to children and older relatives. This is clearly speculation, perhaps even grandiose expectation, although the absence of these conditions seemed to have been associated with considerable family unrest and economic hardship for women.

However, it would be fair to say that if older women of the future develop skills not necessarily restricted by traditional views of women, have the freedom to enter the work force with those skills and be paid well for their work, and are not consigned exclusively to the home role (in fact, had equal sharing with their husbands of home tasks), then the negative consequences of the current situation discussed earlier in this chapter might less likely appear to plague them. They would be less likely to be valued for just the home role, and their worth to society would be more apparent, starting from their early work life and continuing through their retirement. They would have more practical resources for those retirement years as well as skills for independent living. Their worth would not be determined primarily by their meeting family expectations, and they would be less likely to feel obsolete and discarded when the family role has ended.

Spakes' (1988) call for a National Women's Policy to substitute for a National Family policy coincides with the above future scenario. Her proposal calls for attention to women's needs as individuals first—for education, employment options, adequate pay, and choices about family life. She quarrels with the emphasis on family policy because such a pronatalist stance is predicted on women being in the family role essentially. This chapter has argued that relegating women to that role has had harmful consequences for the economic, social, and emotional condition of the present cohort of older women. If the future is to be changed for the next cohorts, then basic expectations of women and economic policies that devalue them need to be changed.

CONCLUSION

This discussion has contained both bad news and good news for older women. The bad news is that the present cohort of women in their 60s and older suffer from the consequences of a society that has defined women primarily in their family role. The result is that, on the whole, they are less apt to have the skills and self-enhancing attitudes, as well as the practical resources, to live a fulfilling older life. Many of the women in this current cohort are being denied the opportunities to lead productive lives past their family responsibilities.

The good news is that the situation appears to be changing for the cohorts of older women who are to follow. There appears to be a gradual but inexorable movement toward other views of women's place in society, views that have the promise of changing not only women's own attitudes and behavior but providing them in their younger adult years with practical resources for the work they do both inside and outside the home. The more positive consequences for their later years will be clear. As health care advances have made it possible for women to live longer lives, political and social advances can make it possible for older women to live those years fruitfully.

Considerable changes in the current realities of family life may help society to develop a different view of women. It no longer makes practical sense to consider as an examplar the family in its traditional form — husband at work and wife at home with the children. In addition to the wife's labor force participation, there are myriad family forms — for example, the blended family following divorce or death of a spouse, the single-parent household, homosexual partners with or without children, the household of siblings, and cross-generational families formed purposefully, not by blood ties. The varieties of families runs parallel with the loosening of gender-specific home responsibilities. The more the gender constraints are blurred, the more likely it will be that women will have increased practical and inner resources to lead productive later lives.

Even in the present cohort, older women have displayed remarkable resilience and innovativeness in the face of adversity (Riley & Riley, 1986). Added to these qualities, there is a growing interest in the changes that individual older women can make well into very late life.

The tasks of those of us concerned about older women today are twofold. We need to attend to the needs of the current cohort of older women and recognize the negative impact of our ageist, racist, and sexist stereotypes and policies. It is particularly important to see both the negative and positive effects on women of the roles they play in their families and to help these women see the potentials in their later years, even in view of a previous restrictive life. Many women have led satisfying family-oriented adult lives, and many are fortunate to have lifetime partners, to have enough income, and to be in good health. The problem for most women is a lack of synchrony between their earlier and later adult years. Those family years, probably accompanied by some experiences in and out of the paid workforce, do not provide enough of what women on their own need in the last third of their lives — enough income, enough autonomous traits, and enough support systems. For most, the earlier ingredients are not there to provide what is needed later on.

In understanding the basis of many older women's current difficulties, we can take on the second task of working to bring about another scenario for later cohorts. It is possible that through different socialization (or at least consciousness about a changing socialization process), through family policies, and through family-oriented workplaces, we can create more self-enhancing family and work lives for younger women, which can result in their experience of more satisfying aging years.

REFERENCES

Almquist, E. (1984). Race and ethnicity in the lives of minority women. In J. Freeman (Ed.), *Women: A feminist perspective* (pp. 423-453). Palo Alto, CA: Mayfield.

Archbold, P. (1982). All-consuming activity: The family as caregiver. *Generations, 7*, 12-14.

Arling G. (1976). Resistance to isolation among elderly widows. *International Journal of Aging and Human Development, 7*, 67-84.

Atcherson, E. (1987). The politics of equality for women. *AFFILIA: Journal of Women and Social Work, 2*, 20-33.

Barnett, R., & Baruch, G. (1978). Women in the middle years: A critique of research and theory. *Psychology of Women Quarterly, 3*, 187-197.

Baron, J., & Bielby, W. (1985). Organizational barriers to gender equality: Sex segregation of jobs and opportunities. In A. Rossi (Ed.), *Gender and the life course* (pp. 233-251). New York: Aldine.

Bart, P. (1980). The emotional and social status of the older women. In *No longer young: The older woman in America* (Occasional Papers). Ann Arbor, MI: University of Michigan Institute of Gerontology.

Beckman, L., & Houser, B. (1982). The consequences of childlessness on the social-psychological well-being of older women. *Journal of Gerontology, 37*, 243-250.

Bernard, J. (1976). Homosociality and female depression. *Journal of Social Issues, 32*, 213-237.,

Block, M. R., Davidson, J. L., & Grambs, J. D. (1981). *Women over forty, visions & realities*. New York: Springer.

Braito, R. & Anderson, D. (1983). The ever-single elderly woman. In E. Markson (Ed.), *Older women* (pp. 195-225). Lexington, MA: Lexington Books.

Briar, K., Hoff, M., & Seck, E. (1987). Women and work. In D. Burden & N. Gottlieb (Eds.), *The woman client* (pp. 195-208). New York: Tavistock.

Brinson-Pineda, B. (1984). Hispanic women: Toward an agenda for the future. In A. Sargent (Ed.), *Beyond sex roles* (pp. 252-257). St. Paul, MN: West Publishing.

Brody, E., Johnsen, P., Fulcomer, M., & Lang, A. (1983). Women's changing roles and help to elderly parents: Attitudes of three generations of women. *Journal of Gerontology, 28*, 597-608.

Broverman, I., Broverman, D., Clarkson, F., Rosenkrantz, P., & Vogel, S.

(1970). Sex-role stereotypes and clinical judgments in mental health. *Journal of Consulting and Clinical Psychology, 34,* 1-7.

Burden, D., & Gottlieb, N. (1987). Human behavior in the social environment: The knowledge base for practice. In D. Burden & N. Gottlieb (Eds.), *The woman client* (pp. 41-52). New York: Tavistock.

Campbell, S. (1979). Delayed mandatory retirement and the working woman. *The Gerontologist, 19,* 257-264.

Cancian, F. (1985). Gender politics: Love and power in the private and public spheres. In A. Rossi (Ed.), *Gender and the life course* (pp. 253-264). New York: Aldine.

Candy, S. (1977). What do women use friends for. In L. Troll, J. Israel, & K. Israel (Eds.), *Look ahead* (pp. 106-111). Englewood Cliffs, NJ: Prentice-Hall.

Chow, E. (1984). The acculturation experience of Asian-American women. In A. Sargent (Ed.). *Beyond sex roles* (pp. 238-251). St. Paul, MN: West Publishing.

Crossman, L. London, C., & Barry, C. (1981). Older women caring for disabled spouses. A model for supportive services. *The Gerontologist 21,* 464-470.

Enrenreich, B., & English, D. (1979). *For her own good.* London: Pluto Press.

England, P. (1984). Socioeconomics and explanations of job segregation. In H. Remick (Ed.), *Comparable worth and wage discrimination* (pp. 28-46). Philadelphia: Temple University Press.

Erdwins, C., Tyler, Z., & Mellinger, J. (1980). Personality traits of mature women in student versus homemaker roles. *The Journal of Psychology, 105,* 189-195.

Fengler, A. & Goodrich, N. (1979). Wives of elderly disabled: The hidden patients. *Generations, 19,* 175-183.

Fiske, M. (1980). Changing hierarchies of commitment in adulthood. In N. Smelser & E. Erickson (Eds.), *Themes of work and love in adulthood* (pp. 238-264). Cambridge, MA: Harvard University Press.

Forman, M. (1983). Social security is a woman's issue. *Social Policy, 14,* 35-38.

Fox, M. & Hesse-Biber, A. (1984). *Women at work.* Palo Alto, CA: Mayfield.

Fries, J. (1983). The compression of morbidity. *Milbank Memorial Fund Quarterly/Health and Society, 61,* 397-419.

Gallagher, D. E., Thompson, L. W., & Peterson, J. A. (1983). Effects of bereavement on indicators of mental health in elderly widows and widowers. *Journal of Gerontology, 38,* 565-571.

George, L. (1982). Models of transition in middle and later life. *Annals of the American Academy of Political and Social Sciences, 464,* 22-37.

Giele, J. (1978). *Women and the future.* New York: Free Press.

Giele, J. (1982a). Future research and policy questions. In J. Giele (Ed.), *Women in the middle years* (pp. 199-240). New York: Wiley.

Giele, J. (1982b). Women in adulthood: Unanswered questions. In J. Giele (Ed.). *Women in the middle years* (pp. 1-35). New York: Wiley.

Gilligan, C. (1982a). Adult development and women's development: Arrangements for a marriage. In J. Giele (Ed.), *Women in the middle years* (pp. 89-114). New York: Wiley.

Gilligan, C. (1982b). *In a different voice*. Cambridge, MA: Harvard University Press.

Gottlieb, N. (1980). The older woman. In N. Gottlieb (Ed.), *Alternative social services for women* (pp. 280-331). New York: Columbia University Press.

Gottlieb, N., Burden, D., McCormick, R. & Nicarthy, G. (1983). The distinctive attributes of feminist groups. *Social Work with Groups, 6*, 81-93.

Greenwood-Audrant, L. (1984). The internalization of powerlessness: A case study of the displaced homemaker. In J. Freeman (Ed.), *Women: A feminist perspective* (pp. 264-281). Palo Alto, CA: Mayfield.

Gutmann, D. (1980). Psychoanalysis and aging: A developmental view. In S. Greenspan & G. Pollock (Eds.), *The course of life: Psychoanalytic contributions toward understanding personality development: Vol. 3. Adulthood and the aging process*. Washington, DC: U.S. Government Printing Office.

Hess, B. (1985). Aging policies and old women: The hidden agenda. In A. Rossi (Ed.), *Gender and the life course* (pp. 319-331). New York: Aldine.

Hess, B., & Waring, J. (1983). Family relationships of older women. In E. Markson (Ed.), *Older women* (pp. 227-251). Lexington, MA: Lexington Books.

Hofferth, S., & Moore, K. (1979). Women's employment and marriage. In R. Smith (Ed.). *The subtle revolution: Women at work* (pp. 99-124). Washington, DC: Urban Institute.

Hoffman, L. (1974). Effects on child. In L. Hoffman & F. Nye (Eds.), *Working mothers* (pp. 126-166). San Francisco: Jossey-Bass.

Hooyman, N. (1987). Older women and the social work curricula. In D. Burden & N. Gottlieb (Eds.). *The woman client* (pp. 263-279). New York: Tavistock.

Hooyman, N., & Gottlieb, N. (1987, March). *The potential of older women*. Paper presented the American Society on Aging Conference, Salt Lake City, UT.

Hooyman, N., & Kiyak, A. (1988). *Social Gerontology*. Boston: Allyn & Bacon.

Hooyman, N., & Lustbader, W. (1986). *Taking care*. New York: Free Press.

Jackson, J. (1980). Categorical differences of older black women. *Generations, 4*, 17, 33.

Johnson, C., & Catalano, D. (1981). Childless elderly and their family supports. *The Gerontologist, 21*, 610-619.

Johnson, E., & Bursk, B. (1980). Relationships between the elderly and their adult children. In M. Fuller & C. Martin (Eds.), *The older woman* (pp. 158-169). Springfield, IL: Charles C Thomas.

Keating, N., & Cole, P. (1980). What do I do with her 24 hours a day? Changes in the housewife role after retirement. *The Gerontologist, 20*, 84-89.

Kline, C. (1980). The socialization process of women: Implications for a theory of successful aging. In M. Fuller, & C. Martin (Eds.), *The older woman* (pp. 59-70). Springfield, IL: Charles C Thomas.

Knox, A. (1979). Perspectives on mid-life. *New Directions for Continuing Education, 2*, 1-6.

Kohen, J. (1983). Old but not alone: Informal social supports among the elderly by marital status and sex. *The Gerontologist, 23*, 57-63.

Lesnoff-Caravaglia, G. (Ed.). (1984). *The world of older women.* New York Human Sciences Press.

Lipman-Blumen, J. (1984). *Gender roles and power.* Englewood Cliffs, NJ: Prentice-Hall.

Livson, F. B. (1983). Gender Identity: A lifespan view of sex role development. In R. Weg (Ed.). *Aging: An international annual (Vol. 1), Sexuality in the later years: Roles and behavior* (pp. 105-124). Menlo Park, CA: Addison-Wesley.

Lloyd, C., & Niemi, B. (Eds.). (1979). *The economics of sex differentials.* New York: Columbia University Press.

Lopata, H. (1977). The meaning of friendships in widowhood. In M. Troll, J. Israel, & J. Israel (Eds.), *Looking ahead* (pp. 93-105). Englewood Cliffs, NJ: Prentice-Hall.

Luker, K. (1975). *Taking chances: Abortion and the decision not to contracept.* Berkeley and Los Angeles: The University of California Press.

Markson, E. (1983). Introduction. In E. Markson (Ed.), *Older women* (pp. 1-5). Lexington, MA: Lexington Books.

Mayer, K. (1985). Some legal considerations in domestic relationships. In H. Hidalgo, T. Peterson, & N. Woodman (Eds.), *Lesbian and gay issues* (pp. 88-91). Silver Spring, MD: National Association of Social Workers.

Neugarten, B. (Ed.). (1975). *Middle age and aging.* Chicago: University of Chicago Press.

Nydegger, C. (1983). Family ties of the elderly in cross cultural perspective. *The Gerontologist, 23*, 26-32.

Older Women's League. (1983). The D.C. Scene. In *Owl Observer.* Feb-March 2, 2-8.

Ozawa, M. (1982). The 1983 amendments to the Social Security Act: The issues of intergenerational equity. *Social Work, 29*, 131-137.

Payne, B., & Whittington, F. (1980). Older women: An examination of popular stereotypes and research evidence. In M. Fuller & C. Martin (Eds.), *The older woman* (pp. 9-30). Springfield, IL: Charles C Thomas.

Piven, F. (1985). Women and the state: Ideology, power and the welfare state. In A. Rossi (Ed.), *Gender and the life course* (pp. 265-287). New York: Aldine.

Powers, E., & Bultena, G. (1980). Sex differences in the intimate friendships of old age. In M. Fuller & C. Martin (Eds.), *The older woman* (pp. 190-208). Springfield, IL: Charles C Thomas.

Quinn, M., & Tomita, S. (1986). *Elder abuse and neglect.* New York: Springer.

Raphael, S., & Robinson, M. (1980). The older lesbian: Love relationships and friendship patterns. *Alternate Lifestyles, 3*, 207-229.

Remick, H. (Ed.). (1984). *Comparable worth and wage discrimination*. Philadelphia: Temple University Press.

Riley, M. W., & Riley, J. (1986). Longevity and social structure: The potential of the added years. In A. Pifer & L. Bronte (Eds.), *Our aging society* (pp. 33-51). New York: Norton.

Rix, S. (1984). *Older women: The economics of aging*. Washington, DC: Women's Research and Education Institute.

Rossi, A. (1986). Sex and gender in the aging society. In A. Piefer & L. Bronte (Eds.), *Our aging society* (pp. 111-139). New York: Norton.

Shanas, E. (1979). Social myths as hypotheses: The case of family relations of old people. *The Gerontologist, 19*, 3-9.

Simon, B. (1986). Never married women as caregivers to elderly patients: Some costs and benefits. *AFFILIA Journal of Women and Social Work, 1*, 29-42.

Spakes, P. (1988, March). *National family policy and feminist social work practice: The incompatible pair*. Paper presented at the Annual Program Meeting, Council in Social Work Education, Atlanta, GA.

Steitz, J. (1981). The female life course: Life situations and perceptions of control. *International Journal of Aging and Human Development, 14*, 195-204.

Stillion, J. (1984). Women and widowhood: The suffering beyond grief. In J. Freeman (Ed.), *Women: A feminist perspective* (pp. 282-293). Palo Alto, CA: Mayfield.

Surrey, J. (1985). *Self in relation: A theory of women's development*. Wellesley, MA: Wellesley College Stone Center for Development Services and Studies.

Szinovacz, J. (1982). *Women's retirement*. Beverly Hills, CA: Sage.

Terrelonge, P. (1984). Feminist consciousness and black women. In J. Freeman (Ed.), *Women: A feminist perspective* (pp. 557-567). Palo Alto, CA: Mayfield.

Timberlake, E. M. (1980). The value of grandchildren to grandmothers. *Journal of Gerontological Social Work, 3*, 63-76.

Treas, J. (1977). Family support systems for the aged. *The Gerontologist, 17*, 486-491.

Trieman, D., Hartman, H., & Roos, A. (1984). Assessing pay discrimination using national data. In H. Remick (Ed.), *Comparable worth and wage discrimination* (pp. 137-154). Philadelphia: Temple University Press.

Uhlenberg, P. (1979). Older women: The growing challenge to design constructive roles. *The Gerontologist, 19*, 236-241.

U.S. Bureau of the Census. (1986) *Money, income, and poverty status of families and persons in the United States, 1985* (Series P-60, No. 85). Washington, DC: U.S. Government Printing Office.

U.S. Bureau of the Census. (1980). A statistical portrait of women in the United States. *Current population reports: Special studies* (Series P-23, No. 100). Washington, DC: U.S. Government Printing Office.

U.S. Senate Special Committee on Aging. (1986). *Aging America: Trends and projections, 1985-1986*. Washington, DC: U.S. Department of Health and Human Services.

Verbrugge, L. (1983). Women and men: Mortality and health of older people. In M. Riley, B. Hess, & B. Bond (Eds.), *Aging in society* (pp. 139-174). Hillsdale, NJ: Erlbaum.

Warlick, J. (1985). Why is poverty after 65 a women's problem? *Journal of Gerontology, 40*, 751-757.

Weitz, R. (1984). What price independence? Social reactions to lesbians, spinsters, widows and nuns. In J. Freeman (Ed.), *Women: A feminist perspective* (pp. 454-464). Palo Alto, CA: Mayfield.

Weitzman, L. (1984). Sex-role socialization: A focus on women. In J. Freeman (Ed.), *Women: A feminist perspective* (pp. 157-237). Palo Alto, CA: Mayfield.

White-Riley, M. (1981). The healthy woman in the year 2000. In *Health issues for older women* (pp. 65-69). Stony Brook, NY: The School of Applied Health Professions, State University of New York.

Sexuality and Intimacy for Aging Women: A Changing Perspective

Susan Rice, DSW

Webster's Unabridged Dictionary (1983) defines *intimate* in five different ways, including (1) inmost; essential; most inward; internal, (2) most private or personal, (3) closely acquainted or associated; very familiar, (4) resulting from careful study or investigation; very close, (5) having sexual relations; a euphemism (p. 962). Furthermore, *sexual* is defined in two different ways; the first being "characteristic of, or affecting the sexes" and the second being the biological definition of "having sex" (p. 1664). Despite the "correct" meaning of these words, our society focuses on the last definition given in each case. Intimacy and sexuality are usually understood to mean having sexual relations or being actively sexual in a physical way. This discussion will operate on the premise that a broader, more universal definition of intimacy and sexuality is applicable, which leads to heretofore unexplored options related to intimacy and sexuality in older women.

Included in the definition will be the concepts of sensuality, closeness, and love and their relationship to interdependence. In later life, most people increase their dependence on other people, whether it is related to an increased need for concrete assistance because of failing physical abilities, or for emotional assistance to fill needs left by interpersonal losses. Montagu (1974) includes maternal love, creative love, sexual love, love of friends, love of mankind, and love of God in his exploration of the elusive nature of

Susan Rice is Associate Professor, Department of Social Work, California State University at Long Beach, 1250 Bellflower Boulevard, Long Beach, CA 90840.

245

love. This definition will allow us to look at sexuality and intimacy in a familial context as well as an individual one. How are relationships with spouses and children part of intimacy and sexuality for older women? The average 65-year-old mother (Cochran, 1985) can look back on intimate relationships with her daughters that include mutual trust, support, and understanding, which can contribute to a long era of good feelings and psychological well-being for both mother and daughter. This, too, is intimacy as part of old age.

Sexual intimacy, perhaps, is a specialized way of expressing the broader spectrums of the emotions we feel when there is a closeness or bonding between two people.

ISSUES THAT AFFECT SEXUALITY IN OLDER WOMEN

A variety of issues prevent women from having a satisfactory level of intimacy and sexuality in their lives as they grow old. The issues that will be discussed have in common their tendency to demoralize a woman and destroy her self-confidence and self-esteem, so that she tends to withdraw from rather than engage with the people in her life. This psychological withdrawal works strongly against the achievement of emotional and physical intimacy and a fulfilled sense of sexuality.

The double standard (Sontag, 1972) toward aging in our society is so pervasive that it becomes incorporated into our sense of selves without our being fully aware of it. Men are thought to gain maturity as they age, whereas women lose the freshness of youth. Last month, one of the new purportedly feminist magazines ran a full 4-page advertisement for a skin cream, in which the copy ran as follows: "I don't intend to grow old gracefully. . . . I intend to fight it every step of the way" (*New Woman*, February, 1988, p. 14). The attitude that smooth skin is equated with self-worth is a wicked example of the ageism that confronts older women today.

Ageism is demoralizing to older people as a group, but its impact on women is especially strong because they have been traditionally viewed primarily in terms of their physical beauty and ability to entertain and amuse other people.

Issues related to traditional perspectives on human development as they affect and are affected by coping patterns are fully discussed in a separate section of this compendium. The effects of developmental issues on sexuality and intimacy relate to the ways in which women see themselves. Most writers agree (Stevens-Long, 1988) that people who are intimate engage in self-disclosure; that is, they confide in each other about personal matters. Therefore, if self-disclosure is a defining characteristic of intimacy, there is also a strong relationship between intimacy and identity. In other words, how can a person tell someone else about who they are if they do not see themselves clearly? Furthermore, if sexuality emerges from intimacy, the ability to be sexual is also stymied if one does not have a clear sense of self-identity.

Research has demonstrated (Maccoby & Jacklin, 1976) that there is much greater variation within genders than between them in terms of actual gender-related psychological differences. However, if women are socialized differently than men from the beginning, adult behavior and cognitions will also be different (Weitzman, 1979) because of the differing sense of self-identity that is fostered. Socialization that encourages girls not to separate from parents and to gain support from parental approval fosters dependency and fear of rejection, which makes it harder for adults to seek out the kinds of intimacy that they want. Specifically, the results of a study of young adults demonstrated (Orlofsky, 1976) that subjects who had adopted the identity outlined for them by their parents were likely to possess only superficial relationships or to develop commitments out of a sense of social convenience rather than mutuality, love, respect, and understanding.

It is important to recognize the tremendous change in sexual attitudes that has come about in the past century. Our society has moved from a climate in which words like "sex," "pregnant," and "menstruation" were not spoken aloud in mixed company, children were told absolutely nothing about sex, and young pregnant women were not expected to appear in public once their pregnancy was obvious (Hancock, 1987). Mary Margaret Sanger was arrested and jailed after opening the first birth control clinic, only a little over 60 years ago (Gordon, 1979). Now every popular magazine, radio and television show, and newspaper discusses "private" or intimate issues in public, which creates a sense that such problems are acceptable for discussion, as well as soluble. Older people to-day, however, are caught up in a tremendous conflict between the societal message of yesterday of prohibition and secrecy and the one of today in which we "let it all hang out." We must be sensitive to the impact of the values with which today's older generation of women grew up with and were inculcated and the pervasive nature of those values in terms of influencing their present-day behavior.

Bereavement affects sexuality and intimacy and is a distinct and different phenomenon depending on a woman's marital status. Feminist theory recognizes (Gilligan, 1978) that a woman's identity is often defined through relationships and caring for others, so that when a woman loses a loved one she also loses a sense of self, which intensifies grief and requires a new identity formation. For a widow, this process may take several years (Glick, Weiss, & Parkes, 1974) and will inhibit any reaching out to new people, unless her definition of intimacy encompasses a nonsexual, non-partner-oriented concept. Even in such a scenario, initial attempts to be intimate will be somewhat diffuse, because of the struggle to know exactly who one is and what one has to give to others in any kind of emotionally intimate encounter.

Of the main psychiatric syndromes seen in the elderly, depression is the most common (Edinburg, 1982), with an incidence of 10% for ages 66 to 75. There is also a high incidence of suicide. One out of two suicide attempts by the elderly is successful, which is a much higher rate than for other age groups (Flaste, 1979). Thus far, elderly men have suffered more than women in this area, as demonstrated by the fact that white males in the 70 to 74 age group commit suicide at a rate nearly 5 times as high as that of all women of the same age. The speculation is that the more successful (in societal terms) one has been, the harder it is to deal with the irreversible losses of work, spouse, family, and friends. For women, the suicide rate peaks at ages 50 to 54, which might be a clue as to when present-day women experience their greatest losses. As our society changes in ways that allow more freedom and potential achievements for women, the losses of those achievements may also be harder for them to deal with.

Reactive depressions arise as a result of a loss or accumulation of losses, such as loss of a spouse, financial loss, loss of hearing or sight, and loss of mobility (Busse & Pfeiffer, 1977). It is, however, important to note that only a minority of older people suffer "clinically significant" depressions (Brink, 1979). The lack of sexuality and intimacy is both a cause and effect of depression. Women turn inward when they feel isolated and alone, and that withdrawal makes it harder for them to fully engage with other people.

Women who have been in abusive relationships reach old age with a scarred view of intimacy, which affects the ability to be intimate with nonthreatening partners. It is estimated that two-thirds of American couples experience violent incidents at some time in their marriages, and about one-third experience violence every year (Straus, Gelles, & Steinmetz, 1981). Up to 50% of all women (Walker, 1979) will be battered at some time in their lives. When sexuality is so commonly coupled with violence, women become reluctant to seek out sexual or emotional intimacy in situations in which they see themselves as frail.

In addition, one in ten elderly people that live with a family member are physically or psychologically abused each year (Lau & Kosberg, 1978). The most likely elderly people to be abused are women with severe physical or mental impairments, because of the fact that such impairments lead to dependence, which makes the elderly person especially vulnerable to abuse (O'Rourke, 1981). Although child abuse is recognized to be a horror of our society, there is much more tolerance for abuse of the elderly. The intention is benevolent—a recognition that the strain and burden on the family leads to stress (Miller, 1981) and a desire not to interfere with personal liberties. However, the result is that elderly women are left with few alternatives to the abuse in situations where they feel dependent upon their families. As with sexual abuse, this situation leaves little surplus emotional or physical resources for searching out satisfactory forms of intimacy.

When a woman enters an institution, in most cases she is expected and forced to live a life of celibacy (Kelly & Rice, 1986). Double beds are almost nonexistent in institutional settings, and even solitary expressions of direct sexuality such as masturbation are unavailable because of the lack of privacy. The psychological effect of ignoring the need for closeness is that women (and men) start to feel as though they are no longer human. Even the social expressions of sexual intimacy, such as flirting, kissing, dancing, hugging, and hand-holding are frowned upon, as if physical desire was completely inappropriate. Even if the concept that touching, whether it be sexual or nonsexual, expresses intimacy is promoted on a personal level, restrictions or disapproval by one's caretakers works directly against the achievement of intimacy.

All of the issues that have been discussed directly affect sexuality in older women because of their impact on self-esteem and on a woman's willingness and ability to seek out the kind of fulfillment that she wants in old age. If these issues are confronted, an opportunity exists. A distinguished, prolific feminist writer (Sarton, 1975, p. 27) says of old age:

> We have greater freedom than ever before to be our true selves. Everything is opening out inside and around us. The walls are dissolving between being and essence, and when they dissolve altogether, when our *selves*, as we have known them, dissolve into death, it will be that we have grown into another dimension.

Many older women suffer from physical diseases that have a direct effect on sexual expression, as well as indirectly affecting self-esteem and self-image. Women who have had cerebrovascular accidents (strokes) or heart attacks frequently stop any sexual activity completely for fear of having a second heart attack or stroke. The actual facts regarding this issue are not clear, but one author (Butler & Lewis, 1982) estimates that only 1% of sudden coronary deaths occur during intercourse. Physicians often encourage their patients to continue sexual activity, as it is thought that the amount of oxygen needed for sexual intercourse with partners of long standing is equivalent to merely the amount needed for climbing a flight of stairs or walking briskly (Puksta, 1977).

Other chronic health problems, including Parkinson's disease and arthritis, make it physically uncomfortable to engage in sexual activity, as well as making women feel that they are no longer desirable. Again, if a woman has incorporated the belief that her physical self is the sum of her self-identity, this chronic physical debilitation exacerbates her ability to be emotionally intimate as well.

PHYSICAL CHANGES IN SEXUALITY

There is a wide measure of agreement that none of the changes in sexual physiology that occur in women necessarily limit the sexual functioning or responsiveness of older women (Masters & Johnson, 1966, 1970).

Most of the physiological sexual changes in women are related to the decline of female hormones such as estrogen following menopause (Butler & Lewis, 1976). A decline of estrogen can produce symptoms including a lessening of vaginal lubrication, which can make intercourse painful. The lining of the vagina itself begins to thin and becomes easily irritated, leading to pain and bleeding during intercourse, especially if it is of long duration or following a long period without sexual contact. Because older men often take a longer time to complete the act of intercourse, the probability of this occurring increases. Sometimes the shape of the vagina itself changes, becoming narrower, shorter, and less elastic. The usually acid vaginal secretions become less acidic, increasing the possibility of vaginal infection, and causing burning, itching, and discharge. However, during one course of "treatment" for all of these problems, hormone replacement therapy, the symptoms are effectively eliminated. There is some concern about the side effects related to receiving too much estrogen, which can include fluid retention and weight gain, headaches, and high blood pressure. Another solution to these problems is the use of topical estrogen creams. Many standard lubricating creams and gels (such as Vaseline) may be unsuccessful in increasing vaginal lubrication because the altered nature of the lining of the vagina leads to an inability to hold moisture when it is applied directly (Weg, 1983). Estrogen cream, on the other hand, is essentially self-lubricating, and can reduce discomfort. The lower dosages minimize the possibility of damaging side effects.

A third solution, paradoxically enough, is increased amounts of sexual activity, which is found to stimulate estrogen production. The paradox, of course, is that when sexual intercourse is uncomfortable and/or the woman feels inadequate in her performance, she is less likely to seek out opportunities to be sexually active, even if such opportunities were potentially available.

The psychological feelings that go along with these physical changes have a much greater impact on women, as do the changes in sexual physiology that accompany aging in men, since most women engage in heterosexual relationships. Therefore, a decline in the sexual functioning of men inevitably produces the same effect in women, although this too, has a basis that stems more from psychological effects than physical liabilities. In our society (Murphy, 1979), romantic love is equated to intense physical desire whose only appropriate sexual expression is characterized by passionate lovemaking and the achievement of sexual union through simultaneous orgasm. Older people (and younger people!) cannot consistently measure up to these expectations, yet through this attitude the belief is fostered that "real" sexual pleasure is only for a privileged few. Older women feel that they are not measuring up and so become reluctant to be sexually active at all, as it is a constant reminder of their inadequacy.

In summary, what are the sexual needs of older women?

> They are exactly the same kinds as those of younger people, with equivalent variations in intensity, kinds of expression, and other persons to express those needs with. As human beings at any stage of life, we long for other human beings to respond to us and to be responsive with whether in touch, in shared pleasures, joys, sorrows, intellectual interchange, or from time to time in sexual responsiveness at many levels including the purely physical. (Calderone, 1971)

SPECIAL POPULATIONS

There are certain groups of women who by virtue of some demographic characteristic are especially vulnerable to the issues that affect sexuality and intimacy in old age. These groups — including lesbians, never-married women, widows, the physically disabled, and minority women — face additional prejudices and pressures that take away available energy for finding personal fulfillment. However, it is also true that these groups have found, out of necessity, more creative solutions than women in the mainstream and in some ways fare better in their achievement of a positive sense of sexuality and intimacy because of the problems they have faced.

For example, it is interesting to note (Berger, 1982) that love relationships between older lesbians are not disrupted as frequently or as early as their heterosexual counterparts are by widowhood. In addition, the participants in the relationship are not devalued by their lesbian partners for being "old."

A study of life satisfaction and single, elderly, childless women (Rice, in press) demonstrated that never-married women had higher degrees of life satisfaction than widows because they had learned to create substitutes for the traditional social support systems of husband and children. These women were the political activists, the travellers, and the substitute aunts for relatives, and they were able to "create" support systems into old age in a way that allowed them to feel continuing satisfaction and intimacy. They had long ago accepted the fact that they did not fit by normal societal standards and had learned to aggressively pursue the things in life that would bring them satisfaction.

The greater longevity of women means that the number of widows exceeds widowers at all age levels. In 1982 (Bureau of the Census, 1982), for 65- to 74-year-olds the ratio of women to men was 6.4 to 1 and for 75 years and over the ratio of women to men was 5.3 to 1. The problem for widowed women in its essence is loneliness (Wyly & Hulicka, 1977). Widowed women miss their husbands as companions, as partners in activities, and as providers of social support. They must change their basic self-identity as a woman, especially if they have been traditionally oriented and have seen the role of wife as central to their lives. It is not usual for these women to think of finding emotional or physical intimacy in other kinds of relationships, and they are more likely to equate the death of their spouse with the simultaneous death of their own sexuality and emotional intimacy.

Physically handicapped women have an additional obstacle in terms of fulfilling their sexual needs because they are not usually perceived as sexual beings (Siemens & Brandzel, 1982). Their problems do not lie so much in the physical achievement of sexual acts but in the finding of a potential partner that would regard them as having sexual interests. They too may accept the societal standard that says that sexuality and intimacy is not appropriate for their situation.

In all of these situations, the lifelong practices of dealing with adversity can be an asset for the aging woman in continuing to engage in fulfilling and intimate relationships or it can have the immobilizing effect of determining that old age is "the last nail in the coffin," that the issue is no longer worth struggling with.

INTERVENTION TO ENHANCE SEXUALITY AND INTIMACY

It is clear that anyone interested in promoting fulfillment related to sexuality and intimacy for older women must intervene in a way that gives a different message to them than does mainstream society. That message has to incorporate elements of freedom, of choice, and of opportunities. In *The Aging Game* (Anderson, 1979), tactics are discussed for improving one's intimate relations, including "developing the alliances that count." Recognizing that all women need to depend on other people (as do all people) allows one to depend on friends without feeling ashamed or inadequate. It allows women to assertively seek out other people, male and female, with whom they would like to become closer. It allows them to count on children and grandchildren for support without feeling that they are a burden.

Pets have also been recognized (Garner, 1985) as an important potential source of love and sharing. They provide unconditional, nonjudgmental love and affection, unlike society, which judges people's worth by factors such as beauty, youth, perceived status, or possessions.

Shared housing is another concept that can facilitate the achievement of intimacy for older women. Shared housing can range from an informal arrangement in which two or more unrelated people decide to share their own home to facilities in which common dining and recreational facilities are provided. There are organizations that assist people in finding other women to share their homes with or locating commercial residential facilities. This can have a strong positive impact on women's sense of intimacy because they become involved in daily sharing and reciprocal relationships. One of the problems with this concept is that independence has been valued so strongly by older adults that they tend to equate sharing with dependence, and so refuse to consider such options until some kind of crisis occurs.

The above interventions are aimed at broadening the opportunities in the environment in which it might be possible to seek more kinds of emotional intimacy. It cannot be forgotten, however, that physical sexuality can also be important. Frank discussion with older women could be helpful in allowing them to recognize and validate their own feelings. It is appropriate to help women become aware of the myths and misinformation that exist about sex, to be informative about the physiological changes that affect sexual functioning, and to be matter-of-fact and accepting about a wide range of variation in sexual behaviors.

Women who are not in an ongoing physical relationship need to be given permission to accept their sexuality in whatever way it exists for them—whether it be enjoying their fantasies and accepting normal coital alternatives such as self-massage, use of a vibrator, caressing, and mutual genital pleasuring, or whether it be controlling their sexual expressions and making peace with an asexual life style.

Annon (1976) suggests a four-pronged approach to intervention in sexual issues that is as applicable for older adults as for any other population. The first level of achieving an atmosphere in which a humanistic, pleasure-oriented (rather than performance-oriented) view of sexuality conveys the assumption that sex is an expression of the self. In order to do this, women might try to become aware of their own sense of comfort and their value systems. The second level is providing information in a limited way to dispel myths and provide key information about sexual anatomy and normal physiological changes that occur in aging. On the third level, specific suggestions might be made as to changes women could make in their own lives, which could include readings, self-stimulation procedures, and alternative sexual positions and activities. The fourth level involves referral to a qualified sex therapist.

It is also important, however, to be ready to accept a value and activity system in which the strongest feeling is one of relief that the physical aspect of sexuality is one that no longer must be addressed. For many women, because of the world they grew up in, physical sexuality was not seen as a pleasure, and it is unlikely for those feelings to change in old age.

PROFESSIONAL CONTACTS WITH OLDER WOMEN

The interventions that have been discussed above can occur only within a context of a relationship between older women and helping professionals, whether it be psychiatrists, psychologists, social workers, doctors, nurses, senior citizen workers, recreation therapists, physical therapists, home health aides, or volunteer personnel in community agencies. Despite the varied work that they do, the commonality that these professionals bring to their interaction with older people is the desire to be a part of a helping relationship and the skills that allow communication about a variety of emotionally laden issues.

What is a relationship? It can be defined (Perlman, 1979) as

a human being's feeling or sense of emotional bonding with another. It leaps into being like an electric current, or it emerges and develops cautiously when emotion is aroused by and invested in someone or something and that someone or something "connects back" responsively. We feel "related" when we feel at one with another person in some heartfelt way.

It is clear to see that, in a relationship, we model intimacy for the people we work with. In our interactions with them, we demonstrate the bonding process and allow our clients to experience intimacy in a safe and nonthreatening atmosphere. This intimacy can be both physical and verbal; although it should be clearly stated that the ethics of all of the helping professions specifically prohibits sexual intimacy in the name of "helping."

For example, when an in-office encounter takes place between a practitioner and an older woman, sitting behind a desk creates barriers and is less likely to lead to emotional intimacy in the interpersonal transaction. On a more subtle level, calling a client by her first name and expecting her to call you by your last name and title erects the same kind of barrier. Technical flexibility (Beaver & Miller, 1985) can relate to all phases of the interventive process, ranging from using different concepts from different theories in establishing rapport with a client, developing a treatment plan and carrying it out, even though the thinking behind one's actions does not form an integrated system. Many practitioners have agreed that it is important for older people to dispense with some of the formalities of "professional" practice. Older women need to feel that there is a personal relationship in order to be intimate with you and to explore their own feelings about their own lives.

The core set of therapeutic conditions that have been identified (Truax & Carkhuff, 1967) by client-centered helping professionals includes a sense of accurate empathy, respect, and genuineness. Empathy is the helper's ability to perceive accurately and with sensitivity the client's immediate feelings and to understand their significance. The worker must then communicate to the client so that the client knows that she is being understood. Thus, as a doctor dealing with an older woman who lives alone, there is the recognition that a physical examination may be the only time in the past weeks that she has physically been touched by another human being. The woman who is seen by a home health aide after weeks of isolation is understood to be especially needy of "small talk." Empathy allows the helping professional to let clients know that their needs are understood, that they are valid and acceptable, and that we recognize the possibility of fulfilling these needs within our professional interactions.

Respect refers to the worker's ability to communicate a feeling of warmth and the attitudes of concern and acceptance to the client. Respect can be demonstrated by being an advocate for a woman who is having a relationship with a younger man of whom her children disapprove. If we nonjudgmentally assist people to assess their own methods of striving for intimacy, we encourage them to expand their capacity for intimacy as well.

Genuineness refers to the worker's ability to behave as an open, honest, and congruent person whose feelings about the here-and-now interactions between herself and the client are real. It may mean that we share personal incidents about our own lives, that we sit down and have a cup of tea with a woman who arrives during lunch, or that we cry with someone who is telling about a sad time in their lives.

There is some fear that the growing dichotomy of "professional" and "personal" in our behavior has diminished our effectiveness in practice. Developing skill in regard to these core areas is a way of reminding us that above all, the key to intimacy is person-to-person relationships.

FUTURE TRENDS

There is room for a great deal of optimism in the future, as people become more aware of and attempt to deal with the issues that relate to problems with sexuality and intimacy in the present. An exploratory study (Junge & Maya, 1985) of a group of women in their forties (the old of tomorrow) suggests that this group, because of the combination of their traditional backgrounds and changed expectations, suffer more conflict in dealing with the age-appropriate developmental tasks than similar-aged women before or since. These tasks include the formation of a separate identity and the attainment of a sense of independence versus being dependent on another person. The achievement of the former is needed for a positive sense of sexuality and intimacy in old age. The fact that this cohort of women is actively struggling with the issue suggests the potential for a greater degree of comfortability with their own situations when they reach old age.

One author suggests (Abu-Laban, 1981) that aging women of the future will have increased access to alternative bases of prestige that go beyond age-linked physical attractiveness or the derived status of a wife, which will diminish the psychological issues correlated with lack of sexuality and intimacy. As has been discussed, contemporary women experience the most prestige or esteem at the stage of life where they are defined as the most attractive, and that esteem declines with age according to society's notions of physical attractiveness. However, because far more young women today are gainfully employed in areas that provide them with other kinds of satisfaction and rewards, that aspect of life will assist in keeping their esteem high. In addition, as more women actively participate in their own financial planning, they will have access to monetary benefits aside from the pension plans or Social Security benefits of a spouse. This lessening of economic dependence will also lead to an increase or sustaining of esteem in old age.

It is also suggested that due to the greater freedom today for women to experiment with different life styles and to explore their own sexuality and intimacy, women will have had many more experiences with transitory living/loving relationships, including living with partners outside a legal marriage, divorce, and a greater number of sexual partners. These experiences teach skills related to beginning and ending relationships and leave women with an enhanced ability to cope with loss and to rely on a more self-sufficient and self-directed life style — in other words, to seek out more aggressively the intimacy that is needed in old age.

A second aspect of the greater societal tolerance of differences in relationships will affect the next generation of older women in another positive way. Younger women today feel freer to have life partners who are disparate in terms of age. Marriages to younger men would mean more of an equalization in terms of death rate in old age, so that fewer women will find themselves widowed. The freedom to engage in relationships that have previously been seen as "deviant" will also promote greater freedom within all relationships to pursue intimacy and sexuality in alternative ways.

Women will also have more access to familial relationships in old age, which is important within our broad definition of intimacy. Demographic trends indicate that women who reach the age of 65-75 in the Year 2000 will actually have more adult children as potential supports than did the women of earlier generations (Neugarten, 1975). As women recognize that they are not necessarily a burden to their family, but a source of pleasure and suppport, they will be freer to spend time with family members and to allow themselves to feel close without feeling simultaneously threatened by their own neediness.

A more pessimistic view of the future for women in terms of sexuality and intimacy considers the fact that conservative religious sentiment has blossomed in the past decade (Kokosalakis, 1974). Some writers (Bellah, 1976, p. 351) predict a return to traditional authoritarianism in American society. Conservative religious beliefs affect sexuality and intimacy for women negatively, because they suggest a return to less liberated ideas about sex role ideologies. For example, growing numbers of older women have relationships outside of marriage, for a variety of reasons. They may have pensions from a spouse who died that would cease if they were to remarry. They may have health issues, or be concerned about health issues of a potential spouse, and may not want to take on the legal ramifications of responsibility that go along with marriage. If those out-of-wedlock relationships become even more unacceptable because of increased religious influences and constraints, the alternatives are to not have relationships at all.

Erikson (1982) has refined his definition of ego integrity in a way that is more consistent with an understanding of women and that eloquently depicts the broader notion of sexuality and intimacy that we are striving for. Integrity

> is a comradeship with the ordering ways of distant times and different pursuits, as expressed in their simple products and sayings. But there emerges also a different, a timeless love for those few others who have become the main counterplayers in life's most significant contexts. For individual life is the coincidence of but one life with but one segment of history: and all human integrity stands or falls with one style of integrity of which one partakes. (pp. 65-66)

"Timeless love," that appreciation of the people who have been significant in one's life, allows for intimacy in old age.

Clearly, it is in our best interests to promote an environment in which sexuality and intimacy are expected to last until old age. The meaning of love and sex includes (Butler & Lewis, 1978) the opportunity for expression of passion, affection, admiration, loyalty, and other positive emotion, an affirmation of one's body and its functioning, a strong sense of self, a means of self-assertion, the pleasure of being touched or caressed, and a defiance of the stereotypes of aging. It is a reciprocal process, in which the greater degree to which women can be intimate, the greater degree to which they will retain their capacity for further intimacy.

And yet, there is some reluctance on the part of this author to leave an impression that if the environment and attitudes that surround older women change, sexuality and intimacy will absolutely be expressed in a fulfilling way. If one listens to older women, in clinical, community, and personal settings, the negative effects of the physical aches and pains that accompany old age cannot be underestimated. While the terminology in regard to arthritis is confusing and physicians use the terms rheumatic disease, arthritis, and rheumatoid arthritis interchangeably, it is a documented fact that nearly every individual over 60 has arthritis to the extent that it can be identified on X-rays (Freese, 1978).

When a woman aches when she gets out of bed in the morning, the first message that bombards her senses and sense of self is "I'm old," rather than "I'm a sexual person who is capable of intimacy." When she has lunch with a friend and finds herself not wanting to be close, because she doesn't want to hear about the other woman's problems as it reminds her of her own, the message is apparently that comfort is more important than intimacy. We academicians, theoreticians, and clinicians must keep in mind that we are writing, studying, and thinking about the ideal. In the real world, physical discomfort is often more overpowering than any ideological striving to be a more complete human being. It is excruciatingly painful to grow old, to see friends and family die, to feel unable to keep up with younger people, to feel less and less a sense of why one's life is continuing, and to combat constant and chronic physical pain. In our attempt to improve conditions for older women, it is also important to be realistic. One of the most valuable gifts a woman can be presented with is the chance to express her feelings about her life, without any preconceived notions of what those feelings ought to be.

Perhaps our goals need to be expanded to allow the expression of the ambivalence described in the preceding paragraphs. As well as understanding that we can only imperfectly affect the human condition, we can improve the environment in a variety of ways to allow the opportunity for enhanced intimacy. We can work with human beings in ways that allow them to recognize the unlimited potential within themselves and to succumb less often and less completely to the pressures that make older women feel worthless and incapable of intimacy.

As an example, the travel industry has made a quantum leap forward in understanding that people's desires do not change as they age, but the ways that they fulfill their desires need adaptations. Growing numbers of cruise lines, hotels, and restaurants recognize that older people still want to experience new adventures. They slow down the pace and make it affordable enough so that a 75-year-old woman can go down the Nile, although it may be on a large boat rather than in a canoe, and she may have an air-conditioned bus waiting at the end of the trip rather than a donkey. As helping professionals, we can also broaden the arena in which intimacy and sexuality can be expressed and assist women in finding creative solutions to the issues that they face.

REFERENCES

Abu-Laban, S. (1981). Women and aging: A futurist perspective. *Psychology of Women Quarterly, 6*(1), 85-98.

Anderson, B. (1979). *The aging game: Success, sanity, and sex after 60*. New York: McGraw-Hill.

Annon, J. S. (1976). *Behavioral treatment of sexual problems*. Hagerstown, MD: Harper & Row.

Beaver, M., & Miller, D. (1985). *Clinical social work practice with the elderly*. Homestead, IL: Dorsey Press.

Bellah, R. N. (1976). New religious consciousness and the crisis in modernity. In C. V. Glock & R. N. Bellah (Eds.), *The new religious consciousness* (pp. 333-352). Berkeley: University of California Press.

Berger, R. (1982). The unseen minority: Older gays and lesbians. *Social Work, 27,* 236-242.

Brink, T. L. (1979). *Geriatric psychotherapy*. New York: Human Sciences Press.

Bureau of the Census. (1982). *U. S. Department of Commerce: Statistical abstract of the United States* (103rd ed.) Washington DC: U.S. Government Printing Office.

Busse, E., & Pfeiffer, E. (1977). Functional psychiatric disorders in old age. In E. Busse & E. Pfeiffer (Eds.), *Behavior and adaptation in late life* (2nd ed.) (pp. 158-211). Boston: Little, Brown.

Butler, R., & Lewis, M. (1976). *Sex after sixty: A guide for men and women for their later years*. New York: Harper & Row.

Butler, R., & Lewis, M. (1978). The second language of sex. In R. L. Solnick

(Ed.), *Sexuality and aging* (pp. 176-183). Los Angeles: University of Southern California Press.

Butler, R., & Lewis, M. (1982). *Aging and mental health: Positive psychosocial and biomedical approaches* (3rd ed.) St. Louis: Mosby.

Calderone, M. (1971). *Sexuality and human values: The personal dimension of sexual experience*. New York: Association Press.

Cochran, M. (1985). The mother-daughter dyad throughout the life cycle. *Women & Therapy, 4*(2), 3-8.

Edinburg, G. (1982). Women and aging. In C. Nadelson and M. Notman (Eds.), *The woman patient: Volume 2: Concepts of femininity and the life cycle* (pp. 169-194). New York: Plenum Press.

Erikson, E. (1982). *Life cycle completed*. New York: Norton.

Flaste, R. (1979). Research begins to focus on suicide among the aged. *The New York Times*.

Freese, A. (1978). *Arthritis: Everybody's disease* (Public Affairs Pamphlet No. 562). New York: Public Affairs Committee.

Garner, D. (1985). The search for intimacy: Relationships and sexuality in later life. *Proceedings: Social Work Clinic* (pp. 1-10). Toronto: Baycrest Center for Geriatric Care.

Gilligan, C. (1978). *In a different voice*. Cambridge, MA: Harvard University Press.

Glick, I., Weiss, R., & Parkes, C. (1974). *The first year of bereavement*. New York: Wiley.

Gordon, L. (1979). Birth control and social revolution. In N. Cott & E. Pleck (Eds.), *A heritage of her own*. New York: Simon & Schuster.

Hancock, B. L. (1987). *Social work with older people*. Englewood Cliffs, NJ: Prentice-Hall.

Junge, M., & Maya, V. (1985). Women in their forties: A group portrait and implications for psychotherapy. *Women & Therapy, 4*(3), 3-19.

Kelly, J., & Rice, S. (1986). The aged. In H. Gochros, J. Gochros, & J. Fischer (Eds.), *Helping the sexually oppressed* (pp. 98-116). Englewood Cliffs, NJ: Prentice-Hall.

Kokosalakis, N. (1974). The contemporary metamorphasis of religion. *The Human Context, 6*, 243-249.

Lau, E., & Kosberg, J. (1978). *Abuse of the elderly by informal care providers: Practice and research of issues*. Paper presented at the 31st annual meeting of the Gerontological Society, Dallas, TX.

Maccoby, E. E., & Jacklin, C. N. (1976). Summary and commentary from *The Psychology of Sex Differences* (1974). In S. Cox (Ed.), *Female psychology: The emerging self*. Chicago: Science Research Associates.

Masters, W. H., & Johnson, V. (1966). *Human sexual response*. Boston: Little, Brown.

Masters, W. H., & Johnson, V. (1970). *Human sexual inadequacy*. Boston: Little, Brown.

Miller, D. (1981). The "Sandwich" generation: Adult children of the aging. *Social Work*, *26*, 419-423.

Montagu, A. (1974). *The meaning of love*. Westport, CT: Greenwood Press.

Murphy, G. (1979). Human sexuality and the potential of the older person. In D. Kunkel (Ed.), *Sexual issues in social work: Emerging concerns on education and practice* (pp. 72-88). Honolulu: University of Hawaii, School of Social Work.

Neugarten, B. L. (1975). The future and the young old. *The Gerontologist*, *15*, 4-9.

New Woman, (1986, February 14-17), Miller, P. (Ed.), Advertisement.

Orlofsky, J. L. (1976). Intimacy status: Relationship to interpersonal perception. *Journal of Youth and Adolescence*, *5*, 73-88.

O'Rourke, M. (1981). *Elder abuse: The state of the art*. Paper presented at the National Conference on the Abuse of Older Persons, Boston, MA.

Perlman, H. H. (1979). *Relationship: The heart of helping people*. Chicago: University of Chicago Press.

Puksta, N. (1977). All about sex . . . after a coronary. *American Journal of Nursing*, *77*(4), 603.

Rice, S. (in press). Single, older, childless women: A study of social support and life satisfaction. *Journal of Gerontological Social Work*.

Rice, S., & Kelly, J. (1987). Love and intimacy needs of the elderly: Some philosophical and intervention issues. *Journal of Social Work & Human Sexuality*, *5*(2), 89-96.

Sarton, M. (1975). Toward another dimension. *Women: A Journal of Liberation*, *4*(4), 26-28.

Siemens, S., & Brandzel, R. (1982). *Sexuality: Nursing assessment and intervention*. Philadelphia: Lippincott.

Sontag, S. (1972, September). The double standard of aging. *Saturday Review of Literature*, *95*, 29-38.

Stevens-Long, J. (1988). *Adult life: Developmental processes* (3rd ed.). Mountain View, CA: Mayfield.

Straus, M., Gelles, R., & Steinmetz, S. (1981). *Behind closed doors: Violence in the American family*. Garden City, NY: Anchor Press/Doubleday.

Truax, C. B., & Carkhuff, R. (1967). *Toward effective counseling and psychotherapy*. Chicago: Aldine.

Walker, L. E. (1979). *The battered woman*. New York: Harper & Row.

(1983). *Webster's deluxe unabridged dictionary* (2nd ed.). Cleveland: Dorset & Baber.

Weg, R. (1983). *Sexuality in the later years: Roles and behavior*. New York: Academic Press.

Weitzman, L. J. (1979). Sex role socialization. In J. Freeman (Ed.), *Women: A feminist perspective* (pp. 157-237). Palo Alto, CA: Mayfield.

Wyly, M. V., & Hulicka, I. M. (1977). Problems and compensations of widowhood. In I. M. Hulicka (Ed.), *Empirical studies in the psychology and sociology of aging*. New York: Crowell.

Group Work with Older Women:
A Modality to Improve
the Quality of Life

Irene M. Burnside, RN, MS, FAAN, FGSA

So I still care. At my age I care to my roots about the quality of
women, and I care because I know how important her quality is.

Florida Scott-Maxwell (1968, pp. 104-105)

Groups have been used as a treatment modality since World War
II. Groups are a valid therapeutic modality because they have the
advantage of economy and socialization as well as validation from
the group members (Hartford 1980). A variety of groups may be
designed for elders to improve their functioning as well as the quality of life: reality orientation, remotivation, reminiscence therapy,
art, poetry, bibliotherapy, exercise/movement, and psychotherapy.

Many of the studies and reports in the literature are about groups
conducted in nursing homes. These groups were undoubtedly comprised predominantly of frail older women. That assumption is
based on data indicating that 71% of institutionalized residents are
women (George, 1984).

The purpose of this article is fourfold: (1) to locate and describe
articles about group work with older women, (2) to emphasize the
need for prevention and health promotion in elderly women, (3) to
present perspectives on teaching group work with this select group,
and (4) to suggest, in a brainstorming mode, ideas for future group
work.

Why should one consider group work as a modality designed

Irene M. Burnside is a doctoral student, University of Texas, 4210 Red River,
#116, Austin, TX 78706.

265

specifically for aged women? It is easy to build a case for the modality. The first reason is the obvious one — the population explosion. The female population age 85 and over will *triple* between 1980 and 2030 (Davis, 1986). The Social Security Administration's 1980 data indicated there were 15,528 centenarians (11,132 females and 4,126 males); white females have more than any other group (1 in 9,677) followed by black females (1 centenarian in 13,260; Pieroni, 1984, p. 8).

It has already been noted that 71% of those in institutions are women (George, 1984). Clearly, there is a growing need to improve the life quality of the frail old and old-old women. Second, we continue to ignore the abilities, talents, and contributions of elderly women; older women have not made it to the top very often. For example, Bearon (1984) listed 63 celebrities aged 65-74 as of 1981. Out of the list of 63, there were only 15 (23%) women. A list of 32 celebrities aged 75 or over as of 1981 included five women (15%). Hagestad (1986) puts it succinctly, "there is a striking lack of perception of the old as *constituting a resource*, a lack that ignores economic as well as psychological realities" (p. 15).

A third reason is to begin to identify the differences between all-female groups and all-male groups. It is quite rare for the searcher to find accounts of single-sex groups, and different issues do come alive during the reading of such accounts (Middleton, 1987).

A fourth reason is sheer self-interest; we are investing in our own years ahead, and our contributions in the present may make a difference in our own futures. Pifer and Bronte (1986) remind us that "The future is not preordained. Population of aging holds within it the promise of a much better society for all of us, or paradoxically, a far worse one. The choice is clearly there, and it is ours to make" (p. 13).

Last, if we pay attention to a parable, perhaps we can even change that parable. There is a Moroccan parable that says at birth each boy is surrounded by 100 devils. However, each girl born is surrounded by 100 angels. With each year of life, one devil is exchanged for one angel. So men who live to be one hundred will be surrounded by angels, but the women centenarians will be surrounded by devils (Livson, 1983). We will need to help surround the women with angels.

OVERVIEW OF THE LITERATURE

Because the computer of a large university library was not very helpful, a hand search was done using available reference lists of articles/chapters about group work, as well as a hand-check of gerontology journals. No dissertations or theses were included in the search. However, theses about group work with older women are reported in the field of nursing. Because this article is an endeavor to explicate the state of the art, and to trace the beginnings of group work with elderly women, no projects or studies were eliminated because of inadequacy, incompleteness, or lack of sophistication of research methods.

The following overview is in no sense an integrative review (Copper, 1984) of group work with older women. The paucity of research reported on these specific groups forced the author to include anecdotal writings and descriptions. No attempt is made here to analyze any of the data, methodologies, or conclusions in the research articles. Rather, the focus is on pointing the reader to available writings to indicate the dire need for improvement, both quantitative and qualitative, in the uncharted area of group work with this population.

A literature search can be frustrating, and the search for materials about group work with older women was no exception. Rarely did the indexes of books on aging include "women," "females," or "gender." Publications about such group work were not only scant but scattered in diverse publications. However, it was consoling to think that the *Journal of Women & Aging* may help in the future to consolidate literature specific to aging women.

Studies reviewed were especially deficient regarding important data about the sample. Age, sex, and ethnic background of subjects often was either missing or lacked specificity. The terms *elderly* or *geriatric* are poor substitutions for the mean age. Early group work also ignored the cultural diversity of members. Note in Table 1 that early group work did include two groups of Italian women. No reports were found about groups of black, Hispanic, Asian, or Native American members. The literature search did reveal many disciplines conducted groups with elders: nurses, physicians, social

TABLE 1. Group Work with Older Women 1953-1987

Date	Author	Type of Group	Group Size and Age of Member	Ethnic Background
1953	Linden, M.E.	Psychotherapy (Research)	Mean age=70 Mode=69 3 persons younger then 60, 1 member aged 89	Not stated
1973	Stange, A.Z.	Reminiscence (Project)	8 women aged 39-87	1 black, 7 Caucasian
1973	Morrison, J.M.	Directive-Verbal (Here and Now Project)	54-72 M=64.3 8 members	4 foreign-born
1976	Hennessey M.J.	Reminiscence Resocialization Directive-verbal (Project)	16 women (ages not stated)	Not stated (affluent members)
1978	Nickoley & Leavitt	Support	65-83; 11 members one group; 12 members	Not stated
1979	Borus & Anastasi	Support	Aged 55-70 One group growing to 50 members	Italian-American

Setting	Length of Group	Goal of Group	Outcome
State hospital	2 years	1. Resolution of depressive affect 2. Increase alertness 3. Diminish confusion 4. Improve orientation 5. Replenish memory hiati	
State hospital	1 hour weekly 11 weeks	Resocialization	Cohesiveness of group emerged
Outpatient clinic	Weekly, 4 months	1. Help members let go of past 2. Help members form new relationships	Members resumed social contacts Engaged in outside activities Physical complaints decreased Ability increased to discuss feelings
Intermediary care unit in a retirement community	1 hour weekly for 3 months	1. Facilitate communication 2. Increase resocialization	Group cohesiveness emerged
Senior citizen high rise complex	Twelve one-hour sessions twice weekly followed by one-half hour socializational refreshment period	See Table 3 for needs addressed	Descriptive, observable but not measurable outcomes
Community health center	Weekly meetings for six years	1. Provide meaningful role in community 2. Increase socialization 3. Increase peer network 4. Sharing experiences about aging 5. Health education	Increased activity in their community

TABLE 1 (continued)

Date	Author	Type of Group	Group Size and Age of Member	Ethnic Background
1979	Borus & Anastasi	Preventive/ Support/ Reminiscence	75-90+	European born; Italian speaking
1980	Blackman, J.E.	Reminiscence (Research)	8 members age 70-87 Mean=80.75	3 European born; all Caucasians
1981	Michelson, S.	Reminiscence	Fifteen women aged 64-81 (14 were nuns)	Not stated
1983	Hawkins	Support and therapy	12 members aged 75-93	
1984	Waller & Griffin	Discussion/ Therapy	One group of 25 women (ages not stated)	Not stated
1987	Holland	Life review/ communication Repeated measures design	10 71-86 Mean age=77.8	Caucasian
1987	Engels & Poser	Social skills training	6 members 62-70	Not stated

Setting	Length of Group	Goal of Group	Outcome
Community health center		1. Reminisce 2. Mourn the losses and cultural traditions 3. Discuss here and now	1. Increased the social network 2. Increased the health habits 3. Relocation to housing centers
Senior day care center	Twice weekly 1 hour, 13 weeks	1. Increases verbal reminiscence 2. Resocialization 3. Increase self-esteem	Questionnaires did not indicate a high level of interpersonal social behavior
Nursing home	Twice weekly for 3 weeks	Reduce depressive state	Downward trend in reminiscent group's score noted
Adult day			Themes of Group: Anger Struggle for leadership Housing Independence Health Relationship with children Stereotypes
Senior center	Weekly	1. Prevent depression 2. Enhance or maintain adaptive capacities	1. Attendance increased groups 2. Fluctuating pattern in participants' depression using Hamilton Depression Inventory over 18 months
Nursing home	Six weeks; 1 hour weekly	1. Short term language therapy 2. Assess the effectiveness of the treatment	Treatment efficiency was demonstrated (unless health status had deteriorated)
Community	Nine sessions over 5 week period; each session 90 minutes	1. Increase interaction 2. Express opinions in group 3. Increase assertiveness	All behaviors improved for each member

workers, psychologists, geropsychiatrists, and occupational therapists. Table 1 indicates group articles located in the literature.

The first article in the literature appeared in 1953. This classic
about group work and older women was written by a renowned
geropsychiatrist, Maurice Linden (1953). He led a group of 40 state
hospital elderly women suffering from dementia. His perseverance
and dedication is to be commended: He led that group for two
years! He is one of the first writers to discuss the use of humor as a
strategy to be skillfully implemented by the leader and to describe a
style of leadership. The article is also the first research effort directed toward the understanding of older women in group.

Books on group work with elders are few. The first book on
group work appeared in 1953 and focused mainly on socialization
groups in a senior center in New York City (Kubie & Landau,
1953). It was interesting to note that crafts were the focus of many
of the groups described.

The most common types of group modalities used with elders are
described in the next section.

TYPES OF GROUP MODALITIES

One of the first types of group modalities to be reported after
Linden's work was reality orientation (Taulbee & Folsom, 1966).
The literature contains a number of articles about reality orientation
(Gubrium & Ksander, 1975; MacDonald & Settin, 1976; Taulbee,
1984). It was widely used in long-term settings in the '60s and '70s,
and used as a 24-hour one-to-one intervention plus as a group process (Taulbee & Folsom, 1966). Gubrium (1975) described reality
orientation as a "drill-like procedure that presumably teaches time
and place to disoriented residents" (p. 189). He was speaking about
reality orientation conducted in nursing homes. There is little consensus in the literature about the therapeutic value of these groups
(Donahue, 1984), but it must be acknowledged that this has been a
popular modality with demented elders in institutions (Taulbee,
1984). No reports were located on reality orientation groups designed exclusively for elderly women, although they very likely
existed for the reason stated earlier.

Reality orientation is used with confused, disoriented individuals and therefore the leader should keep the group small, perhaps four to six members. The rationale for a small group is to reduce the stimuli, to keep anxiety minimal, and also to reduce the work of the leader. Group work with demented individuals can be very draining on the leader.

It is difficult to predict if reality orientation groups will continue to be used. The expected benefits for older women would be to decrease confusional states and to offer increased chance to socialize and to improve the quality of their lives.

REMOTIVATION THEORY

Remotivation groups were begun at Pennsylvania State Hospital by a volunteer, Dorothy Smith (Dennis, 1984). The groups were designed for chronic schizophrenics, and the leader was trained in the method of using a structured format. This group modality never gained the wide popularity that reality orientation did. Perhaps these are some of the reasons: (1) the focus was not on reducing confusion and disorientation; (2) publications about the modality were minimal; (3) the structured, locked-in steps may have discouraged the creative person who wished to be innovative as a leader. Because the goal was to return the patient to the community, the method has to be modified if used with frail elders, especially those who are institutionalized. No studies in remotivation therapy using only women subjects were located.

Remotivation therapy would be the next level of group work after reality orientation. There are more members in a remotivation group, but the group is designed for confused, usually institutionalized elders. The five basic steps of this group must be adapted for elders. One such step is "appreciation of the kinds of work of the world," which seems quite inappropriate for elders, especially for elderly women who have never worked.

This modality uses themes or motifs for each meeting, which create interest for the members. Dennis (1984) has described an excellent format that could be used by a new group leader.

Women could expect to enjoy their peers in such a group, be able to use the group leader as a role model, and have added opportunities to communicate and socialize with other women.

REMINISCENCE THERAPY

The theoretical basis for reminiscence therapy lies in the seminal work of Butler, who described the "life review" (1963). His definition is commonly quoted in the literature on reminiscence therapy, "a naturally occurring, universal mental process characterized by the progressive return to consciousness of past experiences, and, particularly the resurgence of unresolved conflicts; simultaneously, and normally, these revived experiences and conflicts can be surveyed and reintegrated" (p. 65). His use of the word *reminiscence* in the title of his classic article may have created confusion for subsequent group leaders, because there are no clear distinctions between *life review* and *reminiscence* in the literature; the words are commonly used interchangeably. It would be helpful if all the researchers in the area of reminiscence would clearly define their terms. The type of group this writer has most often observed is reminiscence therapy—not life review therapy groups (Burnside, 1988). Haight (1988) notes that "Clinical case studies, reminiscing groups, autobiographical experience, life histories, and multiple other forms of reminiscing have all been placed under the banner of life review" (p. 40).

A year after Butler's seminal article on life review, the first study on reminiscence therapy was published (McMahon & Rhudick, 1964). They took a different approach and defined reminiscence as "The act or habit of thinking about or relating past experiences" (p. 292). This study included elderly male volunteers, all of whom were Spanish-American war veterans. It would be interesting to repeat this landmark using older women as subjects.

An important rationale to consider for conducting reminiscence groups comes from Polster (1987) who reminds us to recognize ". . . the healing effect that comes to people as they learn how remarkably interesting they are." It has been the author's experience that many of the frail elderly women do not view themselves as interesting. A common putdown heard in groups is, "I was *just* a housewife." Other reasons to conduct reminiscence groups are indicated by Sherman (1987) who stated "It appears that reminiscence groups not only lead to new friendships, but that they can also be an effective means for the development of ongoing, peer support groups among community elderly" (p. 572). That has been observed by the writer. One should encourage out-of-group meetings and activities to further the development of friendships and confidants.

The clientele for a reminiscence group can vary from the somewhat confused to the intellectual. However, in regard to those with high intellect, one must remember that they may balk at joining such a group if they believe that reminiscing is a sign of approaching dementia (or "senility" as they may call it).

The modality can be used with a specific purpose: for example, reducing anxiety, depression, loneliness, or alienation, or to improve the quality of life because one of the goals could be to increase networking, friends, and confidants.

Reminiscence is beneficial to frail elders; its purposes can be noted in Figure 1.

The benefits of reminiscence are multifaceted. No one has stud-

FIGURE 1

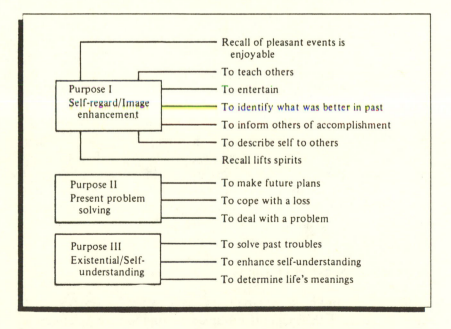

Based on: Romaniuk, M. and J. Romaniuk (1981). Looking back: An analysis of reminiscence functions and triggers. *Experimental Aging Research*, 7:477-489.

ied the value of humor in reminiscence (or even in other groups) and yet, the author has had the pleasure of enjoying the wit and the fabulous storytelling of humorous events by elderly women. Some of their stories about their first lemon pie or the first time they baked bread have been highly entertaining.

The leader should begin with a group of six or eight, especially if there is no co-leader. Try to encourage reminiscence that will boost the self-esteem and help restore the identity of the individuals. Use props, photographs, and memorabilia for catalysts. Use trigger events that all would recall, for example, the assassination of John F. Kennedy. You might ask them if they remember what they were doing on that day, and most of them will. Burnside (1988) outlines specific recommendations regarding reminiscence therapy (pp. 671-672).

As yet, there is not enough consistency in the research findings for this writer to feel comfortable about ascribing certain functions to reminiscence in late life, especially when we are not yet even in agreement on the definition of reminiscence!

OTHER GROUP MODALITIES

A variety of group modalities have been used with elders, although the articles reviewed were not specifically geared for women: art (Wolcott, 1978), poetry (Brandler, 1984; Getzel, 1981; Koch, 1977), music (Hennessey, 1984; Moore, 1984), bibliotherapy (O'Dell, 1984), movement (Booth-Buehring, 1984), self-help (Burnside, 1984), family-sculpting (Martin, 1984), and psychotherapy (Altholz, 1984). It is of interest to note that poetry has been a popular group modality since 1953, when Kubie and Landau formed their first group around an interest or theme, rather than a craft. It should be noted that memories and reminiscence can be combined with the above group modalities.

Support and Self-Help Groups

Support groups and self-help groups have become more prevalent since the mid-1970s. Support groups are common for relatives of Alzheimer's patients, widows, cancer patients, alcoholics, and people with life-threatening illnesses. It is not uncommon to begin such a group in a clinic or high-rise senior housing. No articles were found regarding elderly women living in mobile trailer parks. One would think a need for support groups might exist in those environments.

Support groups help an individual become mobilized to handle the loss or the emotional upset. There can be support from the leader, and peers may share experiences and offer suggestions to help cope with the situation(s).

Self-help groups, however, by their very existence, tend to minimize the referrals to professionals or agencies and this may be because there is no self-help to be had (Burnside, 1984). Self-help groups include (1) control of behavior (Alcoholics Anonymous, Weight Watchers, etc.); (2) stress, coping, and support (widow groups, stroke groups); (3) survival-oriented (National Organization for Women); (4) personal growth (Senior Actualization and Growth Exploration [Sage] group). The preceding four categories of self-help groups were delineated by Levy (1976).

Educational Groups

Educational groups or teaching groups are yet another form of important group work with elderly women. Nutrition sites have been amenable to groups, which probably was to increase socialization and interest elders in attending regularly. Sexuality has been a favorite topic, as has health education (e.g., nutrition, exercise, medication usage). The captive audience in the sites certainly facilitates groups for the leader. Most generally it is an open group with members changing from week to week. Education groups are also found in adult day care centers and may be geared to the relatives. These centers are usually excellent placements for group work for students. Day care centers often operate on a shoestring, so the added input, teaching, and group work of the students from a variety of disciplines is generally appreciated.

Group Psychotherapy

Group psychotherapy places demands on the therapist and can be more tiring than individual psychotherapy (Poggi, 1984). The group process according to Poggi (1984) ''is an effort on the part of group members to work together to satisfy leadership needs common to all people.''

A group psychotherapist must be trained in two specialized areas — psychotherapy and gerontology. The therapist must understand group dynamics of elders, the aging process, and countertransference in such groups plus the basics of psychology, psychiatry, social work, nursing, or counseling. Poggi (1984) reminds us that ''The potential for harmful reactions toward the elderly is greatly enhanced for the geroclinician by virtue of the powerful emotional situations confronting him or her in work with older people'' (p. 365).

Depression is common in elders, particularly reactive depression. This group of elderly women would benefit from group therapy. And one has to remember that ''The elderly are frequently denied needed psychotherapy because of professional attitudes toward aging'' (Garner, personal communication, 1988). There can also be depression in the early phases of Alzheimer's disease — which should be treated. And as women continue to live longer, it can be anticipated there will be increases in Alzheimer's disease among them. The ''therapeutic nihilism'' that has existed for so long regarding psychotherapy with elders is, we hope, waning.

One can see that group modality runs the gamut. The leader's imagination and creativity, combined with the elderly members' needs, allows for much creativity and variety. Friedlob and Kelly (1984) remind us that ''Creativity can be explored within a structured program'' (p. 316). However, it is more difficult to explore creativity in the formats of the group modalities (reality orientation and remotivation) because they are so very structured.

Community Setting

The first book about group work in the community was *Group Work with the Aged* (Kubie & Landau, 1953). The book describes groups in a recreation center based on the nine years of experience of the authors. Of the 40 members, 27 were men and 13 were women. In the 35 years since that publication, the noted change would be the ratio of men to women being reversed. Another change would be the movement towards more specialized therapeutic groups instead of only socialization groups.

Groups in community settings could be held in senior housing, mobile parks, day care centers, senior centers, churches, synagogues, and board and care homes (Beckett, 1981; Friedlob & Kelly, 1984).

Beckett (1981) posed the idea that the milieu of the adult foster home is personalized and family-like and may help to decrease or eliminate the many problems that detract from reality orientation as a modality in a large institution. Friedlob and Kelly (1984) have written a pragmatic, detailed description of reminiscence groups in board and care homes, which is recommended to the reader needing basic information about implementing groups.

Day Care Settings

Adult day care centers in the United States have developed in a noticeably brief time (Aaronson, 1983). However, there is currently little in the literature regarding work with confused elderly who attend these centers. There are approximately 1,000 day care centers in the Central States (Hallburg, personal communication, 1988). The author has observed a high enrollment of clients with Alzheimer's disease in such centers. Because of the respite the centers offer family, institutionalization is often postponed for several years. The wide array of groups help to maintain the functioning of participants. The writer once collaborated with the art therapist to do drawings of a clock in a group. The students who worked with the group were surprised to discover how cognitively impaired were many of the elders, who nevertheless had excellent social graces.

The elder who cannot be maintained at home or in a day care center is usually placed in a nursing home, and then often gives up hope of ever living anywhere else. Day care centers are important!

Waller and Griffin (1984) described a therapy group in the community that they co-led for depressed elders. There were separate groups of women and groups of men. They state,

From the outset the women's group has differed from the men's. Self-disclosure comes early and without inhibition. The topics and dialogue tend to be more intensely personal, and related to home and family. . . . The women's attendance at group meetings tend to be short sessions; men attend for longer periods. (p. 310)

Nursing Home Settings

The author was struck with the number of studies and projects about group work conducted in nursing homes — probably because of the captive audience. The need to improve the quality of life of nursing home residents is imperative.

Vladeck (1980) described the typical resident in a nursing home as "an eighty-year old white widow or spinster of relatively limited means suffering from three or four chronic ailments" (p. 13). The average length of stay is over 2-1/2 years, and only a small proportion are discharged because they have been rehabilitated. Furthermore, Garner and Mercer (1980) point out that "many people will live out their lives during a period of potentially declining health, physical separation from significant others, and diminished controls and choices over their entire environment" (p. 77). Group leaders and qualified personnel in nursing homes, can monitor health problems, help create pseudofamilies, increase confidants, and assist elderly women to gain more control and have an impact on the milieu.

PREVENTION: A CONSTANT GOAL

Little attention has been given to preventive strategies in the area of mental health. Garcia and Kosberg (1985) found the presenting problems in descending order for 68 elderly subjects that are noted in Table 2. Some of the possible effects of groups are noted in the table. Risk factors can also be monitored in groups. The group modality can be a vehicle for elders to develop new coping behaviors, to enhance self-esteem during the creative problem-solving process, to increase awareness about health behaviors, and to increase con-

TABLE 2

Identified by Elderly*	Possible Effects of Group on Problems**
1. Life adjustment	1. Reminiscence or life review may facilitate adjustment; peer feedback valuable.
2. Emotional distress	2. Can be monitored by a skilled leader and, if necessary, referred to appropriate resource.
3. Self-esteem	3. Self-esteem may be enhanced by: (a) Performance in group (b) The positive feedback from leader, peers (c) Being in a milieu which encourages individuality (d) Increase in control which may come from the group experience
4. Communication	4. Peers (and especially the leader) can serve as powerful role models. Communication skills often improve noticeably during the life of the group.
5. Marital conflict	5. Unresolved conflicts may be mitigated if the leader, who is qualified, can initiate the life review process.

Identified by Counselor*	Possible Effects of Group on Problems**
1. Unrealistic expectation of self and others.	1. The honesty and candidness of elders in groups often can help level out such expectations.
2. Grief management	2. Peer support and sharing of their management, resolution of grief
3. Adjustment to physical loss	3. Observing other group members facing and coping with same losses can be powerful
4. Power struggles	4. Often these are played out in the group and members gain insight about the problem
5. Communication	5. See #4 above

* Based on Garcia and Kosberg (1985), p. 306.

** Author

formity to acceptable health behaviors through peer pressure in groups (Gioella & Bevil, 1985).

Nickoley-Colquitt (1981) reviewed 18 group interventions, which involved an elderly population or their family members. Group leaders were similar to those described above. Leaders were peer counselors, social workers, psychiatrists, psychologists, and nurses. The group interventions were designed for those "who were experiencing common developmental and situational changes or stresses" (p. 80). The needs that can be addressed through use of preventive group strategies can be found in Table 3 (Nickoley-Colquitt, 1981). There were three groups composed solely of women in the 18 groups surveyed; two of the women's groups consisted of women of Italian backgrounds.

TABLE 3

NEEDS ADDRESSED THROUGH PREVENTIVE GROUP INTERACTION

- Knowledgeable about aging process, changes and use of supportive resources
- Management of change
- Development and use of effective coping strategies
- Control and mastery
- Self-esteem
- Continued growth and use of potential
- Communication, feedback, effective interpersonal skills, expression of feelings
- Affiliation, social interaction
- Meaningful roles

Nickoley-Colquitt, (1981). Preventive Group Interventions for Elderly Clients: Are They Effective, in *Family & Community Health: The Journal of Health Promotion & Maintenance*, 3(4):80 February. Reprinted with permission of Aspen Publishers, Inc.

The reader is referred to an excellent in-depth article on the nursing home as a setting for health promotion (Minkler, 1985). This health educator states we must humanize the nursing home environment and place greater accent on rehabilitation and on patient education. Group modalities can help to fulfill those goals and can be part of a rehabilitation care plan. Health professionals will need to continue to fight "therapeutic nihilism" and ageism.

One constantly needs to remember that ageism has not gone away. Ask any older woman who has been ignored at a counter, or treated rudely, or jeered at. Ageism is a problem, and caregivers need to be sensitive to it because, "the harshest description of American cultural definitions of old age is that they do not treat it as a human condition" (Keith, 1982, p. 113).

As we consider group modalities as a means to monitor, prevent, and promote health, we can focus on each individual within the group because "the greatest need of elderly persons is to be recognized as individual human beings with individual feelings, desires and aspirations. It is a need they share with all other human beings whatever their age may be" (Canadian Non-Governmental Organization's Report on Aging, 1982, p. 21).

TEACHING GROUP WORK

Tappen (1985) reminds us that there are problems in designing clinical group experiences for students and the frail elders in institutions. This educator noted that initially students experienced difficulty in selecting appropriate members for their groups and also in accepting the impaired elder's ability to participate in a group. She recommends that "reminiscence group experience be added to direct care responsibilities to improve acceptance and learning in institutional settings" (p. 201).

Burnside (1984) states the need for strong preceptor support for neophyte group leaders and Steffl (1984) recommends that experiential exercises be used to help the new student in gerontology develop empathy. Students at all levels enjoy and learn when they are a member of an experiential reminiscence group. It is also helpful to use experiential sensory exercises that pertain to losses.

One area that students might study is the use of humor. Using humor deftly and effectively is important, but it is a seldom-mentioned component of group work by group leaders and members. Linden (1953) was the first to describe his personal style of leadership, which included humor.

Cousins (1979) was "greatly elated by the discovery that there is physiologic basis for the ancient theory that laughter is good medicine" (p. 40). Many elders have developed a sense of wit that is often delightful (Burnside et al., 1984). The elders should be acknowledged as having a positive healthful habit; caregivers and leaders need to be encouraged, too. Sullivan and Deane (1988) view use of humor as a caring behavior; however, it is not at the expense of the elder—no teasing or mocking that demeans the elder, and no assault to the self-esteem. Instructors need to be knowledgeable about the therapeutic use of humor in group work.

Kurland (1978) noted that theory-building in group work lacks an overall attention to the phases of the pregroup planning needed for group work services. This also applies to the student level and initiating groups. Poorly planned groups may fail and turn the elders against group interactions. In addition, students need successful learning experiences, which they can replicate when they leave school.

There is "a pressing need to develop a conceptual model to account for what is effective and ineffective in group leader behavior" (Stockton, Moran, & Velkoff, 1987, p. 163). Although these authors were not focusing on therapeutic small groups of elders, their words are certainly applicable. Instructors could begin to execute small research designs about leadership in the student group leader.

The instructor would do well to tap the talents of older women—in class presentations, interviews, and group demonstrations—because "the ability of elderly people to learn and to teach is routinely under-estimated and under-used" (Canadian Non-Governmental Organization's Report on Aging, 1982, p. 16). And educators in gerontology could increase their use of elderly women to teach.

THE FUTURE OF GROUP WORK WITH ELDERLY WOMEN

• It will be common in the future to have elderly women included in women's studies classes and lectures. Group demonstrations by a skillful leader could be a powerful teaching technique. Older women—even nonagenarians and centenarians—will be teaching classes with the status and pay of younger teachers.

• Elderly women should be given chances at leadership. Nursing homes could train a cadre of leaders who could co-lead with women residents. (The residents are usually too frail and lack energy to be the prime movers to plan, implement, and conduct a group.)

• A national information center containing research related to all older women's grousp would be available.

• Training courses for group leaders would be available in a national center, which also includes a think tank for scholars dedicated to improving the quality of life for older women.

• A journal on group work with older women would be published so that studies would be found in one publication.

• Funding for research would be available for group leaders who are generating research. For example, what are the qualities of a successful leader? What are the differences in group results when a male leads an all-female group (as Linden did), or a female leads an all-female group, or co-leaders, a male and female, lead (as Linden did later in the group experience)? What modalities of groups are most effective for demented older women? Alert women? Depressed older women? What tools best measure depression in older women? What models of group programs are effective? And for what setting? For example, the group activities designed for a day care center may be quite different from those for a nursing home. And what can be learned about the cultural diversity in groups? What are the therapeutic leader interventions, for example, during depression, anger, monopolizing, hearing impairments, vision loss, and withdrawal? What is the minimum length of group life to be effective? What time of day should groups be held? How do the disciplines vary in their approach to group work? And what are some of the commonalities? What are the gender differences? Waller and Griffin (1984) have suggested a few.

• When a larger body of knowledge is available, there will be meta-analyses of groups of older women so that the effect of size can be determined.

• The dearth of teaching materials will be helped by the national information center, but private funds will be donated for worthwhile group projects. ("The Teaching Nursing Home" is a model of one such national project to improve quality of care and quality of life.)

SUMMARY

The group modality for elders is certainly on the increase, although it has been most difficult to ferret out the growth of women-only groups in the current literature. Miller and Solomon (1980) noted that traditional group work with the aged has consisted of activity, recreation, and entertainment; this is changing as researchers become more sophisticated. Zimpfer (1984), who compiled an extensive bibliography, noted "the creativity, vitality and explosive increase in the use of group in delivering helping services" (p. 1).

Gillman (quoted in Price, 1984) states, "Women are growing . . . braver, stronger, more healthful, skillful and able and free. More human in all ways" (p. 53). But does this hold for older women? Copper (1986) writes,

> I believe that age passing is one of the primary learning arenas of female competition, as well as an apprenticeship to hatred of old women . . . Acceptance of age in women has not kept pace with our increasing life expectancy: It is the quality of that extra time that is important. (pp. 47-48)

Group work is a modality than can improve the quality of extra time for the aging woman.

REFERENCES

Aaronson, L. (1983). Adult day care: A developing concept. *Journal of Gerontological Social Work, 5*(3), 35-47.

Altholz, J. A. (1984). Group psychotherapy with the elderly. In I. Burnside (Ed.), *Working with the elderly: Group process and techniques* (2nd ed., pp. 248-258). Boston: Jones & Bartlett.

Bearon, L. (1984). Famous aged. In E. Palmore (Ed.), *Handbook on the aged in the United States* (pp. 17-30). Westport, CT: Greenwood Press.

Beckett, R. (1981). The use of reality orientation in adult foster care homes: A rationale. *Journal of Gerontological Social Work, 3*(3), 3-13.

Brandler, S. (1984). Poetry: Group work and the aged. *Journal of Gerontological Social Work*, *1*(4), 295-351.

Burnside, I. (1981). Reminiscing as therapy: An overview. In I. Burnside (Ed.), *Nursing and the aged* (2nd ed., pp. 98-113). New York: McGraw-Hill.

Burnside, I. (1983, January). *Reminiscence therapy: An effective modality*. Paper presented at the Aging and Mental Health Conference, Honolulu, HI.

Burnside, I. (1984). Education for group work. In I. Burnside (Ed.), *Working with the elderly: Group process and techniques* (2nd ed., pp. 91-101). Boston: Jones & Bartlett.

Burnside, I. (1988). Reminiscence and the other therapeutic modalities. In I. Burnside (Ed.), *Nursing and the aged*, (3rd ed., pp. 645-685). New York: McGraw-Hill.

Burnside, I., Baumler, J. & Weaverdyck, S. (1984). Group work in a day care center. In *Working with the elderly: Group process and techniques* (2nd ed., pp. 79-88). Boston: Jones & Bartlett.

Butler, R. N. (1963). The life review: An interpretation of reminiscence in the aged. *Psychiatry*, *26*(1), 65-76.

Canadian Non-Governmental Organization's Report on Aging, Canada (1982). Ottawa, Canada: National Advisory Council on Aging.

Cooper, H. M. (1984). *The integrative research review: A systematic approach*. Beverly Hills, CA: Sage.

Copper, B. (1986). Voices: On becoming old women. In *Women and aging: An anthology by women*. Corvalis, OR: Calyx Books.

Cousins, N. (1979). *Anatomy of an illness as perceived by the patient*. New York: Norton.

Davis, K. (1986). Paying the health-care bills of an aging population. In A. Pifer & L. Bronte (Eds.), *Our aging society* (pp. 299-318). New York: Norton.

Dennis, H. (1984). Remotivation therapy. In I. Burnside (Ed.), *Working with the elderly: Group process and techniques* (2nd ed., pp. 187-197). Boston: Bartlett & Jones.

Donahue, E. (1984). Reality orientation: A review of the literature. In *Working with the elderly: Group process and techniques* (2nd ed., pp. 167-176). Boston: Bartlett & Jones.

Friedlob, S., & Kelly, J. (1984). Reminiscing groups in board-and-care homes. In I. Burnside (Ed.), *Working with the elderly: Group process and techniques* (2nd ed., pp. 308-327). Boston: Bartlett & Jones.

Garner, J. D., & Mercer, S. (1980). Social work practice in long-term care facilities: Implications of the current model. *Journal of Gerontological Social Work*, *3*(2); 71-77.

George, L. (1984). The institutionalized in famous aged. In E. Palmore (Ed.), *Handbook on the aged in the United States* (pp. 339-354). Westport, CT: Greenwood Press.

Getzel, G. (1981). Old people, poetry, and groups. *Journal of Gerontological Social Work*, *3*(1); 77-85.

Gioella, E., & Bevil, C. (1985). Management of risk factors. In E. Gioella & C. Bevil (Eds.), *Nursing care of the aging client: Promoting healthy adaptation* (pp. 197-215). Norwalk, CT: Appleton-Century-Crofts.

Gubrium, J. (1975). *Living and dying at Murray Manor*. New York: St. Martin's Press.

Gubrium, J., & Ksander, M. (1975). On multiple realities and reality orientation. *The Gerontologist, 15,* 142-145.

Hagestad, G. (1986). The family: Women and grandparents as kin-keepers. In A. Pifer and L. Bronte (Eds.), *Our aging society* (pp. 141-160). New York: Norton.

Haight, B. K. (1988). The therapeutic role of a structured life review process in homebound elderly subjects. *Journal of Geronotology, Psychological Sciences 43*(2), 40-44.

Hartford, M. E. (1980). The use of group methods for work with the aged. In J. E. Birren & R. B. Sloane (Eds.), *Handbook of mental health and aging* (pp. 806-826). Englewood Cliffs, NJ: Prentice-Hall.

Hennessey, M. J. (1984). Music therapy. In I. Burnside (Ed.), *Working with the elderly: Group processes and techniques* (2nd ed., pp. 198-210). Boston: Bartlett & Jones.

Keith, J. (1982). *Old people as people: Social and cultural influences on aging and old age*. Boston: Little, Brown.

Koch, K. (1977). *I never told anybody*. New York: Random House.

Kubie, S., & Landau, G. (1953). *Group work with the aged*. New York: International Universities Press.

Kurland, R. (1978). Planning: Neglected components of group developments. *Social Work with Groups, 1,* 173-178.

Levy, L. H. (1976). Self-help groups: Types and psychological process. *Journal of Applied Behavioral Sciences, 12,* 310-322.

Linden, M. (1953). Group psychotherapy with institutionalized senile women: Study in gerontological human relations. *International Journal of Group Psychotherapy, 3,* 130-170.

Livson, F. B. (1983). Gender identity: A life-span view of sex role development. In R. Weg (Ed.), *Sexuality in the later years: Roles and behavior* (pp. 105-127). New York: Academic Press.

MacDonald, M. W., & Settin, J. M. (1976). Reality orientation versus sheltered workshops as treatment for the institutionalized aging. *Journal of Gerontology, 33,* 416-421.

McMahon, A. W., & Rhudick, P. J. (1964). Reminiscing adaptational significance in the aged. *Archives of General Psychiatry, 10*(3), 292-298.

Middleton, R. (1987). Book review. *Social Work in Health Care, 12*(4), 119.

Miller, I., & Solomon, R. (1980). The development of group services for the elderly. *Journal of Gerontological Social Work, 2*(3), 241-257.

Minkler, M. (1985). The nursing home: A neglected setting for health promotion. *Family and Community Health, 8*(1), 46-58.

Moore, E. C. (1984). A music therapist's perspective. In I. Burnside (Ed.), *Working with the elderly: Group process and techniques* (2nd ed., pp. 426-440). Boston: Bartlett & Jones.

Nickoley-Colquitt (1981). Preventative group interventions for elderly clients: Are they effective? In *Family & Community Health: The Journal of Health Promotion & Maintenance*, *3*(4), 80 February.

O'Dell, L. (1984). A bibliotherapist's perspective. In I. Burnside (Ed.), *Working with the elderly: Group process and techniques* (2nd ed., pp. 411-425). Boston: Bartlett & Jones.

Pieroni, R. (1984). Centenarians. In E. Palmore (Ed.), *Handbook of the aged in the United States*. Westport, CT: Greenwood Press.

Pifer, A., & Bronte, L. (1986). *Our aging society: Paradox and promise*. New York: Norton.

Poggi, R. (1984). A psychiatrist's perspective. In I. Burnside (Ed.), *Working with the elderly: Group process and techniques* (2nd ed., pp. 358-368). Boston: Bartlett & Jones.

Polster, E. (1987). *Every person's life is worth a novel*. New York: Norton.

Price, S. (1984). *The female ego*. New York: Rawson Associates.

Richman, J. (1985). *Humor in group, family, and individual psychotherapy with the depressed elderly*. New York: XIIIth International Congress of Gerontology, 306.

Romaniuk, M., & Romaniuk, J. (1981). Looking back: An analysis of reminiscence functions and triggers. *Experimental Aging Research*, *7*, 477-489.

Scott-Maxwell, F. (1968). *The measure of my days*. New York: Knopf.

Sherman, E. (1987). Reminiscence groups for community elderly. *The Gerontologist*, *27*(5), 569-572.

Steffl, B. (1984). Group work and professional curricula. In I. Burnside (Ed.), *Working with the elderly: Group process and techniques* (2nd ed., pp. 487-497). Boston: Bartlett & Jones.

Stockton, R., Moran, D., & Velkoff, P. (1987). Leadership of therapeutic small groups. *Journal of Group Psychotherapy, Psychodrama and Sociometry*, *39*(4), 157-165.

Sullivan, J., & Deane, D. (1988). Humor and health. *Journal of Gerontological Nursing*, *14*(1), 20-24.

Tappen, R. M. (1985). Student-led reminiscence groups: Preceptor responsibilities and outcomes. In *Book of abstracts* (p. 201). New York: XIIIth International Congress of Gerontology.

Taulbee, L. (1984). Reality orientation and clinical practice. In I. Burnside (Ed.), *Working with the elderly: Group process and techniques* (2nd ed., pp. 177-186). Boston: Bartlett & Jones.

Taulbee, L., & Folsom, J. C. (1966). Reality orientation for geriatric patients. *Hospital and Community Psychiatry*, *17*, 133-135.

Vladeck, B. (1980). *Unloving care: The nursing home tragedy*. New York: Basic Books.

Waller, M., & Griffin, M. (1984). Group therapy for depressed elders. *Geriatric Nursing, September/October, 5*, 309-311.

Wolcott, A. (1978). Art therapy: An experimental group. In I. Burnside, (Ed.), *Working with the elderly: Group process and techniques* (pp. 292-310). Belmont, CA: Wadsworth.

Zimpfer, D. (1984). *Group work in the helping professions: A bibliography.* Muncie, IN: Accelerated Development.

Women and Aging: Perspectives on Public and Social Policy

Lou Ann B. Jorgensen, DSW

This article addresses the benefits and limitations of policy in relation to women—specifically, to the aging female population. The framework is similar to that used by David G. Gil to analyze and develop social policy. According to Gil (1973), social policies constitute a system of interrelated but not necessarily logically consistent principles and courses of action that determine the nature of intrasocietal relationships. They regulate the development, allocation, and distribution of statuses and roles and their accompanying constraints, rewards, and entitlements among individuals and social units in a society, and they determine the distribution of resources and shape the quality of life. Economic measures are viewed not as a separate domain, but as an important means for realizing the objectives of social policy (Baumheimer & Schoor, 1977). Two indi-

Lou Ann B. Jorgensen is in the Graduate School of Social Work, University of Utah, Salt Lake City, UT 84112.

viduals who have played prominent roles in the development of social policy in the United States are Eveline M. Burns and Charles I. Schottland. Burns has been a leading analyst of social policy since the early thirties and views it as: "the organized efforts of society to meet identifiable personal needs of, or social problems presented by, groups or individuals"; whereas Schottland, who has also served as Commissioner of Social Security, suggests the following broad and general definition:

> A social policy is a statement of social goal and strategy, or a settled course of action dealing with the relations of people with each other, the mutual relations of people with their government, the relations of governments with each other, including legal enactments, judicial decisions, administrative decisions, and mores. (Gil, 1973)

These policy definitions will further guide the analysis of policies in this discussion as they relate to aging women.

HISTORICAL OVERVIEW

Aging women appear today in many publications to be victims, but is this a true characterization? This presentation looks at women and aging as they relate to policies. Rather than identify aging women as victims, it will address this population as one with special characteristics and problems, one that contributes as an active segment of society, and one that is asking to be recognized as valuable now and in the future.

Aging women have always been an integral part of all societies. The status, roles, and position of older women in some societies have been revered and highly respected over the years. Many cultures have had a special place for their female population as they have aged. They were the cared-for population in the past and, in some cases, continue to be so today. Their place has been in the home, first as a daughter, then as a wife, a grandmother, and often a great-grandmother. The family has flocked around the dinner tables of these special citizens, gained knowledge and skills from them, and anticipated continuing to give loving care as these women aged.

Has the picture changed? Why would this population be different than before? Have social scientists, social workers, and human resource persons found life different for aging women today, or are aging women becoming different? Some authors say the primary conflict in recent years has been that the social environment is changing faster than social policy can respond and that it is changing for a population that was socialized to expect traditional sex roles (Smith, 1979). It may be that a growing segment of our population has spoken out in concern for its own well-being. If this is true, the picture has changed, and it is time we address the needs of a group we have basically ignored or found no reason to treat in a special manner.

In the 1980s statistics show that aging women are the fastest growing segment of today's population. Women represent 59.7% of the U.S. population age 50 and over. For every 100 men over age 65 there are 127 women, increasing to 220 women for every 100 men by age 85 (Markson, 1983). Thus it appears that the aging woman's perspective is becoming too important to ignore. We need to understand first just how the lives of women have changed as they have moved outside the home, and how society has responded to these changes. Sara M. Evans has developed a chronological review highlighted in *The American Woman, 1987-88*, edited by Sara Rix (1987), which shows how the lives of women have been shaped and changed since the beginning of the 20th century. Through this review we can identify how changing policies have had a marked effect on the lives of women.

In the late 19th century, women had expanded their domestic sphere far beyond the home be creating thousands of voluntary associations ranging from temperance societies to settlement houses. These associations served women as training grounds for political activism in the interest of social justice. As women began to work through these associations to change society in the name of domestic values, they developed skills, self-confidence, and a new sense of their own rights as individuals.

In 1900 about one in five women worked outside the home; most of them were young and single. Both women and their employers presumed that their employment would end with marriage. As a consequence, women were segregated into the least-skilled, lowest-paying jobs, and women's self-sufficiency was clearly to end when marriage took place. Evans found few women attending college at these times; however, those who did were not allowed to consider male professions such as engineering, medicine, and law. The women who did attend college had a significant impact on the development on what was then termed the female professions, such as nursing, teaching, and social work.

It appeared that of educated women, few practiced their profession outside the home for long periods of time. Urban black women were the only group of married women who presumed a lifetime of work away from the home. Family survival and a high priority on their children's education dictated that black women contribute to the family income. By 1910, middle-class white women were forming increasingly effective alliances with black and working-class women around the issue of women's suffrage.

After the right to vote was won, veteran suffragists split over the Equal Rights Amendment introduced by the National Woman's Party in 1923. Many suffragists with a background in the social reform movement believed strongly in female differences and feared that the ERA would preclude legislation protective of women. This split is one that appears to duplicate the split we continue to see in many states in the 1980s. The impact of the ERA has a history we have not yet experienced.

Next came the Depression—a time when married women who sought work, even those whose husbands were unemployed, faced a hostile backlash that blamed them for taking men's jobs. Although pervasive sex segregation in the labor force meant that women and men rarely competed for the same jobs, many states, cities, and school boards passed laws prohibiting or limiting the employment of married women. This fear did not support the competitive spirit but often demobilized those who controlled economic development for both sexes.

The concept of social security and other New Deal programs that evolved in the mid-thirties can be traced to the previous activities of private charities and settlement houses. The irony of the New Deal for women is that it institutionalized "civic housekeeping," redefining the "public arena" away from its roots in local communities and towards a massive and impersonal bureaucracy. The union drive of the 1930s is seen as serving workers of both sexes but as accepting lower pay scales for women. Both employers and unions presumed that women "belonged" in the home rather than in the labor force, and that working women's income was nonessential.

The outbreak of World War II ended the Depression and began an economic boom. By 1943, severe labor shortages convinced government and industry to reverse prejudices against married working women, and six million women who had never before worked outside the home entered the labor force during the war years. Women themselves were pleased with the opportunity for employment and although many planned to continue this pattern when the men returned home from the war, the gains working women had made in entering new fields of employment were quickly wiped out.

The expanding postwar economy, however, continued to fuel trends toward the employment of older, married women. Not only had the war removed some of the legal and cultural barriers to the employment of married women, but the number of young, single women seeking employment had decreased because of better educational opportunities and a rising propensity to marry. Although women provided the most important source of new workers for an expanding economy, the postwar era dissociated women and private life from politics. The "feminine mystique" defined women's place in a family-centered life style base on new abundance.

By 1960, there were 20 times more clerical workers than there had been in 1900; 96% of these workers were women. One of three women in the labor force was in clerical work. Having married younger and having had children earlier than women of preceding generations, women in their 30s and 40s found themselves at home with numerous "labor saving" appliances and without children to care for during the day. Educated middle-class married women were in the vanguard of the army of women who went to work outside the home in the 1960s and 1970s.

Also during the '60s and '70s we saw the rebirth of a feminist movement and the enactment of legislation, including the Equal Pay Act and Title VII of the Civil Rights Act, designed to prohibit discrimination against women in employment. By 1980 more than half of all adult women were working outside the home (Rix, 1987).

Thus, according to the Evans overview, we have seen women's lives in the 20th century changed and shaped through suffrage policies where women, through creative volunteerism, found a sense of their own rights; through policies that determined cessation of employment when marriage took place; through education governed by the policies that women were not acceptable for certain professions; through social security policies that were accepted by massive bureaucracies as programs to take care of all; through World War II where women's place was redefined and seen as a group expanding the economy; and through policies that provided for equal pay and prohibited discrimination against women. Throughout we see policies that fostered dependency of women in many cases and that definitely controlled them in other cases. The overview shows that policies relating to women are really family policies.

CHANGING ROLES

The emergence of women as independent individuals in society came about as activities developed outside the shelter of the home. The need for employment as part of that independence became evident, leading to a need for change in the underlying value and belief system.

The view that a woman's place is in the home informs women about their proper work and family roles. Also known as the "cult of domesticity" (Epstein, 1976) and the "feminine mystique" (Friedan, 1963), this familiar social norm (referred to in *Feminist Visions for Social Work* as the "family ethic") says that "proper" women marry and bear and raise children while being supported by and subordinated to a male breadwinner. Since the industrial revolution the family ethic has told women not to engage in paid labor outside the home but to work without wages, maintaining family members, managing household affairs, and providing emotional nurturance (VanDenBergh & Cooper, 1986).

Policies that treat women differentially according to their compliance with the family ethic result in poorer services and lower benefits for many women and their families. These policies also create distinctions between women on the basis of family status, race, and class (VanDenBergh & Cooper, 1986). As homemaking and motherhood became the centerpieces of 19th-century femininity, which also defined a woman as frail, pure, and idle, the many women who worked for wages outside the home were excluded from the only acceptable definition of respectable womanhood (VanDenBergh & Cooper, 1986).

The women of this period appeared to have had little concern for how society planned or implemented policies or programs that might affect them. Their overall goal was to fit into societal norms of the time, never anticipating that as they aged life could change and they would find themselves caught in situations they had taken no part in developing or trying to change.

In 1972 Congress approved the Equal Rights Amendment — the proposed amendment to the U.S. Constitution providing that "equality of rights under the law shall not be denied or abridged by the United States or by any State on account of sex." Thirty-five states ratified the amendment, but approval was needed by three more states before 30 June 1982 to make the ERA part of the Constitution. Such ratification failed to occur, and today legislators are still making an effort to draft a new Equal Rights Amendment to submit to Congress (Utah Women and the Law, 1986). Many proponents of the ERA felt that all women would have a stronger base for equal opportunities with the passing of the Equal Rights Amendment. Others felt no difference would be made, and that the passing of the Equal Rights Amendment would be a disadvantage for the advancement of women. This is an issue still under debate; however, it did have an impact on women's goals to experience independence and gain economic power.

WOMEN TODAY

Since 1900 older women have consistently become a larger proportion of the female population. Between 1960 and 1974 the number of older women increased 42% as compared to 18% for the total population and 32% for the older population. Projections for the Year 2000 indicate that although the number of older women will continue to increase, the distribution among separate age groups will decrease for the 65 to 69-year-olds, remain stable for the 70 to 74-year-olds, and increase for those in the over-75 age groups (Block, Davidson, & Grambs, 1981). The fact that women are living longer means that we will see an increasing number of women living beyond the age of 75, thus presenting a new set of difficulties since older women in recent studies are poorer, less educated, less employed, and more alone than older men. Eighty-five percent of women over 65 can anticipate some kind of chronic health problem (Black et al., 1981). This will continue to be a source of much concern for the older woman and will place increasing importance on the need for health services to maintain her and her peers.

Projections for the Year 2000 show a decrease in the percentage of women over 65 who have never married, while indicating that a much larger proportion of older women will be divorced (Gander, 1988) and that women over age 65 have better than a 50% chance of being poor. The economic conditions of women across all ages are related to their marital status. The real income of married women during 1968 to 1975 rose 17%, whereas the real income of widowed, separated, or divorced women declined by more than 10% (Corcoran, 1979). Weitzman's (1985) research showed that, on the average, divorced women experienced a 73% decline in standard of living during the first year following divorce.

Despite rapidly growing continuing education programs, few older women complete college. The median number of school years for women over the age of 65 is projected to increase from 9.4 in 1975 to 12.1 in 2000. As women's level of education increases, so does the likelihood that they will seek work (Black et al., 1981). Nearly half of all middle-aged women were employed in 1976; in 1988, 51% of all women over 50 are employed (U.S. Census Bureau Report, 1988).

Block, Davidson, and Grambs (1981) reported data showing that there are five times as many widows as widowers over age forty. Half of American women are widowed by age 65; by age 75 the incidence has increased to 68%. An equal number of older women live either alone or with a spouse. Of the remaining percentage of women over 65, most live with other family members. Only a small percentage of older women are institutionalized at any one time.

The demographic realities of the plight of older women are becoming an increasingly acute problem. Since the turn of the century, the average life expectancy in the United States has risen from about 50 years to 75 years. Experts predict that changes in life styles and advances in medicine could push that figure to 85 by the Year 2050.

A greater understanding of demographic changes and their future impact on women is critical. As these economic, educational, and employment inequities are understood and rectified, a less dismal picture will be painted for women of the future.

POLICIES AND PROBLEMS
AFFECTING AGING WOMEN

The problem of the aging woman, no matter what status she has, is reflected in the resources available to her. For the poor this is reflected in the lack of financial resources; in the sick, in the lack of medical care; in the homeless in lack of adequate housing; and on and on.

The phrase "feminization of poverty" is used to define the state of many women both young and old—women who have never had resources and women who have recently found themselves without adequate resources to function. This definition also encompasses the many social programs and policies that do not benefit women, thus placing them into more advanced stages of poverty at an earlier age. Members of the general population of aging women today are not the women who at a younger age have ever been AFDC mothers, victims of abuse, or even women who have asked for public assistance. They are women who, as they move into their advanced years, find they are facing problems of poverty that reflect not being prepared for an independent state of existence. They may be women seeking employment without the skills and experience necessary to get or hold a position in the work world; or they nay be displaced homemakers who find themselves divorced or widowed with few community resources available to them. Among families headed by working women, over one third have incomes below the poverty level. They may also find themselves far from family members who can assist or support. The mobile society does not build in family supports for the aging women of today. Whatever circumstances they find themselves in, it appears many of their problems would be solved if the needed resources were available to them. But what resources are available to support aging women?

A common resource for all, Social Security, was initially enacted to assist this kind of population. But does it really assist aging women? Social Security legislation has increasingly been attacked for discriminating on the basis of sex. Although this discrimination results in inequities that can affect both men and women, the inequities, in fact, fall primarily on women. This is largely because Social Security legislation was enacted at a time when women were assumed to be financially dependent on their husbands and marriage was assumed to be a lifetime arrangement. Today half of all marriages break up and half of all married women work, yet Social Security legislation remains substantially the same as when it was enacted forty years ago (Utah Governor's Commission on the Status of Women, 1987).

An example of discrimination against women under the present Social Security laws is the fact that a person can claim benefits both as a wage earner and as a dependent; yet Social Security is structured so a person, either a man or a woman, cannot get both a full benefit as a wage earner and a full benefit as a non-earning dependent. This may result in a two-income family paying more Social Security taxes on their combined wages yet receiving fewer overall benefits than a couple with only one wage earner but the same income. Unless a wage-earning wife is entitled to more than half of her husband's primary benefit amount in her own right, she will not receive any additional benefits as a result of her own Social Security earnings and contribution. Although more women are active in the labor force, large numbers of women do not receive significant benefits from their contributions (Utah Governor's Commission on the Status of Women, 1987).

Further discrimination against women as a consequence of Social Security law comes from the current practice of averaging earnings to determine benefit amounts. Social Security benefits are based on the worker's average earnings in a specified number of years. Because of this, inflation and typical salary increases throughout a career can combine to create a situation in which the average salary is significantly smaller than the preretirement salary. Although this problem exists for both men and women, the consequences for women are much greater, partly because of employment discrimination. In addition, women often spend a period of time bearing and raising children when they may earn very little or nothing. Women who work part time or part of a year will have low annual earnings. A pattern of absences from the labor force seriously affects women's rights to disability benefits. Since the law does not currently view housework and homemaking as a valid occupation, a woman who spends years of her life in such labor may end up with little or no security in her old age (Utah Governor's Commission on the Status of Women, 1987).

Pension adequacy, the phenomenon of retirement, and retraining of older workers for employment all relate directly to the work experience of older people and all feed into the scenario of poverty being the main issue as women experience the many phenomena of aging. For untrained, unemployed, aging women, poverty becomes a way of life to which most of them have not been previously accustomed.

Other issues of importance for aging women are related in one way or another to the resources available to them. The availability of adequate housing, social supports, and health care all become a part of the policy inadequacies affecting the aging woman. Housing for women, particularly aging women and particularly public housing, has not grown or developed adequately. As the population of women has grown, many women find themselves with inadequate housing. The priority for community housing authorities, especially those supported by grants from HUD, has been housing for families (Jorgensen, McCollum, & Pedersen, 1986-87). An examination of how housing is considered by the authorities who govern public policy reveals that when housing for younger single women is addressed, members of Housing Authority Boards often reflect their own biases and do not support housing that is too attractive or comfortable because they fear the women will never get married and will never move out; when plans for housing for older women are discussed they then question these women's ability to maintain themselves in the facility and the availability of additional kinds of care and services that may need to be established to serve this population. Most Housing Authority Boards who set classifications specify housing as being for young, married, or nonmarried women under 35 or for older individuals as housing for divorced or widowed women over 60 (Jorgensen et al., 1986). The middle-aged or aging women are not considered to be in the client population unless they are public assistance clients or handicapped individuals; thus there is little housing for this specific population.

Another problem related to housing for aging women is that women who are in the process of aging often have housing facilities that they may have lived in for many years. The main problem for some aging women is keeping their facility in adequate living condition, since costly repair bills would be another route to poverty. Once again, because women have not learned skills to maintain themselves by being able to take care of home repairs, replacements, or maintenance, they must resort to hiring the services performed. This is another cost the low-income, near-poverty-level person cannot afford.

Aging women also face the problem of lack of adequate food resources. Aging women often look at food as a means of cutting corners, and if financial resources are not available, diet may be another problem area for aging women. A woman short on income can locate many food items that may not be appropriate to the nutritional needs of older people. Women are probably more guilty than most of not eating the right proportion of food as well as not eating a nutritionally balanced diet. This problem may affect the present or future health of aging women and should be seriously addressed by those who work with this population. Generally, a healthy diet is more common when financial resources are available to subsidize planning and development of nutritional menus. Often the more nutritional menu is less expensive, but it takes knowledge of how to plan and use food appropriately to ensure lower costs while including nutritional items in the menu.

As they age, women need direction on the importance of caring for themselves. Often women alone tend to neglect themselves when they no longer have family members around to care for or involvement in a purposeful set of activities. Community support systems are most important to aging women, not only as a resource but to assist them in using their leisure time pleasurably and productively.

In some cases, health and medical care become much more necessary. In a recent magazine article on aging, the author stated that with the baby boomers heading for Golden Pond, increased longevity is a medical time bomb. By the Year 2050, nearly 22% of the U.S. population will be 65 or older. And the elderly already account for 40% of the nation's health care bill. Health problems can also stem from inadequate care of oneself at a younger age and an inadequate knowledge of how to care for oneself earlier in life. Many of these health problems hit aging women at a much younger age than 65.

The availability of health insurance for the older woman becomes a problem if she has no resources for adequate coverage. Many women who have not worked, are not presently employed, or who no longer have a spouse who has family insurance find themselves without insurance to assist them with health and medical costs. As such costs rise, we may be seeing a steady increase in the number of women in our population who will have no assistance if a chronic health problem does occur. Women who are not or have not been employed must depend on someone else to cover their health care.

Another way to support the older dependant women is through help from younger family members; although when the time comes many families may find themselves unable to assist these aging women. Yet for those who do receive family support, another policy dilemma must be addressed: How far does the responsibility of the family member go in the case of health care? We may be looking at a generation of young people who could be bankrupted by having parents, especially mothers, who need medical care.

Policymakers would find it impossible to ignore these specific needs of aging women. Informally, as we see policymakers look at aging women as a population concern, the attitude appears to be one of lack of sacredness of person. Accusations are implied, such as "Shame on you, you aren't making it because you are not staying in the roles identified for you" or "You could take care of yourself if you had character," suggesting that women, and especially older women, must have a character flaw (Jorgensen, 1988).

Many women have become accustomed to enjoying the affluence of society today. The philosophy and attitudes of these women are based on early learned values and experiences. When this life plan does not work out, women become less able to care for themselves and are often referred to as exhibiting "learned helplessness."

There was a day when husbands could have their wives confined to institutions when they did not function as they should by the standards of the male in the home. Many aged chronically mentally ill women in institutions today fall into those categories. We must not allow women to lose their independence to the the point where they do not have control of their own lives and the health care they need.

We find, informally, that women are often treated like children, and because of their lack of knowledge and sophistication they allow this to happen. No one has had a clear vision of women's rights, and women do not have a universal vision themselves; thus in many instances they do not act in an appropriate, rational way on their own behalf.

Employment is one means for women to find recognized places in society and to enable them to acquire adequate resources needed to function more independently. Today over 50% of women are in the work force, but many more could be if aging women could find their places in that important part of society. Programs to retrain and assist aging women to be employed are small, but there is a beginning in this area. Governmental job training services are making available courses for women over 40; they are providing testing services to assist women to know where their present skills and past experiences will best fit; they are providing classes on job interviewing, development of appropriate vitae, dress-for-success classes, and rules on accepting and keeping a job; and they are developing follow-up evaluations to assist those who do not get employment as well as those who acquire jobs. These supports become important assets for women seeking employment.

If women are adequately prepared for employment, they could begin to have some impact on the employment policies of women. Those who enter the work force could affect the salary base of all women in their specific area of employment, thus raising the salary level. This needs to be done to alleviate the poverty levels experienced by aging women. Permanency planning, work incentives and demonstration of cost effectiveness could begin to change the employment picture for aging women. Jobs definitely lead men out of poverty, but often they do not do the same for women. Studies on comparable worth and pay equity for women must be supported, and society must take seriously the results of these studies. Changes can come much more rapidly than we have experienced up to now, and we must ensure that this will happen.

POLICY CHANGES, ENTITLEMENTS, CONSTRAINTS, AND REWARDS

Neugarten (1974) stresses that during middle age there is a heightening sensitivity to one's position within a complex social environment and a theme of reassessment of self. The difference in the time perspective and recognition of the finiteness of time are frequently cited themes of aging. Time left to live becomes an important concern rather than the infinite sense of time of youth. Entitlements become more important; constraints become more of a nuisance than true roadblocks.

Aging women have found employment to be necessary to maintain self, but they are also starting to view employment as an entitlement that allows them the independence sought throughout life. We have seen each year a substantial number of "displaced homemakers" with a long job tenure (at home) looking for paid employment. Low-wage jobs may be inappropriate for many of these women, especially well-educated women and women with usable skills. Where displacement results from marital disruption, there is typically inadequate support from former husbands. As of 1981 only about 15% of divorced and separated women had been awarded alimony; fewer than half received the full amount of child support they had been awarded (Blau & Ferber, 1986). Unfortunately, these women must sometimes support others as well as themselves.

Policy responses should build on these women's prior education and previous work experience as homemakers, recognizing the substantial skill development entailed in household administration. Their financial needs as household heads or important contributors to family economic resources must also be recognized. Policies to support women as their work roles change have been and will continue to be hampered by the lack of data on the household economy comparable to our data for the paid labor market. The initiation of a data collection project for the household sector is long overdue and should be high on the policy agenda for those interested in the economic status of women (Rix, 1987).

Women must find their place in the work force to raise their economic stability. They are entitled to employment that is not a constraint on their ability to improve their status. Not only is work in the paid labor force an important factor in the economic well-being of women and their families but studies also show that employed women also tend to be physically healthier, have less emotional disturbance, exhibit greater life satisfaction, and live longer than women in traditional homemaker roles (Beele, 1982).

The hypothesis that women may be more vulnerable than men to life stresses and strains has been increasingly invoked as one explanation for the depressive symptom excesses frequently reported by women in community surveys. The findings of a recent study by Joy P. Newman show that women are more likely than men to be exposed to hardships associated with the absence of a spouse, deprivation of living companions, inadequate financial resources, and chronic health problems. However, Newman found no evidence to support the hypothesis that women are more vulnerable to a depressive syndrome in response to any of these sources of life strains than are men. Indeed, the data suggest little support for the widely held view that women are more prone to a depressive syndrome than are their male counterparts (Newman, 1987). Other studies and reports also support the premise that women clearly can and do in many cases act equally with their male counterparts. We must not choose to support or reinforce the ideas that women are not physically or mentally capable for any reason to act independently in society.

Policy changes addressing the needs of the aging must then be viewed only in relation to the constraints society places on this group of women. Betty Friedan, 25 years after she sparked the women's movement, was recently featured in a popular magazine. It was reported that when she was speaking to groups of college students she often asks them, "How many of you have ever worn a girdle?" She says that in the era of pantyhose and aerobic exercise, this opener raises titters but only a few hands. She argues, "how can you know what it felt like when being a woman meant wearing a girdle not only here (pointing to her tummy) but here (pointing to her head)?'' (Furth, 1988).

Aging women of today experienced the constraints Betty Friedan so graphically depicts in her speeches. The girdle on the head was an accepted policy 25 or more years ago, and today's aging woman then accepted that constraint. These are the same women who today are asking to be recognized for the changes they believe are necessary if they are to experience equality.

Friedan's worst fear is that economic bad times could bring about a resurgence of women's-place-is-at-home feeling. ''The second paycheck in the family has been one of the real resources of the prosperity of the past 20 years,'' she says. ''It would be disastrous for the family if anyone even thought that women could go home again.'' Much still needs to be done for working families. For example, Friedan stated:

> We are the only industrial country besides South Africa without a policy of parental leave. The difficulties women are having with putting it all together are treated as each woman's own individual problem. So it's back to either kids or career — and that's where I came in! Either-or is no-win. (Furth, 1988)

With the historical impact of women like Betty Friedan, women have come a long way, and employment has provided one of the tracks or patterns to make that possible. Changing roles must address any constraints that may affect change. Giele (1982) states that the realities of women's changing roles have already forced a paradigm shift in the social sciences. Crossover theory better accommodates women's participation in the labor force than traditional theory that justifies a women's place as being entirely in the home. Similarly, new social policies mow support the crossover model of sex roles and the life course. Arrangements that once tacitly segregated men's and women's duties are presently subject to question; flexibility and interchange are instead in vogue — at least among the visionaries and activists who seek change. Consistent with greater diversity in life patterns and family forms, Giele (1982) sees the new programs as representing an emerging policy agenda that covers employment, family education, community, and security throughout the life courses. Giele breaks down these patterns into the following five areas of concern:

> The first is equal employment opportunity: antidiscrimination in hiring; flexible scheduling; reevaluation of comparable worth.
>
> The second, supportive family policies: pro-choice family planning; expansion of child care facilities; encouragement of men's participation in the family; recognition of homemaker contribution.
>
> The third covers equal educational opportunities: expansion of career options; vocational training; apprenticeship; continuing education; women's centers.
>
> Fourth, community supports for women's multiple roles is addressed: better housing design; integration into social networks, credit and encouragement for volunteer and political activity; integration of social services.
>
> And fifth, security throughout life course: equitable distribution of family income between women and men and accumulation of credits for Social Security; supports for the displaced homemaker; adequate pension and benefit coverage regardless of occupation or marital status. (Giele, 1982)

What is interesting about these proposals is that they seek to promote greater choice, not only by encouraging women's entry into new roles but also by lending support and giving recognition to women's traditional occupations. This recognition at an earlier age will make many changes and support having fewer constraints on aging women.

Giele's last proposal recognition of the homemaker, addresses the greatest need of aging women. It is one of the newest and in some ways the most surprising addition to family policy initiatives for changing women's status (1982). Rather than merely devaluing women's family work in an effort to broaden their options, feminists have recently learned to appreciate the unpaid contributions that women have made to family and community life. Some educational institutions will now give older women college credit for life experiences. This has enabled some women, particularly those without advanced education, to complete some sort of degree or certificate program that will assist them in obtaining meaningful employment or advance them in their present employment situation. In 1982 Giele further reported continual concerns about giving recognition and protection to homemakers.

Through the concerns and research in the 70s of various authors (Giele & Kahne 1978; Sommers & Shields, 1978; Houserman, 1980) we would anticipate that these policy changes would reap rewards for aging women in the late 80s. This may not be true, especially if once again we refer to what was reported in *The American Woman 1987-88: A Report in Depth* (Rix, 1987). One of the report's major conclusions is that despite important strides, the American dream of equality remains elusive for the nation's 53 million women in the labor force today. Although there are now about 28 million more women workers than there were a generation ago, including many women who fall into the aging category, they face many of the same barriers their mothers and grandmothers did.

One of the authors of the report, Nancy Barrett, Chair of the Economics Department at American University, concludes that women are in the work force to stay; thus it is essential to have an economic-policy agenda for all women. And although no single policy or program can address the needs of all women workers, women have many needs in common. She further states that women's workplaces having been shifted from the home, makes them similar to displaced workers. Nevertheless, former full-time homemakers are not lacking in skills, and their training needs have to be addressed by the public sector—the private sector can't do it all (Rix, 1987).

Leadership roles must be taken by women of all ages to give the aging woman the support and resources to assist her in making necessary adjustments in her life style. We must anticipate the changes needed by the Year 2000, when over 60% of the population of women will be over 40 years old.

FUTURISTIC VIEWS

The emerging national policy agenda for aging women must reflect a new paradigm. The social structure and the social consciousness surrounding issues affecting aging women must change. Each woman is an individual, and although there are many commonalities there are many differences in women's needs.

Lack of resources has clearly been identified as problematic for aging women. How resources can be acquired to alleviate this problem must be looked at creatively. New ideas must be developed and new policies implemented to ensure that resources are available to maintain a quality of life acceptable to this special population.

As changes in employment, social security, educational opportunities, health care options, and community supports provide for a more secure future for aging women, they will in turn trigger societal changes that will affect men's futures. Longitudinal research will need to be developed to determine if the changes in aging women's life patterns will also affect families, the economic climate, and the overall quality of life for those who interact with these women.

Will the basic self-awareness and self-esteem of women change? Some authors (Gottlieb, 1980; Masi, 1981) support independence as a means to a higher level of self-esteem for aging women. There is a need to apply the independent, self-sufficient theory to aging women in all status levels, including those who have little or no resources, those who have had resources but lack the understanding of how to use them most effectively and efficiently. For many women, the theory of independence is still an alien concept, and enormous tradeoffs are required for them to achieve even moderate success for themselves.

Above all, aging women must be comfortable being women. They must be in touch with their own strengths and courageous enough to use the abilities they have to make things happen for them. Women must find their own styles and their own voices as individuals. They must have confidence in their own opinions and be assertive enough to express them for the betterment of all women as they face the portion of their life where they are viewed as the aging population—no longer bound by girdles of the mind, but finally free to create, to plan, to organize, and to enjoy.

To achieve recognition they must strive to become represented equally by policymakers. Only if aging women of today make a firm effort to become involved as independent citizens in the political process can they make a difference for their younger sisters who are progressing through the life cycle into a period where they will also be identified as aging women. Incremental change must be started immediately. Change in the status of women in society is our only hope for equality for all.

As we approach the Year 2000, the author visualizes a time when aging women will not be identified as a population separate from the mainstream of the professional, business, or educational world — or any other world of which they choose to be a part. Let us hope that public and social policy will have been adapted to both genders; that both women and men will be addressed equally on all issues, and that both will have equal power and political clout in all issues of importance. If this dream could become reality, things would be very different for aging women after the turn of the century.

Aging will, of course, continue to grow stylish as more women reach the later years and as their own dissatisfaction with their circumstances will have forced them to become individually and collectively involved in the policies that affect them. Hopefully we will see women who have learned to mobilize themselves and who are willing to accept the power that will allow them to empower others. They will have recognized that they are no longer limited in their range of choices and will proceed to make decisions for themselves that will lead national policymakers to endorse epochal change, possibly on the order of the Great Society.

The male perspective will no longer be the main one; thus because all women, even aging women, will be equally accepted, no longer will society identify specific roles for specific genders. Services that have been discriminatory will no longer be so. For example, Social Security policies will be revised to identify employment in different ways so that both men and women will be rewarded for the work they have chosen to do throughout their lifetimes. Or, possibly, to avoid putting unbearable burdens on the children of baby boomers, the Social Security system will be abolished and an equalized pension provided for all. This could possibly be supported by organizations other than government or by government in a different way than it is today.

After the turn of the century, education should take a new focus. If our world is to become more egalitarian, education — one of the most powerful elements in change — must be made available to all. Women will be introduced to an educational system that will benefit them throughout their lifetimes. They will be encouraged, trained, supported, and expected to follow some educational plan that will provide them with a means to live independently. The livelihood of women will no longer depend on a male mate or companion or by the rules set down by the same. All women will be encouraged to choose careers of their liking; thus their emerging talents will be more productively recognized independent of one another. There will be no barriers to their becoming anything for which they are willing to strive; and this will be an accepted and expected pattern for women to follow. This concept will be introduced and supported from kindergarten or nursery school days into adulthood. Equality will happen when each woman knows her own capabilities and limitations and can use this knowledge to develop strengths and talents that will benefit herself and those around her.

The educational system of the future will ideally assume the responsibility of allowing each person individual choice and of providing understanding regarding how these choices may affect his/her future. We will expect the educational system, which touches everyone's lives during some period of time, to be prepared to accomplish this task.

Persons who make policies are people with power — active members of society who find a place for themselves in the mainstream of life. Aging women will be these people in the 21st century, as they will have had the opportunity to develop expertise throughout their lifetimes. They will enjoy good health; they will know what type of housing they need and will ensure its accessibility to them; they will be aware of financial resources available to them; they will be well-educated and trained in professions of their choice; they will hold public and social policy positions and offices; and they will be persons of power.

Natasha Josefowitz in *Paths to Power* (1983) states that an active, involved older woman is a wonderful role model for all people of all ages. She says that

> Women must begin to look with new eyes, to hear with new ears, to think thoughts that until just a generation ago were unthinkable. We are in the process of attaining a new status — a new "place" — in the world, fostered by expanded freedom

and a deeper understanding of what women are, want, and can do. We are learning that successful self-realization does not mean giving up our qualities of womanhood, it means adding to them. By celebrating our knowing as well as our knowledge, we can be feminine and powerful. (p. 233)

As utopian as the preceding statements may seem, they are by no means out of reach. As aging women of the next century look at materials written in the 80s, they will see our visions of women corporate heads; they will see human service agencies directed by women; they will see political offices held by women — legislators, mayors, commissioners, governors, and even U.S. presidents and vice-presidents. And these will not be visions to them; they will be living in a time of accomplishments.

To make the changes needed today in public and social policy, we must see changes in attitudes, values, and ethics of all people. Women must be comfortable with not waiting to be discovered, to be hired, to be promoted, to be loved. It will be up to women to take the initiative to open up opportunities for themselves. And, of course, as they do this we will no longer see public and social policies that put roadblocks in the way of their becoming independent, acceptable citizens. We will see more egalitarian policies that will provide strong support for aging women on their own terms. At long last, the true worth of aging women will be understood and appreciated, both by themselves and by others.

REFERENCES

Baumheier, E. C., & Schorr, A. L. (1977). Social policy. In *The encyclopedia of social work* (Vol. 2, Issue 17, pp. 1453-1462). New York: National Association of Social Workers.

Beele, D. (Ed.). (1982). *Lines in stress: Women & depression*. Beverly Hills, CA: Sage.

Blau, F., & Ferber, M. A. (1986). *The economics of women, men & work*. Englewood Cliffs, NJ: Prentice-Hall.

Block, M. R., Davidson, J. L., & Grambs, J. D. (1981). *Women over forty, visions & realities*. New York: Springer.

Epstein, B. (1976, April). Industrialization and femininity: A case study of nineteenth-century New England. *Social Problems, 23,* 389-401.

Friedan, B. (1963). *The feminine mystique*. New York: Dell.

Furth, J. (1988, February). *Life Magazine*, pp. 97-98.

Gander, A. (1988). *Divorced women*. Unpublished doctoral dissertation, Salt Lake City: University of Utah.

Giele, J. Z. (1982a). Future research and policy questions. In J. Z. Giele (Ed.), *Women in the middle years* (pp. 199-231). New York: Wiley.

Giele, J. Z. (1982b). Women in adulthood: Unanswered questions, In J. Z. Giele (Ed.), *Women in the middle years* (pp. 1-36). New York: Wiley.

Giele, J. Z., & Kahne, H. (1978). Meeting work and family responsibilities proposals of flexibility. In U.S. House of Representatives, *Women in midlife— security & fulfillment*. Washington, DC: U.S. Government Printing Office.

Gil, D. G. (1973). *Unraveling social policy, theory, analysis & political action toward social equality*. Cambridge: MA: Schenkman.

Gottlieb, N. (1980). The Older Woman. In Gottlieb, N. (Ed.), *Alternative social service for woman* (pp. 280-331). New York: Columbia University Press.

Houserman, N. R. (1980). The American homemaker; policy proposals. In D. G. McGuigan (Ed.), *Women's lines: New theory, research and policy*. Ann Arbor, MI: University of Michigan, Center for Continuing Education of Women.

Jorgensen, L. B. (in press). The phenomenon of women as they age.

Jorgensen, L. B., McCollum, L., & Pedersen, T. (1986-1987). Women residents in public housing: victims of self-sufficiency programs. *The Journal of Applied Social Sciences*, *11*(1), 48-63.

Josefowitz, N. (1983). *Paths of power*. Menlo Park, CA: Addison-Wesley.

Markson, E. (1983). *Older women*. Lexington, MA: Lexington Books.

Masi, D. A. (1981). *Organizing for women, issues strategies & services*. Lexington, MA: Lexington Books.

Mayer, R. R., & Greenwood, E. (1980). *The design of social policy research*. Englewood Cliffs, NJ: Prentice-Hall.

Neugarten, B. L. (1979). Time, age and the life cycle. *American Journal of Psychiatry*, *136*(7), 887-894.

Neugarten, B. & Daton, N. (1974). The middle years. In S. Arieti (Ed.), *American handbook of psychiatry* (vol. 1, 2nd ed., pp. 592-608). New York: Basic Books.

Newman, J. P. (1987). Gender differences in vulnerability to depression. *Social Service Review*, *61*(3), 447-468.

Rix, S. E. (Ed.). (1987). *The American woman 1987-88, A report in depth*. New York: Norton.

Smith, R. (Ed.). (1979). *The subtle revolution: women at work*. Washington, DC: Urban Institute.

Sommers, T., & Shields, L. (1978). Problems of the displaced homemaker. In U.S. House of Representatives Select Committee on Aging, *Women in midlife—Security and fulfillment* (Part 1, pp. 86-106). Washington DC: U.S. Government Printing Office.

U.S. Bureau of the Census. (1988). *Census bureau report*. Washington, DC: Department of Commerce.

Utah Department of Employment Security. (1987). *Utah affirmative action information, 1986* (Monograph.) Salt Lake City, Utah: Author.

Utah Governor's Commission on the Status of Women. (1987). *Utah women and the law*. Salt Lake City: University of Utah Press.

Van Den Bergh, N., & Cooper, L. B. (Eds.). (1986). *Feminist visions for social work*. Silver Spring, MD: National Association of Social Workers.

Weitzman, L. J. (1985). *The divorce revolution*. New York: Freedom Press.

The Double Standard of Aging and Older Women's Employment

Kathleen E. Nuccio, PhD

The status of older women's employment remains a neglected area of interest and research by both the gerontological and women's studies fields (Congressional Quarterly, 1981: Shaw & Shaw, 1987). The preponderance of studies on "older workers" focuses on men, and interest in the employment problems of women centers on the dilemmas of combining work and family life (Fox & Hesse-Biber, 1984; Voydanoff, 1984). Yet in a patriarchal society that values youth, older women bear unusual economic penalties that increase with age. This article provides an overview of the special status of the older woman worker, her economic vulnerability, and the effects on her of the double standard of aging, both in employment and in pensions and retirement. It also reviews the available legal remedies and their limitations.

BACKGROUND

Employment discrimination against older women is not a recent phenomenon, although it was not illegal until 1967. It has played a role in the labor market throughout the industrial age, although documentation of age discrimination prior to World War II is difficult to obtain. Where data on women's earnings and other factors of employment do exist, they are not broken down by age; similarly, when data are available by age, they are not categorized by sex.

During the Great Depression of the 1930s, many states adopted

---

Kathleen E. Nuccio is Assistant Professor of Social Work and Women's Studies, Ohio State University, Columbus, OH 43210.

laws and regulations to exclude married women from public employment, and Congress enacted legislation that restricted federal civil service jobs to one to a family. Of course, the pressure was greatest for wives to resign their posts. The prevalent mindset of the 1930s was that a job that was held by a woman was stolen from a man (Daniel, 1987).

The Women's Bureau was created within the Department of Labor following World War I, and its establishment, along with that of the War Production Board at the onset of World War II, made data on the status of women in the labor force more available and reliable. War production has historically necessitated women entering the labor force in expanded roles. The broader range on nontraditional jobs open to women and the higher wages associated with industrial jobs offer attractive opportunities for women. However, even in times of war, sex and age discrimination remain persistent factors that account for women's depressed wages, and, in the case of age, their exclusion from the workforce altogether.

Foner (1982) documents the age discrimination that was rampant in the war industries. The average maximum age for women applicants was 30 to 35 in the defense industries. And according to 1944 census data, over 75% of the women in the labor force were under 45 years of age. Age-related hiring policies made a significant mark on the labor force participation of older women during this time period, as is evidenced by the fact that of the 6.5 million women who entered the labor force after Pearl Harbor, over 80% were under the age of 45.

Hartmann (1982) notes that although war-related labor experiences of employers with women eroded long-held biases against married women, prejudice against black women and older women diminished less readily. Even a worsening labor supply in 1943, which expanded some opportunities for older women, did not counteract employers' preference for youth.

Ironically, the advice given by proponents of older women workers, intended to encourage their hiring, was contradictory, at best. Margaret Hickey, chairman [sic] of the Women's Advisory Committee to the War Manpower Commission, observed that whereas older women might get sick more often than younger women, they were more responsible. And *Newsweek* concluded that though they worked less rapidly, older women workers were more efficient (Daniel, 1987).

The years after World War II saw the forced exodus of thousands of women from the labor force. If women had made economic gains in wartime, they are not apparent in the data reflected in Table 1. The wage data presented in Table 1 demonstrate a sex-based wage gap in which women's earnings peak earlier and lose ground more quickly than do those of men in the same age categories.

Although the 1950s are regarded as a time of the generation of home and family, and of the inculcation of the "feminine mystique," these years provided a harsh reality for older women in the workforce. A 1957 report by the Women's Bureau of the Department of Labor noted that not only was age discrimination operating in the labor market, but it had a greater impact on women than it did on men (U.S. Department of Labor, Women's Bureau, 1957).

Although the decades of the 1960s and 1970s are described as times when women entered the labor force in unprecedented numbers (Daniel, 1987), the data in Table 2 demonstrate that the labor force participation of women in their 50s has been around 50% for nearly the last 20 years.

Despite stereotypes to the contrary, women have always worked out of economic necessity (Marshall & Paulin, 1987). Rather than earning "pin money," women have worked to support either themselves or households that they headed. If married, they worked to complement a spouse's income in order to insure a standard of living above the poverty level (Daniel, 1987; Marshall & Paulin, 1987). Concurrent with the increasing participation of women in the labor force has come the steady rise of the proportion of women in poverty. The "feminization of poverty" is a phrase that describes the disproportionate presence of women among the poor (Pearce, 1978). This pattern exists across the life span and is clearly evident within the elderly population.

Among those aged 65 and over, 17% of the women are poor, compared to only 10% of men (Shaw, 1986). The risk of poverty for elderly women is strongly correlated with marital status and race, an important finding in view of the fact that over 60% of white women (and nearly 75% of black women aged 65 and over) are not married (Shaw, 1986).

Table 1

Median Year's Earnings of Women and Men, Full-Time
Workers
by Selected Ages: 1946

Age Group	Women	Men
25-34	$1,698	$2,493
35-44	1,809	2,837
45-54	1,719	2,823
55-64	1,543	2,558
65+	1,188	2,129

Source: U.S. Department of Labor, Women's Bureau,
(1948).   Handbook of Facts on Women Workers, Bull.
225, p. 21.

Due to the preponderance of women who live near or below the
poverty line, who work for depressed wages, and who participate in
income assistance or insurance programs, the linkages among sexism, employment, poverty, and welfare require further exploration
(Pearldaughter & Schneider, 1980). Any examination of the economic status of women over the life span must take into account the
additional interactive effects of ageism (Russell, 1987).

PUBLIC PROGRAMS

Considerable notoriety has been given to the fact that women and
children make up the largest percentage of the Aid to Families with
Dependent Children (AFDC) category of public assistance (Pearce,
1978; Sidel, 1986), but it is less widely publicized that women con-

Table 2

Labor Force Participation Rates By Women in Their 50's
1955-1983
(selected years)

Year	Age 50-54	Age 55-59
1955	41.5%	35.6%
1960	48.8%	42.2%
1965	50.1%	47.1%
1970	53.8%	49.0%
1975	53.3%	47.9%
1979	56.5%	48.7%
1980	57.8%	48.6%
1982	58.0%	49.6%
1983	58.5%	48.8%

Source: Older Women's League. (1984) Statement of the
Older Women's League on Older Women in the Labor Force
Before the Joint Economic Committee, June 6, 1984,
p. 7.

stitute the largest percentage (67.2 in 1983) of the aged category of the Supplemental Security Income (SSI) program (U.S. Department of Health and Human Services, Social Security Administration [Social Security], 1987). Funding levels of both these programs are notoriously low. AFDC payments, for a family of three, range from a low of $118 per month in Alabama to a high of $740 per month in Alaska (Children's Defense Fund, 1987, p. 262). The average monthly SSI payment for the aged category was $164 in 1985 (U.S. Bureau of the Census [Census], 1987B, Table No. 619).

DISPLACED HOMEMAKERS

The problems of late entry and reentry into the labor force are especially important for women, who are disproportionately represented among "reentrants" and "new entrants" in the statistics on unemployment. About 25% of the women who are now middle-aged remained out of the workforce for periods up to 15 years following the birth of their first child (Dex & Shaw, 1986). This makes the inclusion of displaced homemakers particularly germane to any discussion of the older woman and the workplace. Among women who were unemployed in 1985, over 50% were classified as reentrants or new entrants, whereas fewer than 33% of unemployed males are similarly classified (U.S. Bureau of the Census, 1987, Table No. 663).

Middle-aged women entering the job market for the first time, or reentering after an absence, face a double-edged sword of discrimination. The *lack* of experience, which often serves as a ruse to veil age discrimination, can eliminate the former category, whereas exclusion from employment due to being "overqualified" serves to discriminate against the latter category of older women. The Older Women's League describes a case in which a school district restricted teaching applicants to those with less than five years experience (Older Women's League, 1982).

Women who rely on marriage for financial security confront the transition of that institution from one of relative stability to its current state in which the probability of divorce is 50% and rising (Bergman, 1986; Hewlett, 1986). Divorce is a source of major economic hardship for women (Peters, 1986). Remarriage and employment are two channels that can improve the economic hardship of divorce, but, paradoxically, remarriage rates for women who are not in the labor market are lower than for those in the labor market (Peters, 1986), and the probability of remarriage declines with age (Nestel, Mercier, & Shaw, 1983).

The information in Table 3 illustrates the economic vulnerability for women over the age of 40 that is created by child support.

Awards of child support are not guaranteed, and once awarded, the level of support they afford is minimal. Moreover, women whose sole support is AFDC or child support face destitution once

Table 3

Child Support Awards and Payments

Women 40 years of age and over

Number of Women (Thousands)	Percent Awarded Support	Percent Receiving Support	Mean Annual Support
Above the Poverty Line			
2,298	60.9	31.8	$2,968
Below the Poverty Line			
506	42.9	14.8	$1,692

Note. Includes women with own children under 21 years of age present from an absent father.

Source: Taken from data presented in U. S. Bureau of the Census, (1986). Statistical Abstract of the United States: 1987 (107th Ed.). Washington, D.C., Table No. 627.

their eligibility for this support is terminated when their children reach majority.

LABOR-FORCE PARTICIPATION

Middle-aged women already present in the workforce, as well as displaced homemakers entering the job market for the first time or following a hiatus of many years, face age discrimination in addition to the sex discrimination faced by younger women (Pearl-daughter & Schneider, 1980). Older women experience longer periods of unemployment than their younger counterparts. In 1980, the average period of unemployment for women aged 20 to 34 was 10.1 weeks, whereas for women aged 35 to 54, it was 13.2 weeks (U.S. Department of Labor, Bureau of Labor Statistics, 1981, Table 18).

Women who join, or remain in the labor force suffer economic loss from sex-based wage disparity across the life span, but the disparity increases with age. Women over the age of 45 who are employed full-time earn even less than younger women, relative to the earnings of men. According to a 1987 census report, women between the ages of 21 and 29 earned 83 cents to every dollar earned by males of the same age group (U.S. Bureau of the Census, 1987, p. 3). Every age cohort thereafter shows a decline for females, until the disparity widens for the age group 45 to 64 years old to a point where women earn 60 cents to every dollar earned by their male counterparts (U.S. Bureau of the Census, 1987a, p. 3).

AGE DISCRIMINATION IN EMPLOYMENT

If we heed the conclusions of the several studies recently assembled by Sandell (1987), no discussion of employment discrimination and older women would be necessary. Although Sandell notes that employment problems are exacerbated by present or past discrimination, he minimizes the consequences of the economic dislocation of older women:

> The pattern of declining rates and rising duration of unemployment applies to all groups, but it is most pronounced among white men. Women are more likely than men to drop out of the labor force when they lose a job, and the duration of their unemployment is less on average. For blacks and other minority groups the pattern holds, but always at higher levels of unemployment. This implies that the labor market problems of some members of minority groups are *reduced* . . . by age and experience. (Sandell, 1987, p. 9, emphasis added)

The notion that earnings are tied to factors such as experience or education (human capital theory), job crowding, or worker preferences are explanations that are commonly used to argue against discrimination as the cause of the male-female earnings differential (Stromberg & Harkess, 1978). Theories that overlook the effects of discrimination ignore the persistence of wage disparities that persist even when factors such as experience, education, and skill level are taken into account.

A frequently cited reason for the wage gap between males and females is the fact that women experience more interruptions of their work careers than do their male counterparts (Baruch, Barnett, & Rivers, 1983). The overwhelming reason for these interruptions is "family responsibilities." Of full-time workers, aged 21 to 64, 42% of females experienced a period of six months or longer without a job, whereas only 12% of full-time male workers experienced a similar interruption. For female workers, aged 45 to 64, the percentages climb to 65.5, while it hovers at 12.5 for males in the same cohort (U.S. Bureau of the Census, 1987, p. 2).

The issue of work interruptions can be expected to become more problematic as increasing numbers of middle-aged women take on caregiving roles for elderly parents. This phenomenon, known as the "dependency squeeze," describes the dilemma faced by older women who must juggle work and caregiving responsibilities, or who are forced to leave the labor market to assume this role (Gibeau & Anastas, 1987; Older Women's League, 1984).

Although it is true that women experience more work interruptions than men, what role does this factor play in explaining the earnings gap? In comparing hourly earnings of full-time workers who have experienced any work interruptions with those who have not, the wage gap not only persists, but widens with age. For full-time workers *with* work interruptions between the ages of 21 and 29 years old, the males earn $6.95 per hour, and females earn $5.56. For workers 45 to 64 years old, the earnings for males and females are $9.90 and $7.52 per hour, respectively. For workers with *no* work interruptions the gap persists as male workers aged 21 to 29 earn $8.23 per hour to their female counterpart's $6.96. In the 45- to 64-years-old cohort, males earn $12.78 per hour, whereas females earn $7.98 (U.S. Bureau of Census, 1987, p. 17).

In a recent analysis of sex-based earning differentials, the U.S. Bureau of the Census (1987) constructed a model that would take into account a variety of factors commonly used to explain earnings differentials, including job interruptions and the gender composition of the job. The findings of this study demonstrated that 65.5% of the variance in the earnings gap could be explained by the characteristics typically associated with human capital and other wage theories. A residual of 34.5% (for workers who were college graduates) was unaccounted for and may be attributable to discrimination. For high school graduates, the residual rose to 39.9% and for workers without a high school diploma the residual was over 40% (U.S. Bureau of the Census, 1987, Table K, p. 10.).

LEGAL PROTECTIONS

Although there is some evidence that age discrimination against women can begin in the late 20s (Older Women's League, 1982), the federal age discrimination statute protects persons age 40 to 70. Sex-based employment discrimination is barred by Title VII of The Civil Rights Act of 1964, which outlaws employment discrimination based on race, religion, sex, and national origin. To combat widespread age discrimination in employment, Congress passed the Age Discrimination in Employment Act (ADEA) in 1967. Both statutes are now enforced by the Equal Employment Opportunity Commission (EEOC).

Title VII and the ADEA share some common limitations. Both share developmental histories that reflect short-sighted understanding of the depth of the discrimination they intended to obviate. One of these areas is in the characterizations of the scope of the problem. In its consideration of the ADEA, Congress operated on the naive notion that age discrimination in employment was due to lack of information rather than malicious intent (Biek, 1986).

The EEOC has come under fire recently for mishandling more than 900 age-discrimination complaints filed in the past few years. The statute of limitations ran out on these cases before the agency took any action. Its stance on issues such as early retirement and employee waivers has forced several interest groups to appeal to the courts and Congress for assistance. Congress recently suspended an EEOC rule that attempted to legalize waivers of age discrimination rights executed without the EEOC's involvement. Employers had been asking workers to sign these waivers to prevent age discrimination suits upon termination or early retirement.

More recently, the Internal Revenue Service (IRS) intervened to override the EEOC's narrow interpretation of a law regulating how many years of service should be taken into account in determining retirement benefits in "defined-benefit" employee plans. Although the law seemed to require that a retiring employee receive credit for *all* years of work, the EEOC refused to interpret the law to include all years of service. The IRS ruling insures that 300,000 older workers will now receive some $3 billion in pension benefits, and it raises serious questions about the motives of the EEOC (Pressman, 1988).

AGE AND SEX DISCRIMINATION

In an analysis of charge data from 1980 to 1984, conducted by its Office of Program Research, the EEOC found that discrimination charges have dramatically increased (U.S. Equal Employment Opportunity Commission, EEOC, 1985). While in Fiscal Year 1980, 7.2% of all bases for charges were cited as age, by 1984 age discrimination complaints had increased to 17%, and represented the third most frequently cited basis of charges.

More men file age discrimination claims than do women (McConnell, 1983), and one study (Schuster, 1982) notes that the greatest amount of litigation activity involves men between the ages of 50 and 59 who are drawn from professional and managerial occupations. Termination of employment was the most frequent cause of the lawsuit, and the employer won in two out of three cases.

These findings are being cited as evidence that age discrimination in employment may be more of a problem for men than it is for women (Shaw & Shaw, 1987). The fact that the modal category for discrimination complaints is men aged 50 to 59 has led to charges that the Age Discrimination in Employment Act is a "white man's refuge" (Older Women's League, 1982). But is this assertion accurate? As the data in Table 4 demonstrate, a reanalysis of charge data controlling for the number of men and women in the labor force *for each age category* shows that although the number of claims per se is higher for men than for women, it is not disproportionately so.

Table 4

EEOC Age Discrimination Complaints

Percentaged by Age Group and Labor Force Participation

1981

Age	Men		Women	
	Complaints	Labor Force	Complaints	Labor Force
40-44	59.0%	59.2%	41.0%	40.8%
45-49	60.7%	60.2%	39.3%	39.8%
50-54	60.7%	61.2%	39.3%	38.8%
55-59	65.0%	60.7%	35.0%	39.3%
60-64	70.1%	59.9%	29.9%	40.1%
65-69	69.1%	62.9%	30.9%	37.1%
70+	65.0%	60.2%	35.0%	39.8%
Totals	5,797	11,058	3,302	7,253

Note. Labor Force Participation is in thousands

Source: (McConnell, 1978, p. 167); Census (1983).

When the number of complaints is adjusted by the distribution of men and women in the labor force, the proportion of claims filed by men and women is comparable to their distribution in the workforce for the 40 to 44 age category. For ages 45 to 49, the number of complaints filed by women slightly exceeds what would be expected given their numbers in the labor force. It is the upper age categories in which men have higher complaint rates than women (U.S. Bureau of the Census, 1983).

Age discrimination complaint patterns are different for men than for women and may reflect the fact that age discrimination affects older workers differently based on their sex, both in terms of the reason for discrimination and the age range during which it occurs.

Shuster and Miller (1984) found that women are most likely to file complaints on account of hiring, promotion, wages, and fringe benefits. Men more frequently file on account of termination and involuntary retirement. These findings support the conclusion of the Older Women's League that "older men and older women are not in the same boat when it comes to age discrimination" (Older Women's League, 1982, p. 5).

Not only is the basis of discrimination different for men than for women, but women experience discrimination at a younger age (Older Women's League, 1982; Pearldaughter & Schneider, 1980), as the complaint pattern suggests. Age discrimination against older women is more insidious than that which men experience, because it is based on standards of "youthful appearance," which are very difficult to uncover (Buchman, 1985).

The "double standard of aging" describes society's different attitudes and treatment of older people, based on their sex. Women are viewed as becoming older at an earlier age than men (Sommers, 1981; Sontag, 1979). In a youth-oriented society, the phenomenon of age discrimination in employment is not surprising. The additional emphasis on sexual attractiveness, and the narrow definition for women of what constitutes sexual attractiveness, increases the vulnerability of older women who seek to secure and to hold on to employment.

In addition to appearance-related discrimination, which puts women at a special disadvantage, negative stereotypes are associated with the biological changes middle-aged women experience (Barnett & Baruch, 1978; Berun, 1983). Despite evidence to the contrary, many myths surrounding the productive potential of older workers persist. Research on cognitive performance, which includes problem-solving tasks, learning performance, and thought processes, indicates that older people perform at about the same or better levels as younger people. Myths about physical decline are unfounded and should also be dismissed (Mowsesian, 1986).

THE DUAL BURDEN OF SEX AND AGE

One barrier to an effective legal strategy for discrimination against older women is the fact that relief is available under two separate statutes, Title VII of the Civil Rights Act of 1964, and the

Age Discrimination in Employment Act (ADEA), passed in 1967. These statutes contain significantly different provisions related to jury trials, forms of damages, guidelines regulating class actions, and statutes of limitation.

The combination of procedural hurdles, proof problems, stated exceptions, and lack of enforcement powers has reduced the potential of Title VII to ameliorate women's secondary employment status (Nuccio, 1987; Pearldaughter & Schneider, 1980). Of all complaints filed under the ADEA, 60% fail to pass on the basis of procedural errors alone (Older Women's League, 1982, p. 12).

The interaction of sex and age places older women in a special category, a "subclass" that falls through the cracks created by coverage provided by two distinct statutes. The problems created by this division are illustrated by the following scenario, as described by the Older Women's League:

> A 55 year old female job applicant may not have been rejected only because she's a woman, or only because she's too old. Chances are good that it's because she's both older and female: an older woman. She belongs to a discriminated against sub-class which can too often fall through the cracks of the discrimination statutes. For example, she applies to bank after bank for an entry-level position, and is turned away by bank after bank. If she complains to the EEOC on the basis of sex discrimination, the banks may successfully defend by a showing of an abundance of female employees (tellers and clerks under thirty). If she charges discrimination, the defendant will point to a similar abundance of employees over age 40 (the management males). It is a fact that many employers can actively (although not openly) pursue a policy of discrimination against older women, yet escape the sting of the law. (Older Women's League, 1982, p. 12)

The creation of a subclass that would address the special employment discrimination of older women is not a new concept. It has been developed to cover the special circumstances created by the interaction of race and sex. In *Jefferies v. Harris County Community Action Association*, 615 F.2d 1025 (5th Cir. 1980), the plaintiff, a black woman, filed a complaint after failing to be promoted.

The successful candidate for the position was a black male, a fact that led a lower court to rule that race discrimination was not a factor in the employer's decision. Since the organization was predominantly female, there was allegedly no sex discrimination.

On appeal, a higher court reversed the lower court and required the employer to show adequate numbers of black women, not just women (white), or blacks (male). The court wrote that "discrimination against black females can exist even in the absence of discrimination against black men or white women" (615 F. 2d 1025, at 1032).

This rule recognizes that the interaction of race and sex must be extended to older women, so that the interaction of age and sex can be addressed. The development of a sex/age subclass would facilitate crossover suits between Title VII and the ADEA (Buchman, 1985; Older Women's League, 1982).

In summary, the interaction of age and gender in the workplace has serious economic consequences for women. The problem of pay equity, germane across the career span, is exacerbated by discrimination that takes several forms. Older women who are new or recent entrants into the labor force may be penalized for lacking experience, whereas other midlife women who have been in the workforce for some time may be excluded from consideration because they are "overqualified." Middle-aged women cannot expect the earnings curve that men experience, which peaks during their mid-40s, but rather expect earnings that remain relatively static, and peak around age 30 (Pearldaughter & Schneider, 1980). Age and sex discrimination reach beyond the job site and have implications for retirement years, both in social security and pension issues.

RETIREMENT AND PENSIONS

Nowhere is the economic disadvantage of older women more apparent than in the retirement years. Despite gains in the annual cash income of the elderly made over the past generation, income inadequacy remains great and is a more serious problem for women, especially minority women, as Table 5 indicates (Rathbone-McCuan, 1985).

Older women anticipating retirement confront several grim eco-

Table 5

Incidence of Poverty Among Women

Age 55 and Older, by Race, 1981

Percentage of Older Women with
Income Below Poverty Line

	Age 55-64	Age 65 and Older
Females	12.1	18.6
White Females	9.9	16.2
Black Females	33.7	43.5
Hispanic Females	21.2	27.4

Source: U. S. Bureau of the Census. (1981). "Money Income and Poverty Status of Families and Persons in the United States: 1981," Current Population Reports, Series P-60, No. 134.

nomic realities. The sex-segregated labor market, in which women are concentrated into a limited number of occupations and in which their work is undervalued and underpaid, makes it unlikely that most women will be able to amass the capital necessary to support themselves upon retirement (Wolf, 1986). Women who rely on social security retirement find that here, too, the sex-segregated labor market takes its economic toll. Benefit levels that are tied to lifetime earnings result in depressed payment levels for women. In 1987, for example, the average monthly payment was $550 for men and $420 for women (U.S. Department of Health and Human Services, Social Security, 1987, p. II).

When Old Age, Survivor's, and Disability Insurance (OASDI)

was first developed in 1935, and was solely a retirement program, it was sex-neutral. As programs were added, particularly survivor's benefits, this picture changed with preferential treatment going to men in some cases (as was the case with special age-72 benefits) and to women in others (as with survivor benefits). Over the past 50 years, Congress and the courts have intervened to correct many of these suspect policies. Legislation in 1983 removed the last of these inequities (Myers, 1985).

Predictably, the only area where average social security payments for women exceed those for men is in the area of survivor's benefits, a place where benefit levels are more reflective of male earnings. The effects of historical patterns of pay inequity can be staggering for older women, as this testimony from a 1973 hearing on the economic problems of women indicates:

> A woman . . . went down to apply for her social security. She had worked 34 years . . . her husband had died in 1939. He had paid in the social security for 27 months. Under *his* entitlement she got more money than she did under hers after 34 years in the labor force [emphasis added]. (U.S. Joint Committee, 1973, pp. 39-40)

Inequities in pay and benefits have a cumulative, life-time effect in the area of pensions. Prior to the passage of the Pension Reform Act of 1984, pension programs were not required to vest anyone under the age of 25, so that a woman received no credit for employment between the ages of 21 and 25, with the following result:

> In practice, a woman could work for a firm from age 21 to 26; leave for a couple of years to raise a family, and return to work with no vested pension rights whatever. Coupled with lower pay for women overall and the fact that spacing a family may require repeating this pattern, it is easy to see why women's earned pensions are virtually half those of men. (U.S. Senate Finance Committee, 1983, p. 1)

Historically wives have been victimized by pension provisions that eliminated their entitlements to contributions made by their husbands if they died, even within hours of meeting the eligibility age. Divorce or separation could also jeopardize a wife's entitlement (U.S. House of Representatives, Ways and Means Committee, 1983).

In 1984 Congress passed the Retirement Equity Act, which adjusted the Retirement Income Security Act of 1974 in the following ways: It lowered from 25 to 21 the general minimum age for pension plan participation; required credit toward pensions for employee absences due to pregnancy, childbirth, adoption, or newborn care; and required the written consent of a pension plan participant's spouse for any waiver of survivor benefits (Congressional Information Service, 1984).

Even with these reforms, there is need for continuing attention to income security for older women. Many women are at work in occupations that do not provide for pension plans. In 1982, for example, nearly 40% of older men but only 19% of older women had some income from pensions and/or annuities (Heen, 1986).

An additional problem concerns that fact that many annuity program benefits are calculated on sex-based mortality tables. A recent court decision in *Arizona v. Norris* (1983) prohibits the use of sex-based actuarial tables to calculate sex-differentiated employee retirement benefits (Heen, 1985). The problem hers is that the decision in *Norris* affects only employer-sponsored plans, leaving many women who may purchase annuities or insurance plans on the open market subject to lower benefits.

There is considerable work to be done both in terms of the numbers of women who are covered by annuity programs and of the extension of the protections of *Norris* to private plans. Congress has yet to act on these proposals.

CONCLUSION

In a patriarchal society that values youth, women are at special jeopardy as they age. A sex-segregated labor market in which women are concentrated in a few occupations, where the work performed is undervalued and underpaid, is responsible for wage disparities that widen as women age.

The double standard of aging defines women as old at an earlier age than men and has led to speculation that discrimination in employment may be a problem for women at ages younger than 40 years old, the age established by Congress as the lower limit for discrimination protection.

Age and gender interact to create a subclass of workers, that is, older women who are unprotected by current antidiscrimination laws. The conceptual foundation of employment opportunity policies must be reexamined in light of evidence that men and women experience different types of discrimination at different times in their careers.

The effects of sexism and ageism in the labor force interact in a cumulative way to increase the economic vulnerability of older women. Social insurance and assistance programs as well as private pension programs have serious equity and adequacy deficits. Notwithstanding legislative and judicial reforms, pension programs can still provide benefits calculated on sex-based actuarial tables, resulting in lower benefits for women, who are already on the lower rung of the economic ladder offered by OASDI and SSI.

The baby boomers are already working under the protection of the ADEA, and research efforts must become more discerning in identifying how the employment and retirement concerns of men and women differ. Studies on "the aging worker" must acknowledge that older women are a substantial part of the workforce, and our numbers will only increase.

The legislative field is ripe for intervention by coalitions of women's and older women's groups to insure pay equity reform, continued pension reform, and recognition of the special needs of the older woman worker.

Given these circumstances, legal protections against discrimination in employment on account of sex and age are of critical importance to older women. Yet studies in this area overlook the concerns of women workers, and more research is needed to assess adequacy of legal remedies that have been developed by the EEOC.

REFERENCES

Barnett, R. C., & Baruch, G. K. (1978). *The competent woman: Perspectives on development*. New York: Irvington.

Baruch, G., Barnett, R., & Rivers, C. (1983). *Lifeprints: New patterns of love and work for today's woman*. New York: McGraw-Hill.

Bergman, B. R. (1986). *The economic emergence of women*. New York: Basic Books.

Berun, C. S. (1983). Changing appearance for women in the middle years of life: Trauma? In E. Markson (Ed.), *Older women* (pp. 11-36). Lexington, MA: Lexington Books.

Biek, D. L. (1986). The scourge of discrimination in the workplace: Fighting back with a liberalized class action vehicle and notice provision. *Case Western Reserve Law Review, 37*, 103-147.

Buchman, P. (1985). Title VII limits on discrimination against television anchorwomen on the basis of age-related appearance. *Columbia Law review, 85*, 190-215.

Children's Defense Fund. (1987). *A children's budget, FY1987*. Washington, DC: Author.

Congressional Information Service. (1984). *Legislative histories*. Washington, DC: Congressional Quarterly.

Congressional Quarterly. (1981). *The women's movement: Agenda for the '80s*. Washington, DC: Author.

Daniel, R. L. (1987). *American women in the 20th century: The festival of life*. San Diego: Harcourt Brace Jovanovich.

Dex, S., & Shaw, L. B. (1986). *British and American women at work: Do equal opportunities policies matter?* London: Macmillan.

Foner, P. S. (1982). *Women and the American labor movement*. New York: Free Press.

Fox, M. F., & Hesse-Biber, S. (1984). *Women at work*. Palo Alto, CA: Mayfield.

Gibeau, J. L., & Anastas, J. W. (1987, November). *Breadwinners and caregivers: Interviews with working women*. Paper presented at the Annual Scientific Meeting of the Gerontological Society of America, Washington, DC.

Hartmann, S. M. (1982). *The home front and beyond: American women in the 1940s*. Boston: Twayne.

Heen, M. L. (1985). Sex discrimination in pensions and retirement annuity plans after *Arizona Governing Committee v. Norris:* Recognizing and remedying employer non-compliance. *Women's Rights Law Reporter, 8*, 155-176.

Heen, M. L. (1986). Sex discrimination, mortality tables, and pensions: Improving the economic status of older women. *Women & Health, 11*, 119-131.

Hewlett, S. A. (1986). *A lesser life*. New York: Morrow.

Jefferies v. Harris County Community Action Association, 615 F.2d 1025 (5th Cir. 1980).

Marshall, R., & Paulin, B. (1987). Employment and earnings of women: Historical perspective. In K. S. Koziara, M. H. Moskow, & L. D. Tanner (Eds.), *Working women: Past, present, future* (pp. 1-36). Washington, DC: Bureau of National Affairs.

McConnell, S. R. (1983). Age discrimination in employment. In H. S. Parnes (Ed.), *Policy issues in work and retirement* (pp. 159-196). Kalamazoo, MI: W. E. Upjohn Institute For Employment Research.

Mowsesian, R. (1986). *Rusted realities: Work and aging in America*. Far Hills, NJ: New Horizon Press.

Myers, R. J. (1985). *Social security* (3rd ed.). Homewood, IL: Irwin.

Nestel, G., Mercier, J., & Shaw, L. B. (1983). Economic consequences of midlife change in marital status. In L. B. Shaw (Ed.), *Unplanned careers: The working lives of middle-aged women* (pp. 109-125). Lexington, MA: Lexington Books.

Nuccio, K. E. (1987). *The Equal Employment Opportunity Commission, 1964-1984: A cycle model analysis.* Unpublished doctoral dissertation, Bryn Mawr College, Bryn Mawr, PA.

Older Women's League. (1982). *Gray Paper No. 8: Not even for dogcatcher.* Washington, DC: Author.

Older Women's League. (1984). Statement of the Older Women's League on Older Women in the Labor Force, Before the Joint Economic Committee.

Pearce, D. (1978). The feminization of poverty: Women, work, and welfare. *Urban and Social Change Review, 11,* 28-36.

Pearldaughter, A. M., & Schneider, V. (1980). Women and welfare: The cycle of female poverty. *Golden Gate University Law Review, 10,* 1043-1086.

Peters, E. (1986). Factors affecting remarriage. In L. B. Shaw (Ed.), *Midlife women at work: A fifteen-year perspective* (pp. 99-114). Lexington, MA: Lexington Books.

Pressman, S. (1988, April). IRS overrules EEOC in $3 billion controversy over pension credits. *AARP News Bulletin, 29*(4), 1, 13.

Rathbone-McCuan, E. (1985). Health needs and social policy. *Women & Health, 10,* 17-27.

Russell, C. (1987). Aging as a feminist issue. *Women's Studies International Forum, 10,* 125-132.

Sandell, S. H. (Ed.). (1987). *The problem isn't age: Work and older Americans.* New York: Praeger.

Schuster, M. (1982). Analyzing age discrimination act cases: Development of a methodology. *Law and Policy Quarterly, 3,* 339-351.

Shaw, L. B. (1986). Looking toward retirement: Plans and prospects. In L. B. Shaw (Ed.), *Midlife women at work: A fifteen-year perspective* (pp. 115-134). Lexington, MA: Lexington Books.

Shaw, L. B., & Shaw, R. (1987). From midlife to retirement: The middle-aged woman worker. In K. S. Koziara, M. H. Moskow, & L. D. Tanner (Eds.), *Working women: Past, present, future* (pp. 200-331). Washington, DC: Bureau of National Affairs.

Shuster, M., & Miller, C. S. (1984). An empirical assessment of the age discrimination in employment act. *Industrial and Labor Relations Review, 38,* 64-74.

Sidel, R. (1986). *Women and children last.* New York: Viking Penguin.

Sommers, T. (1981). Women and aging: More on the double standard. In M. A. Suseelan (Ed.), *Resource Book on Aging* (pp. 31-34). New York: United Church Board.

Sontag, S. (1979). The double standard of ageing. In V. Carver & P. Liddiard (Eds.), *Ageing population: A reader and source book* (pp. 72-80). New York: Holmes & Neier.

Stromberg, A. H. & Harkess, S. (Ed.). (1978). *Women working: Theories and facts in perspective.* Palo Alto, CA: Mayfield.

U.S. Bureau of the Census. (1983). *Census of population and housing, 1980: Public-use microdata sample C*. Washington, DC: Bureau of the Census.

U.S. Bureau of the Census. (1987). Male-female differences in work experience, occupation, and earnings: 1984: *Current Population Reports* Series P-70, No. 10). Washington, DC: U.S. Government Printing Office.

U.S. Bureau of the Census. (1987). *Statistical abstracts of the United States: 1987* (107th ed.). Washington, DC: U.S. Government Printing Office.

U.S. Department of Health and Human Services, Social Security Administration. (1987). *Social Security bulletin, annual statistical supplement, 1987*. Washington, DC: U.S. Government Printing Office.

U.S. Department of Labor, Bureau of Labor Statistics. (1981). *Employment and unemployment: A report on 1980*. Washington, DC: U.S. Government Printing Office.

U.S. Department of Labor, Women's Bureau. (1957). *Spotlight on women in the United States, 1956-57*. Washington, DC: U.S. Government Printing Office.

U.S. Equal Employment Opportunity Commission. (1985). *Charge Trend Data (1980-1984)* (Report No. 85-102). Washington, DC: EEOC Office of Program Research.

U.S. House of Representatives Ways and Means Committee. (1983). *Economic Equity Act and Related Tax and Pension Reform Hearings*. 98th Congress, 1st Session, October 25, 1983. Washington, DC: U.S. Government Printing Office.

U.S. Joint Committee. (1973). *Hearings on economic problems of women*. 93rd Congress, 1st Session. Washington, DC: U.S. Government Printing Office.

U.S. Senate Finance Committee. (1983). *Potential inequities affecting women, part 2 of 3 hearings, June 21, 1983*. Washington, DC: U.S. Government Printing Office.

Voydanoff, P. (Ed.). (1984). *Work & family: Changing roles of men and women*. Palo Alto, CA: Mayfield.

Wolf, W. A. (1986). Sex-discrimination in pension plans: The problem of incomplete relief. *Harvard Women's Law Journal, 9*, 83-103.

Women and Aging: Issues of Adequacy and Equity

June Axinn, PhD

There is a new "conventional wisdom" being established in the United States. Where once the elderly had been seen as a deprived group, many now argue that they are economically and politically privileged. Economists, political scientists, sociologists, and general observers of the social scene have pointed out the income changes of the group and contrasted their improved economic situation with the deteriorating position of children in our society. The new aged are politically strong and children are weak. Thus, there has been an emphasis in social policy on income transfers to the old and on neglect of the young (Axinn & Stern, 1985; Kutza, 1981; Preston, 1984; Rochefort, 1985; Schulz, 1985).

True—but false. There is a real sense in which the relative economic situation of the elderly has improved in the past 25 years; their poverty rate at 12% in 1986 was below that of the total population (14%; U.S. Bureau of the Census, 1987a). On the other hand, that of some groups, particularly children, has worsened. Burt and Pittman (1985) in their study of the social welfare policy of the Reagan administration put the matter this way:

> The economic situation of the elderly has improved dramatically in the past two decades and has continued to improve

---

June Axinn is Professor of Social Welfare, School of Social Work, University of Pennsylvania, 3701 Locust Walk, Philadelphia, PA 19107-6214.

339

during the Reagan administration. As late as the 1960s, poverty among older Americans was seen as a very serious concern. Data . . . showed that 6 million elderly . . . had inadequate income. Between 1960 and 1970 this number decreased to 5.7 million; the 1980s have seen it drop to under 4.0 million. Given that the number of persons over age sixty-five has increased 54 percent from 16.6 million in 1960 to 25.6 million in 1980, this decline in the number of elderly living below poverty is impressive. (p. 117)

But all older people have not benefited from economic conditions or from the government policies of the past two decades. Furthermore, many of the elderly, although removed from the poverty group, are still very much at risk. Although only 12% are below the poverty line, 21% are at 125% of the poverty line, just on the edge of poverty; 18% of the total population are counted as "near poor." By this measure, the aging are hardly in a preferred position (U.S. Bureau of the Census, 1987a).

As Burt and Pittman go on to point out, some of the low-income elderly did not share fully in the eased circumstances of their demographic peers. Unrelated individuals, minorities, and in particular women, still suffer unusually high risks of poverty. Furthermore, although the poverty rate for the aged went down, the increased number of older people in the country did not mean that there were fewer poor aged — that depends on the base year you select. Indeed, from 1975 to 1986 the number of older Americans who were poor actually rose 5%; for women it rose 8%.

This article will undertake the following two tasks: (1) It will probe the basis of the improved economic condition of the aging in general and examine the reasons so many women have been left out and (2) it will explore the issue of "affordability." Are we really engaged in intergenerational conflict? Have the number of aged grown so rapidly that we need be concerned about our ability to support all of the dependent populations in society? Can we support older women with minimal adequacy only at the risk of neglect of other groups, or is it possible to be more sanguine about our fiscal future?

THE INCREASED WELL-BEING OF THE AGING

The increased well-being of the aging results from two factors: an improved economy with higher incomes for all and conscious government policy. By 1985, nearly half of all federal domestic spending was on behalf of the aging, the result of a number of program expansions and program innovations.

The Older Americans Act of 1965 helped to provide needed nutrition, transportation, and a comprehensive range of social services. That same year Medicare instituted a national health insurance system to assist the aged with their medical costs. Food stamps, subsidized public housing, Medicaid, and low-income energy allowance programs, further contributed to the economic welfare of the poor, certainly to the aging poor. A host of difficulties arise when calculating the value of these noncash benefits as income substitutes, but it is clear that they reduce the deprivation and severity of economic need for their recipients (Axinn, 1986; U.S. Bureau of the Census, 1986b). Despite the cutbacks of the 1980s in these programs, increased access to health care and improved housing and nutrition have meant reduced mortality rates within older age groups; 34% of all public or subsidized housing, 28% of Medicaid benefits, and 16% of all food stamps go to aging households (U.S. Bureau of the Census, 1987b).

The Social Security Act Amendments of the late 1960s and the 1970s made a major impact on cash income. The five years between 1967 and 1972 were a period of major expansion of cash entitlements. Coverage and benefits both increased in response to a new visibility of poverty among the elderly who had suffered relatively severe inflation losses. Benefit rates rose 58% in that period; Social Security grew from less than 0.05% of the Gross National Product in 1940 to 5.5% in 1973 (Derthick, 1979, pp. 339-368; Rochefort, 1985, pp. 57-98).

In 1972, social insurance benefits were indexed to the cost of living, so that future protection against inflation was insured. Expansion of the program has continued, although at a slower pace. By the early 1980s, over 90% of the aging were getting social security payments, and average benefits were much improved.

Supplemental Security Income — a federalized public assistance program for the poor aged — was introduced in 1972, and by 1975 it too had inflation-proof benefits. But federal benefits have been set at about 75% of the poverty level, virtually guaranteeing an anti-poverty measure with limited effectiveness. In social insurance, on the other hand, the average worker or widow in 1970 received benefits at 76% of the poverty line; by 1981 they were above the poverty line (Burt & Pittman, 1985, pp. 128-133). A major part of the increase in federal social welfare expenditures is for the social security system. Transfer payments to the aging were of most help to those who could benefit from this work-related program.

Poverty, Race, and Gender

Table 1 tells us an important part of the "poverty story." In 1959, the first year for which we have official data, more than one-third of the elderly were poor, compared to one-fifth of the population generally. Men and women both suffered severe deprivation: 36% of all women over 65 and 35% of all men over 65 had incomes below the poverty level.

Ten years later poverty had started to decrease. But the decrease, especially for women, was very slow. By 1970, 29% of older women were poor, and 19% of men. Meanwhile poverty rates for the country as a whole were down to 13%. The next five years saw dramatic changes. The incidence of poverty for older men fell below that of the country (11% compared to 12%), whereas women's poverty risk dropped to 18%. By 1986, the poverty rate for men was down to 9%. The rate for women — at 15% — remained above average and much higher than the poverty risk for men.

Table 2 adds the dimensions of race and ethnicity to the structure of poverty. Hispanics suffer incidence rates more than twice as high as that of whites; blacks almost three times — 31.3% compared with 10.7% in 1986. Over one-fourth of all Hispanic women and one-third of all black women of age 65 or more are poor by official standards.

Table 1

POVERTY RATES, BY GENDER, 1959 to 1986, SELECTED YEARS
(Rates as of March of the Following Year)

Year	ALL 65 AND OVER Poverty Rate	FEMALE 65 AND OVER Poverty Rate	MALE 65 AND OVER Poverty Rate
1959	35.2%	35.6%	34.7%
1970	24.6	28.6	19.2
1975	15.3	18.1	11.4
1980	15.7	19.1	10.9
1981	15.3	18.6	10.5
1982	14.6	17.5	10.4
1983	13.8	16.4	10.0
1984	12.4	15.0	8.7
1985	12.6	15.6	8.5
1986	12.4	15.2	8.5

Source: U.S. Bureau of the Census, Current Population Reports, Series P-60, Characteristics of the Population Below the Poverty Level, U.S.G.P.O., Washington, D.C., selected years.

Table 2

POVERTY RATES, BY RACE AND ETHNICITY, PERSONS 65 AND OVER
(Selected years. Rates as of March of the following years)

Year	FEMALE			MALE		
	HISPANIC	BLACK	WHITE	HISPANIC	BLACK	WHITE
1970	N.A.	52.5%	26.5%	N.A.	41.2%	17.1%
1975	36.0%	40.2	16.1	28.2%	31.0	9.5
1980	34.3	42.6	16.8	27.0	31.4	9.0
1981	27.4	43.5	16.2	23.6	32.2	8.5
1982	31.3	42.4	15.1	19.6	31.7	8.3
1983	22.9	41.2	14.1	21.4	28.4	8.2
1984	22.1	35.5	13.1	20.7	26.0	7.2
1985	27.4	34.8	13.8	19.1	26.6	6.5
1986	25.2	35.5	13.3	18.8	24.2	6.9

Source: U.S. Bureau of the Census, Current Population Reports, Series P-60, No. 152, Characteristics of the Population Below the Poverty Level, Washington, D.C., Government Printing Office, selected years.

Poverty, Age, and Family Status

Table 3 details the relationship between age and poverty. Women receive full social security benefits at 62, men at age 65. Poverty rates are slightly higher before the receipt of social security for each sex than after. Poverty decreases at retirement age but then starts upward. After 65, the older you are, the higher the risk of being poor. At age 62, 12% of all women are poor; by age 72 the incidence of poverty has risen to 18%. The same structure holds for men but at a lower level; 7% at age 65 and 11% at 72 are poor.

The tie between family structure and poverty is well recognized. Those living in families have sharply lower poverty rates than those living alone. And those who are married with a spouse present are much less likely to be poor than widows or widowers.

The overall poverty rate for older women depends on two things: the poverty risk for each subgroup of women (incidence) and the number of women in that group (composition). Not only is the incidence of poverty among those 72 and over higher for women than for men but the composition of the group is different: 41% of women but only 34% of men are in this category. And most men of age 72 live with their families while most women live alone. In terms of marital status, over three-fourths of all older men are married with a spouse present, a low-risk group; that situation is true for less than half of all older women. In virtually every instance, the risk of poverty is greater for women than for men in similar life situations. In addition, a higher percentage of women than men are in the most precarious categories.

Poverty and Source of Income

As Table 3 makes clear, the lowest poverty risk by far is for that small group of women whose support comes from both work and other income such as private pensions, interest, or dividends. The next lowest rate is for women who receive both social security and other income: either second pensions (private or government employee) or income from private assets. In contrast, the group most at risk are those who rely on public assistance — SSI — for their sole support. They have an incidence of poverty of 56%.

The same structure essentially holds for men as for women. For

Table 3

POVERTY CHARACTERISTICS, PERSONS 60 AND OVER, 1984
(Numbers in Thousands. Persons as of March 1985)

Family Status	FEMALE		MALE	
	% of Older Women	Poverty Rate	% of Older Men	Poverty Rate
Total, 60 +	100.0%	14.3%	100.0%	8.8%
In Families	61.9	7.3	83.7	6.6
Unrelated Ind.	38.0	25.8	16.2	21.3
60-61	11.1	13.0	12.3	8.5
In Families	8.6	8.2	10.7	6.8
Unrelated Ind.	2.4	29.5	1.6	19.8
62-64	15.8	12.2	18.6	9.2
In Families	11.8	7.2	16.1	7.0
Unrelated Ind.	3.9	27.9	2.5	22.7
65-71	32.2	11.8	34.8	6.9
In Families	21.4	6.6	30.0	5.3
Unrelated Ind.	10.9	22.2	4.9	16.6
72 +	40.9	17.5	34.3	10.6
In Families	20.1	7.9	27.0	7.0
Unrelated Ind.	20.8	26.8	7.3	23.6

Marital Status	Total	% of Poor Older Women	Total	% of Poor Older Men
Total	100.0%	14.3%	100.0%	8.8%
Single	4.7	17.1	5.3	18.7
Married, Spouse Present	45.1	5.8	77.1	6.2
Married, Spouse Absent	1.8	36.3	2.3	22.4
Widowed	43.1	20.9	11.1	15.5
Divorced	5.3	23.4	4.2	18.7

Source of Income		% of Poor Older Women		% of Poor Older Men
Earnings Only	1.5%	9.9%	3.8%	9.7%
Unearned Income Only	88.8	16.1	64.2	11.0
Earnings & Other	4.3	3.8	31.1	2.7
No Income	5.4	27.5	0.9	56.1
Soc. Sec. Only	30.6	29.9	8.4	28.0
S.S.I. Only	6.0	55.6	0.7	59.6
Soc. Sec. & Non-public Transfers*	26.3	7.6	46.7	4.5
Soc. Sec. & Transfers**	2.2	25.4	1.4	8.3

*   Includes dividends, interest, rent, private pensions, government employee pensions, alimony and annuity income.

** Includes public assistance, unemployment compensation, workmen's compensation, and veterans payments.

Source: Derived from U.S. Department of the Census. Current Population Reports, Series P-60, No. 152, Characteristics of the Population Below the Poverty Level: 1984, U.S.G.P.O., Washington, D.C., 1986.

the most part, the lowest poverty rates are for those who have a good income source in addition to current earnings or social security. For men as for women, reliance on public assistance (SSI) alone means poverty for almost 60% of those in this group.

Again, the composition of the aging population, more than the differential incidence of poverty rates of subgroups of the older population, explains a significant part of the difference between the overall poverty rates for women and men. Only 4% of women over age 60 have money both from work and a second pension or other private source of income; in contrast, 31% of men are in this well-situated group. Looking at the next-best group, those receiving social security in addition to another pension or private source of income, we find 26% of women are in this group, and 47% of men. On the other hand, 6% of women and less than 1% of men are in the poorest group—those receiving just SSI as income. Of women, 31% depend on social security payments alone, compared to only 8% of men.

Economic status in old age depends on work and economic status in midlife. If, in midlife you acquired rights to a second pension, or other assets, your risk of poverty in old age is low. But for the 37% of women who rely solely on one public program, be it social security or public assistance, the risk is high.

A close examination of the data in Table 3 has this lesson: Poverty, or the absence of poverty, depends on age, family structure, and work-life experience.

LIFE EXPERIENCE: THE BASIS OF INCOME IN OLD AGE

A look at the incomes of women and of men over the life cycle highlights the issues at stake. For the total population, the median income of women is 44% of that of men. For full-time workers, the gap narrows to 65%. Table 4 gives us some useful details. Two points in particular are very clear.

In the first place, women workers of age 45 earn only 57% of what men earn; women aged 35, 62%. Given that women who are now aged 35 can expect at age 65 that they will have an additional

Table 4

MEDIAN INCOME OF PERSONS 15 YEARS OF AGE AND OVER, BY RACE, GENDER AND AGE, 1986

	ALL FEMALES		FEMALES WORKING FULL-TIME	
	$ VALUE	% OF MALE	$ VALUE	% OF MALE
ALL	$ 7,610	44.4%	$16,843	65.0%
By Race				
White	7,760	43.0	17,101	64.2
Black	6,566	60.7	14,964	79.7
Span. Origin	6,338	55.0	14,191	83.4
By Age				
15-19	1,854	96.2	8,333	85.6
20-24	6,554	73.1	12,192	86.2
25-34	10,310	53.8	17,087	75.3
35-44	11,064	42.3	18,810	62.3
45-54	10,380	37.4	18,057	57.0
55-64	7,377	35.1	16,983	58.3
65 & Over	6,425	55.7	17,180	62.9

Source: U.S. Bureau of the Census, Current Population Reports, Series P-60, No. 157, Money Income and Poverty Status of Families and Persons in the United States: 1986, U.S.G.P.O., Washington, D.C., 1987.

20 years of life, it is clear that market inequalities will be a basis for major retirement income problems for at least another 50 years.

Second, comparing the female/male income ratio for the total population with that for the aging, the gender gap narrows somewhat. Women over the age of 15 have a median income of 44% of men, for women of 65 or over that percentage rises(!) to 56%. For working women, on the other hand, the percentage remains about the same. It would appear that transfer programs for older age women do go at least a small part of the way towards equalizing income between women and men.

Women, Work, and Social Security Income

To what extent has the improvement in the income status of the aging been due especially to social security benefit increases? For people at the lowest income levels, social security provides basic support; it makes up between 75 and 80% of income (U.S. General Accounting Office, 1986, pp. 3, 22).

Because social security plays such a major role in income support for older women, it is important to understand how benefits are calculated and how they relate to work experience. Basic benefits in social insurance are based on average wages during one's work life. Each worker, upon retirement, receives a percentage of her average wage in benefits. This percentage varies with the level of wages in such a manner that the lowest paid workers get a higher percentage benefit than the highest paid workers, but higher paid workers always receive more in absolute dollars than lower paid workers.

If we compare the social security income of women and men, we discover that the median income from social security for women is only 70% of that of men: $3,876 compared with $5,513 in 1984. This is one major reason for the larger number in poverty. Basing social security income on average wages means that benefits depend on (1) the level of wages and (2) the continuity of work. On both these counts women are at a disadvantage. In calculating average wages, the lowest five years can be subtracted from lifetime earnings for the calculation. This means that if a woman leaves the labor force — perhaps to raise children — for more than five years, these years are counted in as years of zero earnings, bringing the average wage down sharply. Even if she leaves the labor force for only five years, she is at a disadvantage since she has in effect lost the option of dropping her lowest actual earning years from the calculation. Thus, two things bring down average wages, the basis of benefits for workers: (1) the low wages that we have seen prevail throughout the life cycle and (2) the years spent out of the labor force in childrearing.

There is another factor that has long been true for women. Employment for women, much more than for men, is apt to be in service industries, which are notoriously subject to irregular employment patterns. Thus to lower wages for full-time work are added the economic penalties of part-time, part-year work—more prevalent in the services than in manufacturing. In 1984, only 5% of white women who worked full-time all year were poor, compared to 11% of those who worked part-time. Black women paid an even larger penalty for irregular employment: 12% who were in full-time jobs were poor, compared with 32% of those who worked part-time. As our economy improved after 1983, poverty rates were down for all workers, with one dramatic exception: between 1983 and 1985 they rose for workers who were employed full-time but less than full-year (U.S. Bureau of the Census, 1986a). As our economy turns more and more to a post-industrial mode, as work opportunities for both women and men are increasingly found in the service sector, this problem will be intensified. Not only will this serve to lower Social Security income, but other retirement income will be affected as well. Low income during work life means an inability to save for retirement. The acquisition of private assets and annuities becomes less and less possible. Corporate pensions, a major factor in economic well-being in old age, are a fringe benefit of full-time employment, not part-time or occasional work. They will become a smaller part of income in old age. The new labor market structure in the United States foretells increased poverty for some and decreased income security in old age for many.

What part did the increase in government social welfare expenditures play in reducing poverty among older women? To estimate this, Axinn and Stern compared official poverty rates with *pretransfer* poverty; that is, poverty before taxes and before receipt of Social Security, public assistance, and veterans payments (Axinn & Stern,

1988). The difference between official poverty and pretransfer poverty tells us how many women escape poverty because they receive government benefits.

Table 5 compares the official rates with pretransfer poverty (poverty due to private and market factors) and shows the *effectiveness* rate of public programs. It gives us a w..y of analyzing the structure of transfers, by gender, race, and age.

In 1985, 36% of white men, age 65 to 74, were poor before receiving government help and 6% after it; for those over age 75, the results were similar; 52% were poor before, 8% after transfers. Clearly, transfers were highly effective antipoverty measures. White women, however, were less successful; 56% of women age 65 to 74 were poor due to market factors and 18% were still poor after receiving government largesse. Considering those over age 75, the pretransfer poverty rate was 67%, the official rate 24%.

As Table 5 shows, for the black population there is a racial and a gender affect. Black men age 65 to 74 had a 67% pretransfer poverty rate and a 24% official rate; for older black men pretransfer poverty was 80% and dropped to 32% on receipt of transfer income. Black women had the highest rates of all. For those aged 65 to 74, pretransfer poverty was 75%, official poverty 39%; for the over-age-75 group, the pretransfer poverty rate was 80%, dropping to 32% after government assistance.

Social Security was the primary program that helped older people escape poverty. For the "young aged," those 65 to 74, it was 84% effective for white men and 64% effective for black men. For white women, it was 69% effective; for black women, 48%. Effectiveness declined as age rose, except for white men, where there was a slight improvement. The system worked better for men than for women and better for the white population than for the black.

POPULATION SHIFTS AND ECONOMIC STATUS

The demographic shifts since the passage of the Social Security Act have been discussed in detail by other authors in this volume. These changes have important economic implications.

Population aging and the gap between female and male life expectancy combine to mean that there will be an increased number of

Table 5

POVERTY, PRETRANSFER POVERTY, AND EFFECTIVENESS RATE
BY AGE, RACE, AND GENDER OF HOUSEHOLDER, 1985

	Official Rate	Pretransfer Rate	Effectiveness Rate
White Women			
62-64	19.7%	42.6%	54%
65-74	18.1	57.5	69
Over 74	23.7	67.2	65
Black Women			
62-64	40.2	57.5	30
65-74	39.2	75.3	48
Over 74	50.2	83.3	40
White Males			
62-64	7.3	19.0	62
65-74	5.6	36.1	84
Over 74	7.5	51.5	85
Black Males			
62-64	26.1	47.2	45
65-74	23.9	66.7	64
Over 74	31.5	80.4	61

Source: Calculated from U.S. Bureau of the Census, Current
Population Survey, data tape, Washington, D.C., March
1985.

353

single women at economic risk in old age. The fastest-growing part of the aging population—women over the age of 75—is extremely vulnerable. They have fewer personal resources (including private pensions), their public income transfers are less, and their need for health and social services is more than the "young old."

Individuals must plan for longer periods of retirement than ever before, including the potential for at least some years of disability. Savings and planning for old age becomes both more important and more difficult because it is so hard for any individual to estimate personal longevity and health, and the longer the time period, the more magnified any error will become. The problem of familial care for the aging will mean "children" who are themselves past their highest income-earning years trying to help support aging parents. And for society at large, the population changes mean that we now have proportionately more older people to support than in 1930, but fewer youths. We may not have a larger dependent population than the Social Security Act envisioned, but we have a different one. Different age groups have different needs for services and for support. We need to rethink the financing of our social welfare system in light of these changes.

Economic Aspects of Changing Family Structures

The Social Security Act envisioned a typical family made up of a wage-earning father and a homemaker mother, living together for their full adult lives. The expectation was that there would be one wage earner, a long marriage, and a short retirement period. Only 29% of U.S. women, aged 20 to 64, were wage earners in 1940; 66% are today (*Economic Report of the President*, 1987, p. 211). Women are no longer typically homemakers. Nor is marriage as widespread or as long lasting. The number of divorces, the number of widows, and the number of women who do not marry at all is up sharply. All of the basic assumptions of our public pension system have changed.

The design of the insurance system assumes that most women in retirement will be supported through their husbands' entitlement. The further we move away from that reality, the less adequate and equitable has the program become. Widows under the age of 62 do not get benefits at all if there are no dependent children. Women who are divorced after less than 10 years of marriage have no rights to benefits. Increasingly women are having to depend on their own work histories to be the base for their retirement income. But calculations of Social Security depend on steady employment in jobs that provide adequate wages; a poor assumption for today's labor market. In fact many married women who have worked and contributed to the Social Security system never collect their own benefits. They are too low. As we have seen, for women who must rely on these payments, the poverty risk is very high. The Social Security system is the basic building block of income in old age. For women in 1988 it is inappropriately designed.

To summarize, then, the economic status of the aging:

1. In general all of the aging population, including aging women, are doing much better today than they were 50, or even 25 years ago.
2. Our official measure of poverty probably understates the amount of deprivation. The number of "near poor" is higher for the aging than for the total population.
3. Median income is lower and poverty rates are higher for women than for men. This structure holds for divisions by race, by family structure, and for every age group.
4. Poverty hits particularly hard at those who were disadvantaged throughout their work lives. Women, particularly minority women, are most apt to be propertyless, without access to high-paying jobs or steady employment. As a result, they suffer the highest rates of poverty.
5. The risk of poverty is particularly high for the oldest group of women, especially for the part of this group which lives alone. This group gets larger yearly.
6. The relative disadvantages of women are compounded by the design of our transfer programs. The public assistance program, SSI, is funded inadequately, and the Social Security system is poorly designed for today's life situations and problems.
7. A major difference between the aging poor and the rest of the poor is that this is an almost permanent population. The aging

do not "marry out" of poverty, nor do they find more adequate employment. At this stage, solutions depend on transfer programs.

THE OUTLOOK

The permanent nature of the poverty of the aging suggests the need for immediate reform of our income support programs. The over 3 million women who depend on Social Security alone have a 30% poverty rate; the one and a half million who receive a combination of Social Security, SSI, and veterans pensions have a 52% risk of being poor; dependence on SSI alone means a 56% poverty rate for the 330,000 women in this category (U.S. Bureau of the Census, 1986a). Clearly, changes in our major income support programs could bring about significant improvements in the economic welfare of older women. Raising federal SSI payments to at least the level of the poverty line would mean an immediate improvement for this group.

There are a number of changes in the way benefits are calculated for Social Security that would increase the effectiveness of this program. Increasing the number of years that may be excluded in the primary calculation, lowering the eligibility age for widows, and increasing the entitlement rights of divorced women are all proposals that would make the program more equitable and more adequate. There is little argument about the decrease in the poverty of older women that would result.

The question facing us now is whether we can afford these changes. Can we increase social welfare expenditures for the aging? Many people have been concerned with the problem of the costs of supporting an increased aging group in the population. The discussion has centered around the dependency ratio concept, the relationship between the size of the population that needs to be supported and the size of the working population. The dependency ratio appears to be a straightforward concept (the number of dependent people divided by the number of productive people), but there are many interpretations of dependency and productivity. Some social policy analysts and demographers have worked with an age dependency ratio, the proportion of persons age 0 to 17 and over age 65, relative to the total population:

$$\frac{(0\text{-}17) + (65 \ \& \ \text{over})}{(18 \ \text{to} \ 64)}$$

Others have used the following labor-force ratio:

$$\frac{\text{nonworkers}}{\text{workers}}$$

There are other variations. Different age cut offs for entry to the labor market and for retirement lead us to different conclusions. Similarly, some have proposed refining the labor-force concept to acknowledge that productive work occurs outside the workplace. In this view the denominator would include useful work done by non-workers — volunteers and family members and exclude illegal and undesirable activity (Crown, 1985; Adamchak & Friedmann, 1983).

In the first instance, the worry is that the "65 & over" group is increasing (the age dependency ratio); in the second case the number of retirees is rising (the labor-force ratio). In spite of their differences, however, the definitions give us similar views of the future.

In the first case, whereas the number of aging is rising, the number of youths is falling. When we put the two together, the total ratio will fall from now until the Year 2000 and then begin to rise as the baby boom children retire. Note that it will never approach the height of the 1960s, however (see Table 6).

If we consider the labor-force ratio more closely, the decline has been even more marked. The massive entry of women into the labor force has cut almost in half the proportion of midlife dependents between 1950 and 1980. In the future, the labor-force dependency ratio will rise, but at a much slower rate than the age dependency ratio. Declining birth rates should lead to even further increases in female labor-force participation as women have longer periods of their life cycle after their children have left home. Although an increase in dependency may be expected, again, it will not come close to the peak of 1960.

Table 6

AGE DEPENDENCY RATIO

YOUTH, AGED, AND TOTAL COMPONENTS, 1900-2050

(Number of dependents per 100 persons, aged 18-64 years)

Year	Aged Support Ratio (Over 65)	Youth Support Ratio (Under 18)	Total Support Ratio (Under 18 & Over 65)
1900	7.4	76.3	83.7
1920	8.0	67.7	76.7
1940	10.9	51.9	62.8
1960	16.8	65.1	82.0
1980	18.6	45.8	64.4
1990	20.7	41.9	62.6
2000	21.2	40.7	61.9
2025	33.3	37.7	71.0
2050	37.9	36.6	74.5

Source: U.S. Bureau of the Census, Projections of the Population
of the United States, 1982-2050, Current Population Survey,
Series P-25, No. 922 (October 1982) and Estimates of the
Population of the United States, by Single Years, of Age,
Color, and Sex: 1900 to 1959, Current Population Survey,
Series P-25, No. 310 and No. 311 (June and July 1965).

A Basis for Optimism

Most of the discussions about the dependency crisis and the problems of support of the aging have ignored the driving force of our increased standard of living in the 20th century. The expansion of productivity since 1900, not the decline in the dependency ratio, explains the growth in per capita gross national product that we have seen. There is no reason to think that this will not continue to be the case.

Even if we take an extremely pessimistic view of productivity growth and adjust the dependency ratio for only a 1% annual increase in productivity, the age dependency ratio (the most pessimistic index) would fall to 26% lower in 2025 than in 1982. Minimum economic growth means that in terms of our ability to support nonworkers we will be much better off in the future than we are now. More optimistic estimates of economic growth would improve this ratio even further. It is clear that the projected age changes would not mean a smaller total output. Output would expand. The resources will be present to support an increased aging population (Axinn & Stern, 1988).

The composition of the dependent population will be different in 2025 from past experience; we will have more older people and fewer youths to support. Studies on the comparative costs of supporting the two groups yield inconclusive results. Some are concerned that the aging absorb more public resources than children (Clark & Spengler, 1977). Others have argued that, adding together both public and familial costs, children use more resources per capita than the aged (Wander, 1978, pp. 41-69).

The data suggest that total support costs, both public and private, will not necessarily be higher for the aging than for children. But it is true that the source of support has been different for the two groups. It may cost society the same amount of resources to maintain the aging as it does children, but historically, except for education, parents have borne these costs for children. A much larger portion of the cost of maintaining the aging has been borne by the public sector. The problem for the future is to shift resources from the private to the public sector. As midlife adults are freed from some of the financial burdens of raising children, resources will have to be moved for the support of the aging.

There are many unknowns in the situation. The aggregate demand for health and hospital services affects the cost of support; education needs for the postindustrial economy are still largely unknown; the age of entry to the workforce and the age of retirement affect the size of the population to be supported and its age distribution.

It is clear, however, that we will have the resources to support the decreased number of young dependents and the increased number of older people. Working adults will use less of their income to support children and pay more in taxes to support the aging.

Why are women at economic risk? For many it is because the work they do is economically hazardous, their family structures are increasingly unstable, and they are living longer than ever. Demographic forces, social factors, and market operations are all making for more uncertainty and need both during and after work life. As the service economy becomes an even more dominant form on the American scene, and part-time, part-year employment increases, the opportunity structure facing American women is not apt to improve. In the long run, all of these issues must be addressed.

At the point of old age, however, it is the basic income support system — Social Security and Supplemental Security Income — that must be reformed and restructured to meet the crisis of need. These programs were designed for an earlier era — one of more stable marriages and of single-earner families. They need serious review and overhauling to fit current realities.

Two relatively simple and effective antipoverty measures could be instituted rather quickly, however. (1) For SSI, federal payment levels are now set at 75% of the poverty line; raising them to at least the level of the poverty line would mean an immediate improvement in the economic welfare of the very needy group who receive public assistance in old age. (2) Average Social Security benefits received by women are low for many reasons. One change in the direction of upgrading these payments would be to adjust the rules in regard to the calculation of average wages — the base of Social Security payments. Currently, to calculate the average wage one must include all but five years of lifetime earnings. Thus many women have years of zero earnings during the period they were raising children. Maternity leave and childcare leave, which would completely exclude certain time periods from the calculations, would prevent the penalty now imposed on women for raising the next generation. It would not eliminate the entire gap between female and male average benefits, but it would help to lift many women above the poverty level.

The crisis of the next decade is not a crisis of affordability. When we consider the falling youth population and the increased labor-force participation of women, the concerns present in the presentation of traditional dependency ratios recede. When we consider the certain prospect of productivity increases, it disappears. We will have a social surplus; the issue will be to divide it in ways that provide support for *all* needy groups. We do not have to choose to keep any group in permanent poverty. We can maintain all of our dependent population in adequate fashion. Finding a structure for redistribution and reform that will be equitable for all is the challenge now facing us.

REFERENCES

Adamchak, D., & Friedmann, E. (1983). Societal aging and generational dependency relationships: Problems of measurement and conceptualization. *Research on Aging, 5,* 391-338.

Axinn, J. (1986). Value choices in the definition of poverty. In T. Eckhoff, L. Friedman, & J. Uusitalo (Eds.), *Reason and experience in contemporary legal thought* (pp. 363-369). Berlin: Duncker & Humblot.

Axinn, J., & Stern, M. J. (1985). Age and dependency: Children and the aged in American social policy. *Milbank Memorial Fund Quarterly/Health and Society, 63*(4), 648-670.

Axinn, J., & Stern, M. J. (1988). *Dependency and poverty: Old problems in a new world.* Lexington, MA: Lexington Press.

Burt, M. R., & Pittman, K. J. (1985). *Testing the social safety net.* Washington, DC: Urban Institute Press.

Clark, R. L., & Spengler, J. J. (1977). Changing demography and dependent costs: The implications of future dependency ratios. In B. Herzog (Ed.), *Aging and income: Programs and prospects for the elderly* (pp. 55-89). New York: Human Sciences Press.

Crown, W. (1985). Some thoughts on reformulating the dependency ratio. *The Gerontologist, 25*(2), 166-172.

Derthick, M. (1979). *Policymaking for social security.* Washington, DC: Brookings Institution.

Economic Report of the President. (1987). Washington, DC: U.S. Government Printing Office.

Kutza, E. A. (1981). *The benefits of old age: Social welfare policy for the elderly.* Chicago: University of Chicago Press.

Preston, S. H. (1984). Children and the elderly in the U.S. *Scientific American, 251,* 44-47.

Rochefort, D. (1985). *American social welfare policy.* Boulder, CO: Westview Press.

Schulz, J. (1985). *The economics of aging.* Belmont, CA: Wadsworth.

U.S. Bureau of the Census. (1986a). Characteristics of the population below the poverty level: 1984. *Current Population Reports* (Series P-60, No. 152). Washington, DC: Government Printing Office.

U.S. Bureau of the Census. (1986b). *Estimates of poverty including the value of noncash benefits* (Technical Paper 56).Washington, DC: U.S. Government Printing Office.

U.S. Bureau of the Census. (1987a). Money income and poverty status of families and persons in the United States: 1986. *Current Population Reports* (Series P-60, No. 157). Washington, DC: Government Printing Office.

U.S. Bureau of the Census. (1987b). Receipt of selected noncash benefits: 1985. *Current Population Reports* (Series P-60, No. 155). Washington, DC: Government Printing Office.

U.S. General Accounting Office. (1986). *An aging society: Meeting the needs of the elderly while responding to rising federal costs* (Publication No. HRD-86-135). Washington, DC: Government Printing Office.

Wander, H. (1978). Zero population growth now: The lesson from Europe. In T. Espenshade & W. Serow (Eds.), *The economic consequences of slowing population growth* (pp. 41-69). New York: Academic Press.

What's Out There and How to Get It:
A Practical Resource Guide
for the Helpers of Older Women

Cheryl H. Kinderknecht, ACSW

According to an old, wise, and experienced character in *The Velveteen Rabbit*, there is a logical sequence to the maturational process, or that fine art of growing and becoming Real.

> It isn't how you are made . . . it's a thing that happens to you . . . it doesn't happen all at once. You become. It takes a long time to happen. That's why it doesn't often happen to people who break easily, or have sharp edges, or who have to be carefully kept. Generally, by the time you are Real, most of your hair has been loved off, and your eyes drop out and you get loose in the joints and very shabby. But these things don't matter at all, because once you are Real you can't be ugly, except to people who don't understand. (Williams, 1981)[1]

First and foremost, working with aging women means being attuned to and understanding of their needs as individuals, as women, and as older persons. For a woman who lives to senescence in our society, it is with some guarantee that she will be alone, more than a little loose in the joints, and possibly impoverished before she goes, gently or not, into the good night.

Although improvements in mortality rates have been shared by

Cheryl H. Kinderknecht is with Health Care Education Associates, Laguna Niguel, CA.

---

1. This material excerpted from *The Velveteen Rabbit* by Margery Williams, Running Press, © 1981.

both males and females over the last three decades, women have benefited from more rapid improvements for most leading causes of death. Consequently, with their greater life expectancies, most women outlive their spouses and, oftentimes, at least some of their children. Compared to their male counterparts, "proportionately more elderly women are limited in their activities of daily living, visit physicians more frequently, and use more days of hospital and nursing care than men" (Rice & Estes, 1984). In addition, aging women with their average personal incomes of $6,931 are significantly less financially solvent than their male counterparts, who average an annual income of $10,529 (Longino, 1987). Indeed, in 1986, 71.8% of the elderly poor were women (Harrington, 1987). The poverty of women in old age is due to the fact that they must rely on government pensions as their main or sole source of income; all too few have additional financial resources, private pensions, or entitlements (Longino, 1987; Peace, 1986).

Roughly translated for providers, this data means that, as a group, our aging women clients are most likely to share three critical commonalities: they are alone; they are infirm; and they are poor. Consequently, our aging female clients will most likely be in need of the very basic health and financial resources. As providers, we are faced with assisting these women as they navigate the fragmented maze of available services and resources. The "safety net" with which to catch this client group is likely to resemble an old patchwork quilt, with the various resources and services somewhat loosely basted together.

This section will not deal with esoteric services available to older women. Instead, a nuts-and-bolts approach to procuring the essentials for survival will be presented. Federal, state, and common community programs will be presented and additional, selected resources will follow.

THE OLDER AMERICANS ACT:
A VITAL LINK TO SERVICES

In working with older clients, it is essential to have a basic awareness of the Older Americans Act (OAA). Enacted in 1965, this statute (PL 89-73) established the Administration on Aging within the federal government, required U.S. states and territories to set up state units on aging, and is the singly social service statute (PL 89-73) designed specifically for the elderly. The OAA provides an essential stimulus — through a partnership of federal government with state and local governments, the private sector, and older people themselves — for creating a comprehensive and coordinated service system aimed at improving and protecting the lives of older Americans. The assistance it provides has expanded and tied together a wide variety of essential services that directly touch and improve the lives of many of our older clients. Services include health programs, housing resources, community based long-term care, employment programs, and civic, cultural, educational, and recreational opportunities (National Association of the State Units on Aging, 1987). Services are provided locally through grants to local nonprofit and governmental agencies that serve the elderly.

The OAA is the common thread that binds together the aging network. This network consists of 57 state units on aging, some 664 area agencies on aging, and an estimated 15,000 community organizations providing supportive and nutritional services on behalf of the elderly. Your state unit on aging is the hub for program administration, working with both the public and private sectors in meeting the needs of the elderly. The area agencies on aging address the concerns of older Americans at the local level, either offering directly or subcontracting with other organizations to provide a wide variety of direct services to the elderly. Their comprehensive information and referral services are essential to professionals, regardless of discipline, who help the elderly. This agency, more than any other, can help you help your elderly clients directly.

INCOME PROGRAMS

"The proportion of aged who are poor or near poor is larger than the combined proportion of (all other) nonaged who are poor or nonpoor" (U.S. Bureau of the Census, 1985b). Poverty is much more prevalent among elderly women than among elderly men — elderly women have a poverty rate nearly twice that for men (Villers Foundation, 1987). In fact, the median annual income for older women is just $800 over the U.S. official poverty level; therefore, the majority of women are either already living in poverty or perilously close to it (Lewis, 1985). Arendell and Estes (1987) project that well over 50% of older women will find themselves in an impoverished economic situation. A limited number of direct economic benefits or income maintenance programs exist for the elderly in the United States.

Social Security retirement benefits are the most common and available source of income for our aging women clients. Administered through the federal government under the Social Security Act, these benefits are available to those (or their spouses) who have contributed to the Social Security fund for a specified number of quarterly periods. For retirement benefits, one can begin collecting reduced benefits at age 62, or full benefits at the age of 65 years. It often behooves women to collect their benefits under their spouse's claim number, rather than based on their own earnings. In our society, men have traditionally worked longer and for more pay than women; accordingly, men's Social Security retirement benefits will be the greater of the two.

Social Security disability benefits can be collected at any age prior to age 65 in the event of total disability or blindness. Again, eligibility is determined by the amount of contributions to the Social Security fund. Both retirement and disability benefits are figures on a strict and complex schedule based on previous contributions to the Social Security fund.

A third program potentially available to aging women under the Social Security Administration is widow's benefits, with entitlement amounts based on the deceased spouse's earnings record. The widow must be at least 60 years of age or disabled, however, in order to be eligible to apply for these benefits. The average age at which a woman becomes widowed in the United States is about 55, however, and this interim period, referred to as the "widow's gap," is often a period of desperate economic peril for many widowed women (Markson, 1985). This is particularly true of the 55-year-old woman who has been a homemaker or has limited earning potential in a fiercely competitive job market that routinely practices ageism and sexism (Arendell & Estes, 1987). Coupled with the pervasive undercurrent of racism in the workforce, an older woman of color who falls into the widow's gap often finds herself in a position of triple jeopardy.

To apply for any of these benefits, the applicant must contact the closest Social Security Administration Office. The claims representatives at those offices will assist the applicant in choosing the claim under which greatest benefits can be obtained. If there are special circumstances, the claim representative will come directly to the individual's home, to the hospital, nursing facility, or other setting to assist with the application process.

Also available under the Social Security Administration is an important but little-known entitlement program called Supplemental Security Income (SSI). This program provides financial assistance to the elderly (65 years and older), or to the blind or totally disabled under age 65, who must meet strict financial and resource eligibility requirements. Approximately 2 million elderly people receive SSI benefits, but many more are eligible. It has been found that, due to a lack of knowledge, approximately half of the potentially eligible population does not participate in the SSI program (Viller Foundation, 1987). Previous employment contributions to the Social Security fund are not required as a condition of eligibility, thus entitling the many elderly women who played a limited role in the formal workforce. This program can also be vital to those who receive only limited Social Security benefits, in that it supplements low monthly incomes of those who have had a very limited work or earnings history. In addition to cash payments, SSI recipients also receive automatic Medicaid health insurance coverage. This is an important reason to have our clients automatically apply for SSI when applying for Social Security benefits. If their combined income and resources are only one penny below eligibility levels, the Medicaid program will assist in meeting medical expenses. This is an important consideration for women, since older women bear a greater burden of health care costs than men (Arendell & Estes, 1987).

In our society, there is no strict agreement about the magical age at which one is considered to be "aged" or "elderly." Accordingly, it is pertinent to discuss the General Relief or General Assistance Program available through state Departments of Public Social Services. To qualify for General Relief, one can be under age 65 and does not have to be disabled or blind. If the applicant is able to work, most states require work registration. If the applicant is without housing and food at the time of application, emergency assistance is provided until the formal application can be processed. The cash grants provided by this program are generally much less than the entitlements under Social Security or SSI benefits, but food stamps and automatic Medicaid coverage are usually part of the General Relief package. To apply for General Relief, the applicant would need to go to the nearest county office of the state Department of Public Social Services. As with the Social Security Administration, special provisions can be made for the applicant who is, because of an impairment or institutionalization, unable to present to the office for application purposes.

With any federal or state entitlement program, it is essential to advise our potentially eligible clients to go through the formal application process. A phone inquiry or brief interview for eligibility prescreening is not enough to ensure that all vital information has been conveyed and investigated. Furthermore, by going through the formal application process, the applicant is provided with access to the appeal process in the event that the application is denied. Such appeals can involve the recovery of retroactive entitlements back to the time of application, if the denial was erroneously issued.

HEALTH CARE INSURANCE AND SERVICES

Health care costs for the elderly are disproportionately high; people over 65 make up about 10% of the population but accrue 40% of the health care expenditures (Clarke, 1987). Common health insurance available to the elderly includes Medicare, Medicaid, and privately purchased "Medigap" supplemental policies.

Medicare (Title XVIII of the Social Security Act passed in 1965) is a federal health insurance program administered through the Health Care Financing Administration (HCFA) for people 65 or older. Certain disabled people who are under age 65 but eligible for Social Security disability benefits are also covered by Medicare. SSI recipients are automatically eligible for Medicare Medical Insurance (Part B) at age 65 years: Medicare Hospital Insurance (Part A) is available through private purchase arrangements. Medicare payments are deducted directly from the beneficiary's Social Security or SSI benefits. Those over age 65 years who do not qualify for any type of Social Security or SSI benefit may privately purchase Medicare insurance coverage (U.S. Department of Health and Human Services, 1986).

As indicated above, Medicare consists of two parts—hospital insurance and medical insurance. Hospital Insurance, Part "A," helps cover inpatient hospital care, inpatient care in a skilled nursing facility in certain circumstances, home health care for those requiring intermittent skilled care, and hospice care for the terminally ill. Medical insurance, "Part B," helps pay for medically necessary doctors' services, outpatient hospital services, home health care services for those requiring intermittent skilled care, and a number of other medical services, supplies, and tests (U.S. Department of Health and Human Services, 1986).

Medicare does not, however, pay the full cost of most covered services. First of all, there are ever-increasing annual deductibles to be met by the insured party, and second, HCFA has cost caps or allowable chargeds, based on what is a very conservative reasonable or customary charge for any given service. The DRG (diagnostic related groups) prospective payment system limits what a hospital can charge those insured by Medicare, but other health care providers are in no way bound to limit their charges to what HCFA will reimburse. Any charge beyond what HCFA has deemed reasonable or customary is the responsibility of the patient. Recent changes in Medicare have further increased cost-sharing and out-of-pocket expenses for all elderly people receiving hospital and physician services. Furthermore, not all doctors, hospitals, and clinics accept Medicare payment for their services. Those that do not participate in the Medicare program often cite excessive paperwork and what they consider the low rate of Medicare reimbursement (Collins, 1987).

This has staggering consequences to the elderly female, because older women are at a greater risk for chronic disability and economic disadvantage. An elderly married couple paid about 9% of its income on direct, out-of-pocket payments and health insurance premiums in 1986, compared to out-of-pocket expenditures by single elderly women of over 16% of their incomes (Arendell & Estes, 1987). Health care expenditures can be expected to continue to spiral as the woman ages and becomes more firm. Couple this reality with the runaway expense of health care and the effects of inflation, and you have a pretty grim picture. Medicare recipients need to be encouraged to do business with health care providers who will accept Medicare assignment as the full cost of services (Collins, 1988). A list of participating providers can be obtained from the insurance company that handles Medicare in your state. We also need to encourage our low-income patients to inquire, up front, if providers (e.g., physicians, clinics, and durable medical equipment companies) are willing to accept Medicare assignment as full payment.

Available through state Departments of Public Social Services, the Medicaid program (Title XIX of the Social Security Act of 1965) provides vital health care coverage, either as a primary or a secondary insurance, to those eligible. As aforementioned, those eligible for SSI and General Relief automatically receive Medicaid coverage. As a primary insurance, Medicaid meets medical expenses for a wide variety of inpatient, outpatient, home health, prescription costs, and skilled or intermediate nursing facility costs. Certain types of homemaker chore services are also available to the elderly or disabled through the Medicaid program in many states. As a secondary insurance, Medicaid helps pick up the cost of the primary insurance (i.e., Medicare) deductibles, the balance beyond allowable charges, and certain supplies, drugs, or services that the primary insurance may not cover.

Most states also have a Medicaid "share-of-cost" or "spend-down" program for those who have incurred large medical expenses. Such coverage is partial or prorated, based on the medical expenses in relationship to the eligible applicant's income. Although one may be otherwise ineligible for Medicaid coverage, "share-of-cost" Medicaid eligibility is usually figured on a quarterly basis, so it is possible to receive partial coverage within the quarter that excessive medical expenses were incurred, as in the case of a hospitalization.

State- or county-funded "teaching hospitals" are often a good source of discounted, quality care. Such facilities are generally located in highly populated urban areas, however, and are thus not readily accessible to all who are in need. Most counties, however, have a Department of Public Health through which a variety of health services can be obtained at low or no cost. Such services may include, for example, high-blood-pressure clinics, tuberculosis screening, annual flu shots, and certain types of home health care.

On the community level, many large cities have free clinics. Although this service is less common in mid-sized or small communities, there are often a variety of clinics that use an ability-to-pay or sliding-scale fee structure. Other helpful community programs and services include the pharmacies and drugstores that routinely provide lower-cost generic equivalents, if the physician agrees, and "Senior Discounts." Such discounts, which usually run in the neighborhood of 10%, are administered according to the individual pharmacy's policy. Some pharmacies may require customers to register for this service, others may not. Some will designate customers aged 55 years and older as senior citizens, while others may use the age of 60 or 65 years as the determining age.

Many private pay "Medigap" insurance policies are available. These must be carefully and comparatively shopped for, since there are wide variances in coverage. Too many elderly consumers erroneously believe that if they have Medicare and supplemental coverage from a reputable company, they can be worry-free on medical expenses. In fact, many of these policies are keyed or limited to Medicare "allowables." Thus, types of services rejected by Medicare are also waived by the Medigap policy. Studies have shown that, as a group, elderly consumers are not knowledgeable about their health insurance coverage (Cafferata, 1984; McCall, Rice, & Sangl, 1986). Furthermore, consumer knowledge of insurance coverage is lowest among groups at highest risk of serious illness; that is, among the elderly and people of color.

NUTRITION AND FOOD PROGRAMS

Between 1982 and 1987, a total of 77 private and federally conducted studies documented the widespread and serious impact of the increasing hunger in America. At present, one out of 10 Americans does not get enough to eat (Brown, 1988). Whether she is too poor to buy nutritious food, or too impaired to shop for and prepare meals, this is a problem that directly affects the older woman.

In 1972, Congress passed the Nutrition Program for the Elderly (Title 111B under the 1978 amendments of the Older Americans Act), and funds were made available to provide low-cost, nourishing meals, five days a week, to persons aged 60 and over. These congregate meal sites are found in most communities, operating in central locations — schools, churches, community, and senior centers. In large urban settings, such as Los Angeles, that have pockets of significant ethnic populations, you will find diverse menus from center to center (i.e., Kosher, Korean, Japanese, or Mexican food). Whatever the locale, however, the goal is to provide at least one-third of the minimum adult basic nutritional requirements in this meal. The purpose of these programs is two-fold: to provide a nutritious meal and to provide socialization. Participants do not have to meet eligibility requirements, and fees are generally on a suggested donation or ability-to-pay basis. Transportation is generally provided to and from the nutrition site.

Another commonly used federal food program available to the elderly is the Home Delivered Meal Program. Solely funded through the 1978 amendments to the Older Americans Act, there is no charge for this program, which is designed to serve the homebound over age 60. A small contribution may be suggested, but payment is not demanded.

Other senior meal programs, for example, Meals on Wheels, may be supported solely by donations from private individuals, civic groups, community funds, and/or United Way contributions. Some programs may operate on such donations in combination with federal money through Title XX of the Social Security Act. Consequently, these meal programs may vary in price from completely free, to suggested donations only, to sliding scale, or to a standard set fee. Similarly, depending on the funding sources, you will see a wide disparity in how many meals are offered per day, the availability of weekend service, and the age requirements for participation. Still other meal programs may be administered on a for-profit basis and may not be affordable to the average elderly woman.

The best way to find out about the senior nutrition or home delivered meal programs in your locale is to call the closest Area Agency on Aging or the local United Way Agency, which often effectively serves as a clearinghouse for information and referral services.

The Food Stamp Program is another resource available to many elderly women. Food stamps come in booklets of coupons of varying denominations and may be spent in the same manner as cash would be spent in the grocery store. Only food and food products may be purchased with food stamps; they cannot be used for soap, cleaning agents, paper products, tobacco, or alcohol. Although there are specific eligibility requirements, based on income and resources, many with moderate income and limited property and resource holdings are eligible for participation in the Food Stamp Program. Application for this program is through the county office of the state-administered Department of Public Social Services. In some states, (e.g., California), persons receiving SSI do not qualify. Still other states require work registration for Food Stamp recipients under age 65. In emergency situations, a small allotment of Food Stamps or a food voucher can be issued while the formal application is being processed.

Government Surplus Commodity Distribution Centers periodically (usually monthly) distribute surplus food to the low-income of all ages, including elderly SSI and Medicaid recipients. Commonly distributed commodities include cheese, honey, rice, powdered milk, flour, and, on occasion, canned meat. What is available from one time to the next depends strictly on what the government has in surplus. In some cities, a formal distribution site is set up solely for this purpose. In smaller communities, the distribution may occur through the Department of Public Social Services, the Community Action Agency, or through a church or community group. Information regarding the commodity distribution program in your area can be secured through the local Department of Public Social Services.

On a community level, there are a wide variety of emergency food resources. Private and public social services agencies often have an emergency food pantry containing canned and dried food goods. The same is true of many churches and other sectarian groups, and although these groups may have a focus on helping "their own," they will not turn away "outsiders" in need. These resources can be found under the Social Services listing in the Yellow Pages of the phone book.

In response to the burgeoning homeless population over the past ten years, soup kitchens, a phenomenon of the Great Depression era, are once again springing up in many communities, large and small. Operated by social service organizations and churches, the majority of these programs are supported solely through private donations and are offered to those in need at no cost.

HOUSING

As evidenced by the ever-increasing numbers of the homeless in this country, securing affordable housing plagues people of all ages. At this time, the U.S. Department of Housing and Urban Development (HUD) and the Farmer's Home Administration (FHA) show only a minimal interest in this dramatic shortfall (Rathbone-McCuan, 1985). "Since 1981, housing programs subsidized by the Federal government were cut by more than 75%, from $32 billion to $7.5 billion. In most cities, the waiting lists for these programs are so long that they have been closed" (Whitemore, 1988). In 1984, only 16.5% of elderly poor households — or about one out of six in need — lived in federally assisted housing (U.S. Bureau of the Census, 1985a).

Furthermore, in large cities, rent control has spurred landlords to abandon their buildings. These buildings, including the old hotels that provided affordable SROs (single-room occupancy) to the elderly, are sold and then converted to luxury apartments, condominiums, or office space. Conservatively, hundreds of thousands of low-rent dwellings have been replaced in this manner over the past several years. The impact of all of these trends may have the most direct impact on elderly women, because "housing is the single largest budget item for older women" (Porcino, 1983).

Although severely curtailed over the past decade, federal housing subsidy programs do continue to exist. These include Title XX funds for elderly housing services and the limited programs available through HUD and FHA. Additionally, since the 1960s the federal government has funded "some small-scale experiments" in alternative housing for the elderly in Ohio, Georgia, Nebraska, and South Dakota, which are still in operation (Silverstone & Hyman, 1982). More widely available and known are the low-income congregate living sites, senior citizen housing projects, found in towns and cities of all sizes across the country. These congregate living sites often provide a variety of other essential services, such as a congregate meal site, socialization activities, transportation, and shopping services. Residents in these projects are expected to be fairly self-sufficient with basic self-care activities intact, as little or no direct resident supervision is provided. Rent costs are figured on a sliding scale, according to income. Other low-income housing projects subsidized by the federal government are not age segregated but may still offer a limited number of activities or services to the elderly residing in the project. To apply for federally subsidized housing, one must go to the local or county Housing Authority Office.

Today we are more often seeing the concept of subsidized congregate housing for the elderly being adopted and funded by private social service agencies and church groups. Other creative private programs include group homes or "roommate screening and matching" services for the elderly. Programs like these have a two-fold purpose: to cut expenses and to decrease social isolation. Self-contained, nonsubsidized, retirement communities for senior living are also springing up across the country. Developed by private, for-profit corporations, these microcosms of senior living at its finest are often too cost prohibitive for many elderly women.

The best place to find out exactly what federal, state, or community housing programs and resources exist for the elderly in your locale is to phone the Area Agency on Aging or the Housing Authority.

It is also pertinent to explore the tax laws of your own state. Some states — California, for example — offer a variety of tax relief packages for senior homeowners and renters. Individual state programs may include property tax exemptions, rebates, or deferrals. Other states may offer homeowner/renter assistance programs in the form of state income tax credits for the low-income elderly or disabled. To find out what tax relief programs are available to the low-income elderly in your state, call either your local Area Agency on Aging, the state Department of Revenue, or the County Tax Assessor.

EMERGENCY SHELTER

Although the current literature does not reveal that elderly women constitute a significant percentage of the homeless population, they are a group at increasing risk as more and more situationally distressed individuals join the swelling ranks of the homeless. Contributing factors include eviction and, because of rising costs of living, the inability to secure or maintain affordable housing. Furthermore, the link between homelessness and mental illness should not be ignored. Hall (1987) reports that in addition to the scarcity of low-income housing, mental illness represents a primary cause for homelessness.

Although studies of the incidence of physical and mental illness among homeless people have varied greatly in their estimates of occurrence, there is a general consensus that homeless individuals suffer from a large number of severe medical and psychiatric illnesses and that the frequency with which these illnesses occur is far greater than for those who are not homeless (Surber, Dwyer, Ryan, Goldfinger, & Kelly, 1988). In reality, whether these physical and mental illnesses are the cause or the effect of being homeless remains an entangled and often disputed issue.

Although emergency shelters do exist in most cities, there are far too few beds available, particularly for women. Many shelters have limitations on how many nights the individual may stay, and "some agencies have provided clients with one-way out-of-state bus tickets . . . [a procedure] referred to as Greyhound Therapy" (French, 1987). Few shelters or agencies have provisions for assisting the individual in securing permanent living arrangements and other needed services. Furthermore, "homeless shelters are generally located in the slum or bowery district of a city, thereby forcing the homeless into the most marginal and unstable sections of society — those most prone to violence and victimization" (Bussak, Rubin, & Lauriat, 1984).

Sources of emergency shelter for the homeless include time-limited hotel vouchers through the Department of Public Social Services or local civic and church groups, and the emergency shelters operated by the Salvation Army, the Union Rescue Mission, and other church or civic groups. The United Way generally can guide you to the agencies that provide emergency shelter and related services to the homeless.

Aside from arranging for the most immediate need of "three hots and a cot" for our aging women clients who are homeless, it is also imperative that we actively channel them toward the other needed services. Is she eligible for SSI or General Relief? If she is already receiving these funds, is she eligible for, and willing to consider, a Board and Care situation or other permanent living arrangement? Are there acute or follow-up care needs for mental or physical illnesses?

UTILITIES

Federal and state monies are combined to fund the Housing Energy Assistance Program (HEAP), which provides direct payment of utility bills for low-income homeowners or renters. Because of its limited funding, assistance may be limited to the payment of one heating bill per winter and one cooling bill per summer. HEAP applications can be procured through a variety of agencies in the community, that is, the Department of Public Social Services, the local Area Agency on Aging, the Housing Authority, the American Red Cross, or local Community Action Agencies.

The county office of your state Department of Public Social Services also provides limited emergency assistance on utility bills for low-income households. This may take the form of an emergency voucher to the utility company or it may be reflected in an adjusted increase in Food Stamps to compensate for the out-of-pocket expenses for the excessive utility costs.

Many utility companies have become much more attuned to the needs of their low-income customers, offering such services as levelized billing. With these billing plans, annual costs from the previous year are averaged out, and the customer pays a set, average monthly fee. Thus, the customer is not faced with excessive heating or cooling bills, which is particularly helpful for the elderly who are on tight, fixed monthly budgets. These companies also routinely demonstrate a genuine interest in serving and protecting the emergency needs of households that include elderly, disabled, or young individuals. Although the utility company billing clerks have limited authority, a phone call to the Community Relations Representative or the vice president of the company will almost always result in productive arrangements in the case of an emergency.

Many telephone companies now offer a limited-use option for basic services. A reduced monthly rate entitles the customer to a set number of outgoing local phone calls. Fees for long distance calls and any excess outgoing calls are added to the reduced monthly rate. Incoming phone calls are, of course, unlimited and are not billed. Call the billing office of your phone company to ascertain if this service is available to the elderly in your area.

Emergency assistance for utility payments can also be procured through community social services agencies, churches, and sectarian or civic groups. Although all low-income people are served, many of these community groups are especially concerned about meeting the needs of the elderly.

Closely tied to the issue of utilities are the "giveaway programs" to meet the special seasonal needs of the elderly and others in need. A good example of this, in many communities, is the Salvation Army's practice of giving away blankets at the beginning of winter. Another seasonal example is the giveaway of box fans to the elderly during the summer months in many communities. Such programs are usually supported entirely through private donations by individuals and companies and are administered through community agencies such as The Red Cross, The Visiting Nurse Association, local Councils on Aging, or other local social service agencies.

A phone call to the local Area Agency on Aging or the United Way will produce many customary and some obscure resources for assisting your elderly clients with emergency or unusual utility expenses.

CLOTHING

Although the federal and state governments have no formal provisions for providing clothing, most communities have good no-cost or low-cost clothing resources for those in need. Social service agencies and churches often have emergency clothes closets. Upon request, many thrift shops operated by charitable organizations will generally provide basic clothing and blankets at no cost to those in need. Experience has proven that this process is less traumatic for the elderly client if the helping professional eliminates the "red tape" by either making the initial call or writing a letter on the client's behalf.

Again, it is important to watch for any seasonal programs offered in your area. Particularly during the holidays, local businesses and civic or social organizations often band together to provide for the special needs of the low-income and elderly in the community. A good example of this is the winter coat drive sponsored by Scotch Fabric Care Services, a privately owned company in Topeka, Kansas. Winter coats are donated to this company by private citizens. The company's employees volunteer to clean the coats, which are then distributed at no cost to those in need through the local Salvation Army.

LEGAL ASSISTANCE

A wide variety of legal issues directly pertain to the elderly woman. Examples include fighting eviction, drawing up a will, setting up durable power of attorney for health care or property management, conservator or guardianship issues, and management of assets.

In certain cases involving nursing home placement of a spouse, legal assistance may be needed for the separation of assets in order to avoid the impoverishment of the spouse who remains in the couple's home. In some states, Medicaid eligibility regulations allow assets to be split between husband and wife. Because the provisions governing the transfer of assets can be confusing, the assistance of an attorney is recommended for the equitable division of resources. This procedure legally preserves one-half of the community property for the use of the spouse who remains outside of the skilled nursing facility.

Title III of the Older Americans Act, which was designed to develop comprehensive and coordinated delivery of services to the elderly, includes funding specifically earmarked for legal services

(Silverstone & Hyman, 1982). These services are made available to the elderly through the local Area Agency on Aging.

Free or discounted legal advice and services are also available to the low-income elderly through the closest Legal Aid office.

TRANSPORTATION

Although they may have driven a horse and buggy or two in their heyday, many women from our grandmothers' generation were never given the opportunity to learn how to drive an automobile. Still others have been relegated to the passenger seat because of infirmities, vision deficits, or the prohibitive expense of maintaining and insuring an automobile. Traditionally, the elderly have relied on their children, close relatives, friends, and neighbors for their transportation needs. Transportation programs serving the elderly are in short supply, are sometimes limited only to essential medical transportation, and are often nonexistent in many rural and small communities. In our mobile society, the absence of adequate transportation services serves to isolate and restrict the elderly. Fear imposes further isolation and restriction, even when a limited number of transportation resources do exist. "Because they are afraid to go out of the house alone—afraid of getting hurt, getting mugged, getting lost—even semi-independent old people are forced, too soon, to be shut-ins" (Silverstone & Hyman, 1982).

Title III of the Older Americans Act does provide funding to promote access, including transportation, for the elderly. Such transportation and limited escort services are provided through Area Agencies on Aging and Senior Citizen Centers by a limited number of automobiles and wheelchair-accessible vans. Many of these agencies supplement their limited transportation resources through the use of volunteers.

Elderly Medicaid recipients are eligible for cab vouchers through the Department of Public Social Services. Vouchers are limited to medical transportation, however, and must be procured in advance of the appointment date.

On the community level, social service agencies, civic programs, and churches provide some transportation services to the elderly.

Some of these organizations may provide vans with paid drivers, whereas others provide service strictly through the use of volunteers' time and automobiles. In many communities, the American Cancer Society provides transportation to and from radiation and chemotherapy treatment. The American Kidney Fund and local renal dialysis centers have long been active in assisting their patients with transportation to and from treatments.

Over the past decade, city bus companies have made great strides in making buses more physically accessible to the elderly and the handicapped. Most cities offer discount rates for monthly bus passes for senior citizens, and some private cab companies also offer discount rates for the senior citizen, as well.

HOME HEALTH AND HOSPICE CARE

Older women typically have more multiple health problems and are more likely to spend time in a nursing home or to need home care services. Compared to elderly men, elderly women have a greater incidence of illness and chronic, functionally limiting impairments (Verbugge, 1984; Lewis, 1985).

"With the rising cost of health care, the undesirability of institutions, and increased longevity resulting in increasing numbers of frail elderly, home health care is frequently proposed as an alternative to institutional care" (Garner & Mercer, 1982). Home Health Care and hospice programs are available through private, nonprofit or proprietary and hospital-based agencies. Many state and county departments of health also provide these services. Such services are funded through a variety of sources, including Medicare, Medicaid, private insurance companies, donations, and grants.

Medicare covers Home Health Care costs under either Hospital or Medical Insurance. Conditions for eligibility stipulate that the following four conditions be met:

> (1) the care you need includes part-time *skilled* nursing care, physical therapy, or speech therapy, (2) you are confined to your home, (3) a doctor determines you need home health care and sets up a home health plan for you, and (4) the home

health agency providing services is participating in Medicare. (U.S. Department of Health and Human Services, 1986)

The first of these conditions knocks many out of the eligibility arena. Many chronic and debilitating illnesses do not require the technical proficiencies that constitute a skilled level of nursing care under the Medicare guidelines. On the other hand, some complicated illnesses may require around-the-clock or at least ongoing daily care and, as such, would not be limited to the intermittent frequency detailed by Medicare regulations. Stringent homebound requirements further serve to eliminate other potential recipients. To be eligible for home health aides, social work, or occupational therapy services under Medicare home health benefits, one must be receiving either nursing, physical, or speech therapy. The occupational therapist may continue to provide treatments for a short period after other needs have been met. Aide and social work services, however, cannot be provided as autonomous or discrete services.

Medicaid regulations governing Home Health Care are usually much less restrictive regarding the patient's level of care requirements and homebound status. Consequently, an elderly woman whose primary needs may involve the need for assistance with personal care and only periodic nursing supervision would be an eligible candidate for service. Additionally, most states do not impose strict restrictions on homebound status for Medicaid recipients of Home Health Care. Thus, an individual who gets out daily to attend a congregate meal program or to go to dialysis treatment would not be restricted from receiving home visits for personal care and periodic nursing services.

Hospice care benefits for the terminally ill can be provided through the Medicare Hospital Insurance program. Covered services include those rendered by physicians, nurses, therapists, home health aides and homemakers, social workers, and counselors. Other coverage includes medical supplies, drugs, and short-term respite care. Eligibility is restricted by limitations on service duration. Coverage is limited to a maximum of two 90-day periods and one 30-day period. If a patient still needs hospice service after hospice benefits are exhausted, the hospice must continue care unless the patient no longer wants service. This requirement has served as a disincentive to many potential hospice providers who fear the financial ramifications of accepting patients who might outlive their covered benefit periods.

Again, hospice benefits under the Medicaid program are generally less restrictive. In addition, many hospice programs have multiple funding sources that include private and civic donations, government grants, or United Way allocations. Accordingly, the terminally ill elderly individual who has exhausted her Medicare coverage may still receive needed hospice services under Medicaid, a share of cost arrangement, or a fully subsidized care arrangement through the hospice agency.

The home health or hospice programs in your area can be found listed in the Yellow Pages of your phone book. Since federal, state, and county programs are not listed in the Yellow Pages, it is also pertinent to check if your state or county provides these services through the Department of Health.

HOMEMAKER CHORE SERVICES

Most old people living alone or with their spouses are able to care for themselves without too much difficulty. "Yet, there are those who need help in order to remain living within the community, and amongst this minority, women, those over 75-80 years and those living alone, predominate" (Peace, 1986). Older women have more acute and chronic conditions than men and although these conditions are seldom life threatening, they do impose functional impairments that limit activities of daily living (Verbugge, 1984). Providing care for an elderly parent with functional limitations or declining health status has traditionally been a family obligation, with relatives informally providing 80% of long-term care to the dependent elderly (Kutza, 1981). Elderly women are far more likely than elderly men to be in poor health and thus to require assistance from their children (Rix, 1984). "Like other forms of nurturance, caring for elderly parents is predominantly women's work" (Abel, 1986). A recent English study found that women spend nearly 20 times more time than men do in the care of elderly relatives (Walker, 1983).

Public policy has been, for the most part, incredibly myopic in looking at the in-home, long-term care needs of an increasing generation of frail elderly who remain in their homes. Long-term care funding covers a wide range of services ranging from minimal help at home to care in a nursing facility. Yet, institutional care currently absorbs over 90% of the funding earmarked for long-term care (Kutza, 1981). The Reagan administration "views families as the first line of defense" when the elderly need help (Hays, 1984). Because of career opportunities and sheer economic necessity, however, many of these traditional caregivers are found not at mother's bedside, but in the workforce. In addition, 25% of all women around 70 years old have no living children (Lewis, 1985).

Homemaker chore services consist of personal care and household tasks. Depending on the providing agency, these services may also include shopping and transportation. Homemaker chore services are sometimes hospital-based, but more frequently they are community-based, sponsored by private or public agencies. The charges are usually on a sliding scale basis and will vary according to the status of the agency, whether it is public (government funded), voluntary (nonprofit), or proprietary (for profit). Because of funding limitations, homemaker chore services are often very limited and fragmented.

Title XX of the Social Security Act provides block grants to fund an array of social services aimed at increasing the availability of supportive services to vulnerable populations, including the elderly. Funded services do include homemaker chore services (Stone & Newcomer, 1985). In addition, Title III of the 1978 amendments to the Older American Act provides federal funding for in-home services, including homemaker chore services. Most states to some degree supplement federal dollars to provide the nonmedical, in-home supportive services to low-income elders or through a share of cost formula for those who exceed income guidelines but meet low-resource standards. Private contributions and United Way allocations also provide needed funding to these programs in many communities.

To determine the availability of homemaker chore services in your community, call the local Area Agency on Aging, the county office of the Department of Public Social Services, and the state Department of Aging.

MENTAL HEALTH SERVICES

Although the incidence of psychiatric disorders increases greatly with age, only 2% of the elderly consult psychiatrists (Silverstone & Hyman, 1982). The literature reveals that depression is, by far, the most common emotional problem of elderly. Contrary to the beliefs of many health professionals and the general public, "age per se is no bar to effective psychiatric treatment, particularly in the case of depression" (Institute of Medicine, 1986). The literature strongly supports the notion that women in general are more prone to depressive disorders; this is true of situational depression, as well as involutional and endogenous types of depression (Fabry, 1980). Furthermore, more women have organic brain conditions than men because of their longevity and greater numbers (Lewis, 1985).

Old age is generally a time of loss: the loss of loved ones, the loss of health and functional abilities, the loss of income and status, the loss of meaningful and productive social roles and activities, and the possible resultant loss of respect and self-esteem. Considering the fact that women live longer and thus have a very high statistical probability of losing all of these things, how could she not be depressed about her situation and anxious about the future?

Traditionally in this country, the costs of providing mental health care have been borne primarily by the public. Public financing accounts for roughly 70% of mental health care in this country, as opposed to about 20% public funding for all other areas of health care (Harvey, 1975). Public financing includes funding from a wide range of sources including but not limited to research and training grants, National Institute of Mental Health (NIMH) Community Mental Health Centers Program grants, and individual reimbursements for direct service to Medicare and Medicaid recipients.

Because of public support for mental health services in America, there is good access to mental health care for an elderly woman who might be in need of this service, regardless of her ability to pay. State mental institutions, Community Mental Health Centers, Family Service Agencies, and many private mental health practitioners will accept Medicare and Medicaid assignment as full payment for services rendered. Although the psychiatric needs of the elderly have largely been ignored in the past, this area has received more attention over the past decade.

Mental health providers can be found in the Yellow Pages of your local phone book. State- and county-funded programs can also be found in the government section of the phone book. The county medical society, the social service department of local hospitals, and visiting nurse associations are usually good sources for referrals.

SOCIALIZATION

Socialization is essential to life. An isolated existence denies normative, typical experiences and social exchanges that other members of the culture take for granted. As with any other skill, social competencies are diminished through nonuse. Regardless of one's age or limitations, most of us need to be involved, at least to some degree, with others.

Because they are more likely to have mobility problems, older women are more likely to be confined to their homes and thus restricted from social activities (e.g., out-of-the-home visiting, shopping, church or temple attendance, club attendance), 8% report restricted social activities due to health status, compared with 5% for men (Verbugge, 1984). Though less active and more likely to be housebound than men, elderly women are still more likely to see relatives and friends more frequently. They are also more likely than men to be visited and to visit others, especially within the immediate neighborhood (Peace, 1986).

A wide variety of formal and informal opportunities for socialization exists. The more mobile elderly can partake in the activities, field trips, and special events hosted by the Area Agency on Aging and other community programs geared to the elderly. There are also many volunteer opportunities available to the elderly, even in a small community. Examples include civic organizations or local chapters such as the American Red Cross, the American Association of Retired Persons (AARP), the Retired Senior Volunteer Program (RSVP), local hospital auxiliaries, foster grandparenting programs, church-related projects, and nonprofit organizations.

The worth of volunteers has been more widely recognized in this era of program funding cutbacks. Agencies lucky enough to have older volunteers generally capitalize on the volunteers' wide array of skills that have been accrued through years of living and working. Opportunities for political involvement exist, too. More and more, the elderly are speaking out for themselves through their own political pressure groups such as the Gray Panthers, the Congress of Senior Citizens, the American Association of Retired Persons, and the Older Women's League.

Those who are confined to their homes are the most in need of socialization activities. Some Area Agencies on Aging, American Red Cross chapters, and other community programs have escorts and wheelchair accessible vans so the frail and handicapped elderly can also participate in community activities. Because some of these women are receiving Medicare home health care services, however, they cannot jeopardize their homebound status by getting out. Others may be too frail for even a brief outing. Outreach services are provided through the Area Agency on Aging, the American Red Cross, and other volunteer and public programs. Telephone reassurance programs also serve to provide a vital outside link to those who are homebound or have only minimal outside social contacts.

Some of these women may also be excellent home-based volunteers themselves. Through telephone "buddy systems," they can call other elderly women at a prearranged time each day to make sure all is well, or, with materials and supplies provided by local groups, they can sew bedgowns for indigent home health care patients or knit booties for babies at the area Children's Hospital. These practical activities can also serve a therapeutic purpose by providing the homebound elderly woman with the opportunity to provide a meaningful and altruistic service for others.

You can check for socialization and volunteer services and opportunities in your area by calling any of the following: the Area Agency on Aging, the United Way, the American Red Cross, AARP, or RSVP.

INSTITUTIONALIZATION

Older women make greater use than older men of nursing homes. In addition, Butler and Newacheck (cited in Arendell & Estes, 1987) found that persons living alone, whether single, divorced, or separated, have ten times greater probability of being institutionalized than those who are married. "Some 1.6 million elderly persons reside in institutions, three quarters of whom are women" (U.S. Bureau of the Census, 1983). There are multiple reasons for this demographic phenomenon, including

1. Women live longer than men — 5% of all elderly over 65 are in institutions, but of those over 85, 22% are institutionalized.
2. Women outlive spouses, whereas men are usually cared for by their wives.
3. Women have a greater tendency toward multiple and limiting chronic disabilities.
4. Cognitive and behavioral disorders necessitate nursing home placement for many (over 50% of residents have serious organic brain syndromes, OBS), and more women than men have OBS because of longevity and greater numbers.
5. About 50% of U.S. women in nursing homes are childless or have outlived their children.
6. The traditional sources of care, females in their 40s and 50s, are increasingly in the workforce and unable to meet the care needs of elderly relatives. (Lewis, 1985)

Three basic types of institutional care are available: the skilled nursing facility, the intermediate care facility, and facilities that provide board and care arrangements. There are also three different types of sponsorship for long-term care institutions:

1. Voluntary — nonprofit, sectarian or nonsectarian, governed by a lay board
2. Proprietary — private, profit-making
3. Public — federally, state, or county funded (very few). (Silverstone & Hyman, 1982)

According to the Health Insurance Association of America, the average stay in a nursing home is longer than a year (Wasilewski, 1987). The average cost of a year in a nursing home is now around $25,000 (Long Term Care, 1988). Pay sources vary according to the type of facility sponsorship and the type or level of care needed. Private pay is cost-prohibitive, except for the very wealthy. Private insurance plans are expensive and none of them provides full coverage (Long Term Care, 1988). Contrary to popular belief, long-term care is not covered by Medicare: the reimbursement structure for Medicare was designed to pay only for acute, time-limited, inpatient care of a skilled level, rather than for the chronic, long-term care more typically needed by women (Lewis, 1985). Medicaid does cover intermediate and custodial level long-term institutional care and, in fact, annually pays for nearly half of all nursing home costs in the United States (Institute of Medicine, 1986; Wasilewski, 1987). About two-thirds of all nursing home residents depend on Medicaid for payment of some or all of their nursing home costs (U.S. Government Accounting Office, 1983).

Women not already eligible for Medicaid at the time of nursing home admission must spend their overall resources down to the poverty level before they apply for Medicaid assistance. "Ideally, the older woman must time her application for Medicaid to match her last illness before death. If not, her recovery means that she has almost no assets, other than pensions she collects, to live out the rest of her life" (Lewis, 1985).

While it is safe to say "a rose is a rose is a rose" about some things, it is *not* safe to say "a nursing home is a nursing home is a nursing home." It is paramount that both consumers and providers realize that all institutions are not created, or operated, equally. Quality varies significantly from facility to facility. Much has been written on how to go about selecting a nursing home, including checklists and guidelines prepared by periodicals, senior advocacy groups, and the U.S. Public Health Service. Meaningful evaluations of nursing homes by lay persons are difficult (Miller, 1985). Untrained people tend to look at the real estate, the presence or absence of odors, the food, and the recreation programs. Of more importance is the quality of medical and nursing care, the training of the staff, and the attitude of the staff (IOM, 1987; Miller, 1985). Licensure and accreditation of long-term care facilities are carried out by each state. Facilities that accept Medicare reimbursement must also meet certain conditions for participation; these conditions encompass all facets of operation, from staff qualifications to the physical plant itself. In their pursuit of quality, some facilities also voluntarily seek accreditation from private bodies, such as the Joint Commission for Accreditation of Healthcare Organizations.

To find out about a facility's accreditation or to report care problems in the long-term care institutions in your state, contact either the state Office of Long Term Care or the Ombudsman Program through the State Agency on Aging. In 1978, U.S.P.L. 95-478 required every state agency on aging to establish and operate an Ombudsman Program to improve the quality of care in nursing homes. Amendments to this law enacted in 1981 extended the required scope beyond nursing homes to encompass other categories of institutions, including board and care and other group living arrangements.

There are several good sources for assistance with long-term care placement and payment issues, including the local Area Agency on Aging and the county office of the state Department of Public and Social Services. Social workers and discharge planning departments of local and area hospitals are also excellent referral resources. These providers are well aware of the eligibility and pay source requirements for financial assistance for care and can assist the client or the client's family in getting through the bureaucratic maze. In most instances, these providers are also very aware of which area institutions provide good quality care. Although they may not be at liberty to recommend or endorse specific facilities, you can almost always expect an honest answer to the question: "Would you place your mother in this facility?"

WORDS OF CAUTION, WORDS OF COMFORT

That was a great many years ago; but once you are Real you can't become unreal again. It lasts for always. (Williams, 1981)

Old, alone, infirm, and poor, the elderly female has often exhausted all resources by the time she presents or is presented to us for help. To many of these women, we often represent the last thread of hope. This in itself can often be an overwhelming and sobering thought to the helper. As providers, we need to remind ourselves constantly that we can make an impact on the quality of life experienced by our elderly female clients, that we do make a difference, and that our services are of immeasurable intrinsic value.

Since many direct helpers are female (i.e., social workers and nurses), we also need to remind ourselves, as women, to keep demographics in perspective. Seeing the fate that befalls so many of our elderly female clients, we need to remember that our own perceptions of aging are very often negatively skewed by the fact that our practice experience brings into sharp focus only those who need help.

We need to remember to look at the flip side of the coin periodically, to look at those who do not need our help, so that we can bear the reality of our own aging. For example, of all elderly over the age of 65, 95% are not institutionalized. Of these over 85, 78% are not institutionalized. And, although 15% of the elderly in this country do need assistance with self-care activities (Rice & Feldman, 1985), another 85% do not. As helpers, we have limited opportunity or reason to see the 72-year-old woman who still runs her own business, the 80-year-old woman who golfs twice a week, or the 94-year-old woman who still maintains her own household, putters in the garden, and shuns senior citizen programs "because they're for old people." These independent women do exist and flourish. They are merely outside of the provider's customary range of vision.

We will soon welcome in the 21st century, and our country will see its largest numbers of elderly women. In recent years, we have witnessed sweeping and devastating reductions in government funding of social programs. These reductions have been "implemented from a budgetary perspective, with little consideration for how the voluntary sector and individuals and families will cope with the responsibilities the federal government relinquishes" (Schilling, Schinke, & Weatherly, 1988).

Providing services to the elderly female in today's social climate necessitates strong advocacy, brokering, and networking skills. Creativity, coupled with the tenacity of a jackass, cannot hurt either. We do not know how long social policymakers can cast a jaded or blind eye toward the needs of the aging women who represent such a very large and increasing segment of the population. Whatever it takes, we are in it for the duration, basting together the flimsy pieces to create a patchwork safety net.

ADDITIONAL RESOURCES

American Association of Retired Persons (AARP)
    1909 K Street, NW
    Washington, DC 20049

Gray Panthers, National Headquarters
    311 S. Juniper Street, Suite 601
    Philadelphia, PA 19107

National Association of State Units on Aging
    2033 K Street, NW, Suite 304
    Washington, DC 20006

Older Women's League
    1325 G Street, NW
    Washington, DC 20005

Retired Senior Volunteer Program (RSVP)
    5492 La Sierra
    Dallas, TX 75231

REFERENCES

Abel, E. K. (1986). Adult daughters and care for the elderly. *Feminist Studies, 12*(3), 479-497.

Arendell, T., & Estes, C. (1987). Unsettled future: Older women—economics and health. *Feminist Issues, 1*, 3-24.

Brown, J. L. (1988). Domestic hunger is no accident. *Social Work, 33*(22), 99-100.

Bussak, E., Rubin, L., & Lauriat, A. (1984). Is homelessness a mental health problem? *American Journal of Psychiatry, 141*, 1546-1550.

Cafferata, G. L. (1984). Knowledge of their health care insurance coverage by the elderly. *Medical Care, 22*(9), 835-847.

Clarke, J. (1987). The paradoxical effects of aging on health. *Journal of Gerontological Social Work, 10*(3/4), 3-18.

Collins, K. (1987, November 20). Senior forum: Medicare, 'Medigap' policies often not enough. *Topeka Capital-Journal*, Section 2, p. 13.

Fabry, J. (1980). Depression. In R. H. Woody (Ed.), *Encyclopedia of Clinical Assessment* (Vol. 2, pp. 588-601). San Francisco: Jossey-Bass.

French, L. (1987). Victimization of the mentally ill: An unintended consequence of deinstitutionalization. *Social Work, 32*(6), 502-505.

Garner, J. D., & Mercer, S. O. (1982). Meeting the needs of the elderly: Home health care or institutionalization. *Health and Social Work, 7*(3), 183-191.

Hall, H. (1987). The homeless: a mental health debate. *Psychology Today, 21*, 65-66.

Harrington, M. (1987). *Who are the poor?* Washington, DC: Justice for All National Office.

Harvey, E. C. (1975). Financing mental health services. In S. Feldman (Ed.), *The administration of mental health services* (2nd ed., pp. 86-119). Springfield, IL: Charles C Thomas.

Hays, J. A. (1984). Aging and family resources: Availability and proximity of kin. *Gerontologist, 24*, 149-154.

Institute of Medicine (IOM) Committee on Nursing Home Regulation. (1986). *Improving the quality of care in nursing homes*. Washington, DC: National Academy Press.

Kutza, E. (1981). Allocating long-term care services. In J. Meltzer, F. Farrow, & H. Richman (Eds.), *Policy options for long-term care* (p. 127). Chicago: University of Chicago Press.

Lewis, M. (1985). Older women and health: An overview. In S. Golub & R. Freedman (Eds.), *Health needs of women as they age* (pp. 1-16). New York: Haworth Press.

Long Term Care '88. (1988). *Long Term Care: The family issue that no presidential candidate can afford to ignore*. Washington, DC: Author.

Longino, C. F. (1987, December 12). Among the U.S. elderly, men are better off than women. *Los Angeles Times*, p. 36.

Markson, E. (1985). *Older women: Issues and prospects*. Lexington, MA: Lexington Books.

McCall, N., Rice, T., & Sangl, J. (1986). Consumer knowledge of Medicare and supplemental health insurance benefits. *HSR: Health Services Research, 20*(6), 633-657.

Miller, D. (1985). Women and long term nursing care. In S. Golub & R. Freedman (Eds.), *Health needs of women as they age* (pp. 29-38). New York: Haworth Press.

National Association of the State Units on Aging (NASUA). (1987). Linking elderly patients to community resources. *Continuing Care, 6*(3), 12-14.

Peace, S. (1986). The forgotten female: Social policy and older women. In C.

Phillipson & A. Walker (Eds.), *Aging and social policy: A critical assessment* (pp. 61-85). London & Vermont: Gower.

Porcino, J. (1983). *Growing older: Getting better*. Reading, MA: Addison-Wesley.

Rathbone-McCuan, E. (1985). Health needs and social policy. In S. Golub & R. Freedman (Eds.), *Health needs of women as they age* (pp. 17-28). New York: Haworth Press.

Rice, D., & Estes, C. (1984). Health of the elderly: Policy issues and challenges. *Health Affairs, 3*(4), 25-49.

Rice, D., & Feldman, J. (1985). Living longer in the United States: Demographic changes and health needs of the elderly. In M. Janicki & H. Wisniewski (Eds.), *Aging and developmental disabilities: Issues and approaches* (pp. 9-26). Baltimore & London: Brookes.

Rix, S. (1984). *Older women: The economics of aging*. Washington, DC: Women's Research and Education Institute of the Congressional Caucus for Women's Issues.

Schilling, R. F., Schinke, S. P., & Weatherly, R. A. (1988). Service trends in a conservative era: Social workers rediscover the past. *Social Work, 33*(1), 5-10.

Silverstone, B., & Hyman, H. K. (1982). *You and your aging parent*. New York: Pantheon.

Stone, R., & Newcomer, R. (1985). Health and social services policy and the disabled who have become old. In M. Janicki & H. Wisniewski (Eds.), *Aging and developmental disabilities: Issues and approaches* (pp. 27-40). Baltimore & London: Brookes.

Surber, R. W., Dwyer, E., Ryan, K., Goldfinger, S., & Kelly, J. (1988). Medical and psychiatric needs of the homeless—a preliminary response. *Social Work, 32*(2), 116-119.

U.S. Bureau of the Census. (1983). Money, income, and poverty status of families and persons in the United States: 1983. *Current Population Reports* (Series P-60, No. 140). Washington, DC: Author.

U.S. Bureau of the Census. (1985a). *Characteristics of households and persons receiving selected non-cash benefits: 1984* (Series P-60, No. 150). Washington, DC: Author.

U.S. Bureau of the Census. (1985b). *Statistical abstract of the United States, 1984-85*. Washington, DC: National Data Bank and Guide to Sources.

U.S. Department of Health and Human Services. (1986). *Your Medicare handbook*. (Publication No. HCFA-10050, ICN-461250). Washington, DC: Author.

U.S. Government Accounting Office. (1983). *Medicaid and nursing home care: Cost increases and the need for services are creating problems for the states and the elderly*. Washington, DC: Author.

Verbrugge, L. (1984). A health profile of older women with comparisons to older men. *Research on Aging, 6*(3), 291-322.

Villers Foundation. (1987). *On the other side of easy street*. Washington, DC: Author.

Walker, A. (1983) Care for elderly people: A conflict between women and the state. In J. Finch & D. Groves (Eds.), *A labour of love: Women, work and caring* (pp. 117-124). London: Routledge & Kegan Paul.

Wasilewski, C. (1987). Mature customers, immature products. *Best's Review, 8,* 40-46.

Whitemore, H. (1988, January 4). We can't pay the rent. *Parade Magazine,* pp. 4-6.

Williams, M. (1981). *The velveteen rabbit.* Philadelphia: Running Press.

Epilogue

I see you, old woman. I see the YOU, not the old. In your eyes I read the story of the years, of the pain, the sweet delights. I see you, Woman, know your femininity, your graceful movements, your healing tenderness.

. . . If I see you, if I can feel your pain, if I can know your joy, you are not alone. You are not a small "i" far away like a stringless kite.

. . . Look at me, Woman, as I look at you. See . . . we know each other; we are part of the same rainbow. Your colors flow into mine; mine fade into yours. We are the same combination of sun and rain and reflection of life.

There are those who look at you and say, "She is childish." But I view you and I say "she is child-like." To be childish is to be petulant, temperamental, unwilling to endure frustration or punishment or misery of any kind. But the slashes which make parentheses around your mouth show pain long endured and seldom vocalized. Your eyes bear imprints of tears shed and sorrow felt . . . There are traces of laughter, and in your age and your tiring body there still resides the child who can awake to wonder and to the miracle of a light which is just beginning to trace gold lines on the wall of a room.

. . . Old Woman, I do see the you that was and the you that is . . . I see you in the nursery rhyme. You still remember it, "There was an old woman who lived in a shoe . . ."

It wasn't exactly a shoe you lived in, but it seemed crowded like one when the children were young. . . . But now you are an old woman. And the shoe is empty. . . . No sound in the house. Just an old woman and an empty shoe.

You still have so many children you don't know what to do. Mainly because each child has the solution to your old age. And no solution fits you, any more than someone else's shoe can match your foot. Each child want to uproot you, place you in a new shoe, in one which has not been softened to your shape with the passing years.

. . . You will not wither in total loneliness . . . solitary, away. My hands and those of people around me will reach for you in the dungeon of your alienation, will lift you, carefully, into the slanted sunlight of our lives.

Our fires will bring you warmth; our companionship will give you sustenance. We will widen our circles. . . . We will open doors and invite you into the room-brightness of our lives.

I see you, old woman. But even as I look, your face turns into my own. We stand at opposite ends of the same long corridor, reflecting the image of one another.

REFERENCE

Smith, B. K. (1973). *Aging in America*. Boston: Beacon Press, pp. 1-4.

Index